A doctor-patient reflection

FINDING HOPE

WHEN FACING SERIOUS DISEASE

INSPIRING STORIES, HEALING INSIGHTS AND HEALTH RESEARCH

STEVEN J. SOMMER MD

FINDING HOPE

ISBN: 978-0-9954345-0-9

DISCLAIMER

This book has been created to bring hope to individuals (and their families and friends), particularly those people facing serious health challenges. It is not intended in any way to replace other professional health care or mental health advice, but to support it. Readers of this publication agree that neither Dr Steven Sommer nor his publisher, or seller will be held responsible or liable for damages that may be alleged or resulting, directly, or indirectly, from their use of the information shared in this publication. All external links are provided as a resource only and are not guaranteed to remain active for any length of time. Neither the publisher, seller nor the author can be held accountable for the information provided by or actions resulting from accessing these resources.

ALSO BY DR STEVEN SOMMER

Chronic Fatigue Syndrome – a doctor's journey and solutions (soon-to-be-released)
Restoring Balance – meditation/relaxation based stress management MP3 audio recording available at www.drstevensommer.com

Formatting and cover design by The Fast Fingers Book Formatting Service.
Photo of Dr Sommer by Dianne Sommer.

This book is available on Amazon.
See Author page on Amazon Author Central.

To my wonderful wife, Tori my love,
without whom this would not have been possible.

CONTENTS

FOREWORD

Finding Hope is the long-awaited book by acclaimed medical practitioner, Dr Steven Sommer. It was written whilst he was battling chronic diseases during his own personal voyage. My utmost congratulations go out to Steven for creating such an informative, well-researched, and emotionally touching piece. His words will empathize with readers who may be experiencing the inevitable challenges of chronic or life threatening disease, as well as with their healthcare professionals, families and friends.

Steven has seamlessly interwoven over 50 years of aggregated personal and professional experience into this book. It includes reflections on his early childhood, his development as a junior doctor, and later his work as a GP; empowering patients facing the perils of chronic disease. Steven commences the book by extensively recounting the qualities that research suggests help people with cancer who have made remarkable recoveries. Following this pattern throughout the book he evokes strong feelings of inspiration among people living with a wide range of serious diseases. Along the way he provides guidance and strategies for all people to take charge of their health and thus achieve the best quality of care, and most importantly, to never lose hope!

Steven generously relates his incredible life journey, including his own struggles with chronic disease. He shares his persistent search and eventual recovery from chronic fatigue syndrome and life-threatening inflammatory bowel disease through lifestyle and natural therapies. Steven also explores many of the pharmaceutical medications that can make a difference. He continues to search for solutions to Parkinson's disease and remains hopeful that research will bring relief for himself and others with this condition.

Steven describes his difficulties with medication and hospital inpatient care. When doctors experience adversities with their own health and with medical treatments, like many patients, they can experience feelings of helplessness in the medical setting. In addition, the accumulated loss of career and standing can lead to being unsupported or misunderstood by family members. In this way, he gained great insight into the experience of being a patient and is therefore an excellent guide to others in their journey to good health. Steven has articulated his recommendations, supported by evidence, with compassion, honesty, humor and authenticity.

Perhaps the greatest impact of this book for me was the eye-opening and inspirational healing stories by patients Steven was so privileged to know. There is an age-old tradition of storytelling in many cultures. Incorporating this traditional approach by giving space to the patient to tell their story is in itself healing. Patients are empowered when they find meaning in their ill-health; answering the question as to why they became unwell at a particular point in time, or why they were predisposed to their illness. Steven has so eloquently demonstrated this in his book. We know from research that when doctors spend more time with patients, to allow them to talk about their health, not only does it enhance the doctor-patient relationship, but also the healing response. This process allows patients to gain greater insight and meaning through their illness. In this way they can learn and develop from the experience and ask themselves; what in their life journey contributed to their health problems and what actions are required to generate a healing response? The answers to these questions may range from lifestyle changes to forgiveness, to healing relationships with themselves or others. From this, the individual learns to become resilient. Cure is not necessarily the goal. Feeling emotionally in-control, empowered and with an improved overall quality of life, may allow a person the strength to live well with a chronic disease.

Steven was a pioneering medical educator in Australia, teaching doctors about the role of storytelling; linking life journeys and their relation to illness as a way of healing. Steven's strategies and the role of telling healing stories may one day be part of a universally-acknowledged treatment for all patients. The healing and therapeutic potential is enormous. It makes good sense to include this in the training of all health professionals and anyone who wants to help patients on more than just a physiological level. Beyond this, his strategies can be used in every workplace through group sharing. We can learn so much from hearing people's experiences, from the highest highs to the lowest lows.

The stories Steven shares in this book inspired me, they were heartfelt and gave me joy and insight. They taught me how I can better relate to my own patients.

Finally, I am personally indebted to Dr Steven Sommer. When I first met Steven he was a passionate, respected senior lecturer at the Monash University Department of General Practice. He was also a part time general practitioner and president of the Whole Health Institute. He was admired for his work, mentorship and leadership by many students, doctors and the public. He was my early mentor when I first started working in general practice. Steven provided me with the opportunity to speak in a public forum in the early 1990s. There, I was able to share my own life journey and healing process with an audience of health practitioners, and eventually, medical students. It was my first attempt at public speaking, and despite hearing my own voice quiver as I began; the warmth, open hearts and acceptance that exuded from the audience put me at ease. The act of telling my story was a relieving sensation. Moreover, it empowered me as an individual and allowed me to heal.

Steven planted the seed for me to embrace holistic medicine and thereby nurture the doctor-patient relationship in my own clinical practice. I was able to give patients time to share their stories, many of which continue to inspire me to this day. It also enabled me to further the development of holistic and integrative medicine within the medical profession. I am overwhelmed with pride, honor and gratefulness to Steven, my mentor — thank you!

I have no doubt that you too will love and be inspired by this profound book.

Associate Professor Vicki Kotsirilos AM,
MBBS, FRACGP, FACNEM Medical Practitioner

INTRODUCTION

*Hope - the lure of the future that it
may make the present better.*

- TIM COSTELLO, WORLD VISION CEO

It is better to live with hope than to live without it, even if that hope never comes to fruition, for to live without it is to be funneled into resignation, despair and decline. That is my experience, both as a doctor and as a patient.

You may hope for a miracle cure or you may simply hope for a better day tomorrow. You may hope to experience less pain, or you may hope to achieve a greater understanding with a loved one. You may just hope to enjoy a good meal again, or to laugh and play, or to appreciate the blue sky.

Hope keeps us getting out of bed each day, an especially challenging prospect when one is facing serious disease. By serious disease I mean disease that for months or years rocks your confidence in your body's basic ability to keep you healthy. Whether it be cancer, heart disease, autoimmune disease, neurological disease, or a myriad of other diseases, the common denominator is that it's a challenge that has ongoing impacts and consequences. This book is an exploration of finding hope for better health when one is faced with just such a situation or that of a loved one. The principles and information shared will also be of relevance and inspiration to all people who want to stay well.

The origins of this venture began in the mid-1990s. At that time I was working as a GP (family physician), senior lecturer in Monash University's Department of General Practice, stress management consultant, meditation teacher and president of a voluntary non-profit educational organization, the Whole Health Institute. I managed to find one evening free each week to begin writing my ideas. Back then I was trying to help more people beyond my immediate patients. Little did I know it was going to become much more personal.

When my health crashed in 1996, the ideas I wanted to share through my writing were put on the back shelf, as I confronted being on the other side of the desk. I was eventually diagnosed with Chronic Fatigue Syndrome (CFS) and it would take me a further 11 years before I'd be able to return to part-time work. This happened in 2007, at which time my wife Tori and I set up a clinic that operated out of our home. Tori worked as a chiropractor, while I almost exclusively saw patients suffering from CFS. I was also employed to give stress management lectures and tutorials at Deakin University Medical School.

By 2011 further health crises forced the clinic's closure. At this time I was battling with three major illnesses: Parkinson's disease, Ulcerative Colitis and Graves' disease. When moments allowed, I found some time to return to writing, voice-activated software making this possible. Some weeks I was too ill to write at all, or lucky to get one 30 minute session in a day, whilst on my best days, two hour-long sessions were possible.

When I survived a life-threatening bout of colitis in April 2012, I realized that if I'd died any insights or inspirations I'd gleaned from my life would've died with me. It doubled my determination to share these, if at all possible. This project gave meaning and purpose to a day-to-day existence in which my previous work was no longer possible. Writing this book became my work.

If a picture paints a thousand words then a story can illuminate a hundred research papers. For stories open us to possibility, while research helps to explain and define how to make this possible for the many. Stories can also give us clues as to how we might make a difference to our health here and now. They can inspire us to look at new health research and go beyond accepted treatments that may be very important but not give us the full answer. So throughout, true stories are drawn from my patients and friends and from well documented case histories published elsewhere. Vignettes drawn from my own life weave through the text, making it part biography. Along the way I can't resist sharing some ideas of how we might create a healthier health care system. Twenty years of ill health has given me one extraordinary gift, a gift that many doctors don't receive until retirement: time, lots of time, for research and reflection.

The book takes the form of interconnected essays under an overarching theme of finding hope. Part I relates my experiences and explorations in this regard as a practicing clinician and medical educator, while Part II largely refers to my experiences and explorations since I became a patient.

I have included stories and research covering a disparate area of topics: from cancer and heart disease, to mind-body medicine, to epigenetics, to Parkinson's disease, to fecal transplant; topics that reflect my special interests, along with areas relevant to the health issues I've personally been facing. You can pick and choose from the Table of Contents areas of most interest to you (it does not need to be read sequentially), or simply read the book from beginning to end.

We know that a hopeful attitude makes a difference to well-being and recovery from illness. Hope changes us both psychologically and physiologically.[1] Despite this being scientifically validated, patients at times have the rug of hope pulled from underneath them by health professionals. This is often inadvertent, but it happens. There were many times working as a GP where I had the job of restoring this rug to its rightful position. When I became a patient, I felt the full impact of being on the other side of the equation. This occurred when my treating doctors unwittingly suggested or implied that whatever I did for myself would make no or very little difference to my illnesses. It left me having to find hope elsewhere. I found this was not an easy task when one is feeling ill and vulnerable, even with my education and resources.

I discovered as a patient the need to look for hope generally arises when there is a loss of certainty in terms of treatment; unacceptable side effects or risks; or a complete lack of effective therapies. So we enter the realm of uncertainty. Apart from seeking other professional opinions, we can take courage and do some of our own research, tune into our instincts, seek out inspirational stories and remain open to helpful advice. A caveat here, 'Dr Google' can be a great help or hindrance and if at all possible is best combined with the supervision or at least monitoring of a sympathetic GP.

Even with this support, we may need to be prepared to take risks and weigh up potential costs and benefits. Trial and error is inevitably involved and we may be ridiculed by some for our attempts. We need to find supportive people to encourage us as we seek out a plan to instill hope and improve our lot. Keeping a 'hopefulness list' displayed somewhere you can regularly see it, is something I would encourage. As you read this book you might like to jot down any ideas or information that inspires hope in you.

Deep hope is about meaning and purpose.[2] For some this may lie in a full acceptance of one's illness and its prevailing prognosis. One may still hope for the best, but prepare for the worst. There is an opportunity in illness and in dying because we slow down. This can allow us to complete unfinished business and deepen and in some cases heal relationships. For others, who feel it is not yet their time, there may be a combination of acceptance, denial or defiance. This may involve proactively attempting to beat the odds by keeping an eye out for new treatments along with ways of invoking the body's self-healing systems. Seeking out opportunities to continue life's journey is the approach that brings the most hope for these people. It is not a journey that guarantees recovery, but if it is a possibility you wish to explore or simply to seek inspiration, then read on.

Dr Steven Sommer M.B.,B.S FRACGP
January 2017

PART I

Chapter 1

CHANGING THE ODDS

... approaching adversity with a positive attitude at least gives you a chance of success. Approaching it with a defeatist attitude predestines the outcome.

DR BELINDA KIELY, ONCOLOGIST (CANCER SPECIALIST)

...what we can do for ourselves is so much bigger than I think most of us understand.

MATTHEW, CANCER SURVIVOR

Florence Smythe entered my consulting room assisted by her daughter. Thin and bent, her face was gaunt, her skin yellow (jaundiced). At 78, she had been battling bowel cancer for the previous two years. Surgery and chemotherapy had failed to stop the spread of cancer into her liver. She had been told by her oncologist she had, at best, three months to live.

Florence's youngest daughter, Sam, in her 40's, also had a history of cancer, having had a spinal tumor diagnosed 20 years previously. She too had been given a poor prognosis, but had made a remarkable recovery by, in her words, "triggering her body's self-healing systems, by taking a holistic approach." Discovering that I was a doctor open to this possibility, she had tracked me down and brought her mother along.

After initial introductions, I asked Mrs Smythe why she had come to see me.

"My doctors tell me there is nothing more they can do for me, but my daughter believes otherwise," Florence said.

"And what do you believe?" I asked.

"I'm not sure, that's why I agreed to see you."

"Your doctors have said that, because there are no other drugs, radiation treatments or surgery that can help treat your cancer," I said. "However, there are things you can do for yourself, that at best, as your daughter discovered, can make a big difference, while at worst, they may make no difference, but you'll feel better about yourself anyway, because you'll be doing something positive for yourself."

Mrs Smythe sat upright in her chair, "What sort of things do you mean?"

"For a start, what do you enjoy doing?" I asked.

"Well I love ballroom dancing and gardening, but I've been too unwell to do anything like that."

"Do you think you could aim to just sit in on some ballroom dancing and maybe sit in your garden?" I suggested.

She looked at Sam, "I think we could manage that." She looked back at me, "and that can make a difference?"

"Well, when you're feeling happier, your immune system works better and yes, that can make a difference," I said.

Her daughter nodded.

No other pressing medical needs were identified and we arranged to meet again, at which time I would teach her some relaxation/meditation techniques. Sam had nutritional training and was providing her with various nutritional supplements, which I encouraged her to continue doing.

A month later, Mrs Smythe returned a little brighter and steadier on her feet.

"I've been doing what you suggested and feeling better for it."

"Good for you," I said.

"Yes mum's a lot more positive," said Sam.

A month further on, she was steadier again, still accompanied by Sam but no longer requiring her daughters helping hand. We spent some time practicing a meditation exercise and they left smiling.

Two months later, she arrived on her own. Confident and walking easily, her skin color was normal and she had gained two kilograms (4.5lbs) in weight. "Guess what?" she said, "I'm driving my car for the first time in two years and I'm ballroom dancing again."

When she left, my receptionist pulled me aside, "I can't believe that's the same lady who came in with her daughter. She looked like she was dying."

"She was," I said.

Over the next three months, Mrs Smythe continued to be active and well. Then Sam went on a prolonged overseas trip. The rest of her family didn't hold Sam's beliefs and Florence lost this positive support, which may have contributed to her cancer ramping up again. It came in the form of metastases (cancer that has spread beyond the original source) to her ribs. There was one point on her rib cage that she could barely touch without causing her to wince. Apart from painkillers, I suggested we try a visualization method to reduce the pain and she was keen to give it a go.

She lay down and I asked her to close her eyes. After talking her through a brief relaxation I invited her to imagine she was breathing in clear energy through the top of her head, washing it through her body and out through her feet as she exhaled, taking the pain away with it. After 10 minutes we concluded the exercise and she sat up. To my astonishment, she pressed on the previously tender rib several times informing me that the pain was gone.

She continued ballroom dancing and driving her car until her final six weeks, at which time a visiting palliative care nurse was arranged.

Sam had returned and together with the support of the rest of her family, Florence was able to remain at home. She was grateful for the new lease on life she had experienced in her final year. Accepting of her fate now, she continued to manage her pain without medication and died in peace, at home, surrounded by her loved ones. It had been fully 12 months after her initial consultation with me. (Note: we will explore dying well in Chapter 22)

The Bell Shaped Curve

When doctors give a patient a prognosis for a particular cancer, they use statistics that typically take the form of a bell shaped curve to guide them (see figure 1). This graph at its peak, known as the median point, indicates when most people die with a particular cancer. If a doctor quotes a time, it is the median they select, although in truth, around 50% of people will live longer than this and 50% will have less time.[1] In Mrs Smythe's case, three months was the most likely time frame. Importantly, it is a bell shaped curve and not simply an 'n'-shaped curve. This means that there is a tapering at either end, indicating that some people will survive for a shorter time than most, while at the other end there will be people who live for a longer period of time than most. It has been estimated that 10% of patients will have an excellent response to conventional treatment and live 3 to 4 times or longer than their predicted (median) survival time.[2]

The question is, how, with no further conventional treatment, did Mrs Smythe experience a new lease of health and live four times longer than expected? Would this have happened if she had not changed her attitude and approach to her situation?

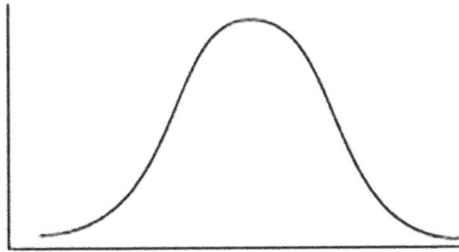

Fig. 1. Bell Curve.

Mind-body influence

The observation that psychosocial factors can influence the progress of cancer is not a new one.[3] Studies of people with cancer who have been randomly assigned to attend support groups that included group psychotherapy and stress management, have found they lived twice as long as those without this support.[4,5] We'll explore potential mechanisms for how this might occur in later chapters. For now, let's consider another example from Dr Tim Oliver, a cancer specialist (oncologist) at the Royal London Hospital, who reports the story of a woman with a terminal prognosis who experienced a remission over a two year period from kidney cancer with metastases to her lung. Dr Oliver found that her tumors waxed and waned not with the inexorable progress of kidney cancer, but with the ups and downs of her relationship with her physically abusive husband. Though she eventually died, her separation from her husband, so far as he could tell, may have been the crucial medicine here.[6] Dr Oliver goes on to say, "It is vital that doctors give patients a minimally realistic, faint concept of hope. I communicate some enthusiasm about at least the possibility of cure in a desperate situation. Regressions tell us there are things beyond our eyes that we cannot know."

Not all doctors agree with this. When I presented Mrs Smythe's story to final year medical students and included a suggestion for a hope-preserving approach to presenting a serious diagnosis, I received a mixed response. While some students seemed to embrace it, others were fearful that it was giving false hope.

American physician and author, Dr Larry Dossey suggests that this is as much to do with the personality of the practitioner as it is to do with any logical reason.[7] Some will naturally see Mrs Smythe's story as 'just a worthless anecdote,' whereas others will see it as a 'valuable case history.' The practitioner's life experience may also play a role. Importantly, most doctors know patients who 'die on time' when given the statistics about their chances of survival. I suspect Mrs Smythe would have followed her three month script if not for Sam's intervention. It could well be that some doctors are unwittingly perpetuating the very statistics they quote. Other people have been known to die suddenly when given bad news. As Dr Dossey suggests, one could question then which is the greater problem, excessive pessimism or false hope?[8]

Hope in uncertainty

It has long been recognized that hope is an essential ingredient for health. That said, breaking bad news can be difficult for anyone, hence, avoiding the removal of hope in the face of a life threatening diagnosis, like cancer, has been an ongoing challenge for doctors. A survey of oncologists in 1961 found 90% approached this problem by simply not disclosing cancer diagnoses to their patients. By 1979, as societal expectations changed and it became clear that most patients wanted to know their diagnosis, 97% of physicians surveyed acknowledged that it was preferable to disclose a cancer diagnosis.[9] How this is done is the critical issue, each situation having its own particular communication challenge.

One of the underlying realities here is that living with uncertainty is not easy. We seek certainty wherever possible. With the increasing array of impressive medical technologies, like Magnetic Resonance Imaging (MRI), there can be an expectation that medicine is an area where we can find exactitude. As a doctor, I have felt this pressure and the temptation to fulfil the role of one who can be so definite. Yet in terms of providing a prognosis, no doctor or machine can tell you exactly where you will fall on the bell-shaped curve of survival probabilities. Whilst acknowledging the seriousness of the condition, we can say that your prognosis with cancer generally improves with each additional year you survive.[10] To add to this uncertainty, the curve itself is a moving feast, ever changing as new treatments are discovered or simply attempted. Cancer Immunotherapy, a conventional treatment which involves the use of various substances to provoke the immune system into attacking tumor cells, is one such promising area.[11] As Mrs Smythe's story helps us to see, the attitude you take and how you live your life, may in the end, be the most important factor of all.

Ignorance can heal

In some circumstances, complete ignorance can have surprising effects:

- In the early 1990s I was working as a senior lecturer at Monash University's Department of General Practice. We were visited by a number of medical professors from China interested to see what we were doing. One of these professors, upon hearing of my interest in how the mind affects health, told me the story of Chen. A peasant farmer and feeling unwell for some months, Chen had visited the city hospital seeking help. After a rigorous assessment, it became

7

clear that he had advanced cancer of the pancreas. This is a notoriously serious cancer and Chen was told he was un-likely to live longer than six months.

- Five years later Chen returned to the hospital. The doctors were surprised, to say the least, to see him. Upon question-ing him, it became clear that Chen had not understood the prognosis given to him five years previously and he had returned to his farm and continued working. It was only after this time that his cancer overcame him. The professor's opinion was that it was Chen's inability to understand his prognosis that somehow led to him surviving way beyond the odds.

The well documented case of Robert Moore presents a similar theme.[12]

- Mr Moore had been a long term smoker. In 1966 at the age of 55 he presented to a hospital in Pittsburg, USA, with shortness of breath. Investigations, including x-rays and a lymph node biopsy, revealed a rapidly progressing small-cell lung cancer. It was decided any treatment would be futile.
- Mr Moore had witnessed his stepmother die of cancer and had said to his family, "If I ever have cancer, I don't want to live." Hence his wife had told doctors not to reveal to him that he had a terminal diagnosis. Instead he was told he had a tumor, which if it caused symptoms, could be treated and that it was best if he returned to work as soon as possible.
- The next time Mr Moore attended the hospital was five years later with an acute shoulder problem. So surprised were staff to see him alive, that a chest x-ray was taken. It revealed no evidence of cancer. A review was also taken of

the earlier pathology slides which confirmed the accuracy of the initial terminal diagnosis.

Robert Moore went on to live to 80 years of age when he died after being struck by a car. A post mortem was performed and no evidence of cancer was found.

Thanks to the research of Caryle Hirshberg and Marc Barasch,[13] who tracked down and interviewed his daughter, we know a little bit about Robert's personality. She described him as indefatigable, "always repairing anything that was broken." He was an affectionate tease who loved to laugh, take her fishing and travel. He was also an avid hunter. He had a repertoire of positive personal mottos which he believed, including: "It's all gonna work out," and "Whatever comes, will come."

They report that there are other cases published in past medical literature that suggest that withholding information can sometimes enhance a patient's survival.[14] Some people drop their bundle and give up when given a terminal diagnosis. On the other hand, a shock like this can cause other people to rally, gather their resources and reprioritize their lives.[15]

Still, Mr Moore's story poses many more questions than we have answers.

How long have I got?

Most people with metastatic cancer indicate they would like an estimate of how long they've got to live.[16] This said, research also tells us that people who respond to a cancer diagnosis with denial, live longer than those who respond with stoic acceptance.[17] This could be because the latter focus more on dying, while the former focus more on getting on with living.[18] Mrs Smythe's story concurs with this.

So how does a doctor help preserve a life affirming attitude in the face of a serious diagnosis like cancer? In an environment of medico-legal concerns around the issue of informed consent, withholding information is nowadays a rarely used approach, even when it might be deemed beneficial to do so. In addition, in an information age most people want to know what they are facing. On the other hand, overwhelming, copious and often frightening information, given to cover any legal comeback, needs a counterbalance. Communicating hopeful possibilities provides this balance. The suggestion of oncologists Belinda Kiely and colleagues is for doctors to include in their provision of information, the fact that around 10% of patients might live beyond three to four times longer than their predicted (median) survival time.[19] One could also contend that the chances of being on this more hopeful side of the bell-shaped curve, may be influenced by non-medical factors.

What of those people who defy the odds completely? As Florence and Sam Smythe teach us, there is more to healing than just Medicine. Let's explore this possibility further.

How common are remarkable recoveries?

A number of patients across a wide variety of cancers defy the odds. The terms spontaneous remission or spontaneous regression have been assigned to such cases where the cancer has been observed to partially or completely disappear, without medical treatment or as a result of therapy that is considered inadequate to treat the disease.[20]

What triggers or pathways allow the body to overcome this out-of-control replication of body cells we call cancer? The mechanism is not fully understood and may differ depending on cancer type. We do know that having a high fever can sometimes trigger this turnaround and that the immune system is involved, as evidenced by the success of

Cancer Immunotherapy for certain tumors.[21]

Some people will suggest that the term spontaneous is misleading as it implies occurrence without a cause, even if that cause is yet to be found. Hence, terms such as 'remarkable recovery,'[22] 'exceptional outcome,'[23] and 'radical remission'[24] have been preferred.

While the rate of spontaneous remission from cancer had been quoted as occurring one in 60,000 to one in 100,000 cases, this was based more on speculation than research.[25] What we did know was that it depended on the cancer type. The frequency of scientific published case reports suggested it was more common with neuroblastoma, renal cell carcinoma, malignant melanoma and lymphomas/leukemias, and less likely with metastatic lung or pancreatic cancers.[26]

The most accurate frequency of remission data for any cancer type was obtained from a review of primary liver (hepatocellular) cancer research.[27] It was found that amongst those patients who received placebo (no therapeutically active treatment) the rate of spontaneous, objective (demonstrated by scans and biopsies) partial remission was 0.406% (16 out of 3941 people) or one in 246 people.

A more recent review of 61 randomized controlled trials involving 18 different advanced solid tumors, found a spontaneous remission rate in those receiving placebo or no treatment of a staggering 1.95% (150 out of 7676 people).[28] This represents close to one in 50 people. Table 1 displays the average percentage of spontaneous remission for these 18 different tumors. In this research review paper this meant partial or complete remission without any effective therapy, demonstrated by biopsy and microscopic examination. Melanoma topped the list with 6.62%, or one in 15 patients, while bowel cancer, Mrs Smythe's tumor type, was found to be the least likely to undergo such a remission, at 0.36%, or less than four in 1000 patients. Even this is far more likely than the often quoted one in 60,000-100,000.

Cancer Type	Spontaneous Remission Rate
Melanoma	6.62%
Ovarian cancer	4.17%
Thyroid cancer	3.72%
Renal (kidney) cancer	3.27%
Gastric (stomach) cancer	2.58%
Breast cancer	2.50%
Head and Neck cancer	1.95%
Hepatocellular (liver) cancer	1.89%
Neuroendocrine cancer	1.84%
Non-Small Cell Lung Cancer	1.84%
Gallbladder cancer	1.79%
Prostate cancer	1.29%
Gastrointestinal Stromal	1.05%
Pancreatic cancer	0.97%
Small-Cell Lung Cancer	0.64%
Urinary Tract	0.58%
Sarcoma	0.42%
Colorectal (bowel)	0.36%
Average spontaneous remission likelihood:	1.95%

Table 1 Overall Spontaneous Remission Rates (complete + partial) by tumor type from Ghatalia et al[29]

The Gawler Foundation, a holistic well-being center, has helped over 15,000 people with a variety of cancers, often at a late stage of their disease. A book published about participants, called *Surviving Cancer*, details the stories of 28 cancer survivors who attended the Foundation's programs and beat the odds.[30] There have apparently been many more than 28, but even this gives a one in 500 complete remission rate amongst program attendees.[31]

So the truth is we are discovering that remarkable recoveries from cancer are far more common than we appreciated. With this in mind, Hirshberg and Barasch suggest that doctors use the term 'ethical hope' rather than false hope, for ethical hope is based on real possibilities not fantasies.[32]

Lessons from survivors

The compelling question is whether these spontaneous remissions are just good luck or can we learn something from these survivors? In their 1995 book, *Remarkable Recovery*, Hirshberg and Barasch report a survey they undertook of 45 remarkable survivors to ascertain if there were common characteristics amongst them. In over 70% of their interviewees the following factors were utilized in actively grappling with their illness. These self-attributed characteristics were a fighting spirit; seeing disease as a challenge; taking responsibility; and belief in a positive outcome (highest score -75 %).[33]

More recently, Kelly Turner, in her book *Radical Remission* broadens our insight further by reporting the findings of her PhD research looking at cancer survivors who have been at death's door and are now thriving against all predictions.[34] She found over 1000 such cases of spontaneous remission published in the medical literature. However, none of these publications reported asking the patient why they thought they had healed. Kelly also interviewed oncologists, all of whom had experience of patients making remarkable recoveries against the odds, but none of whom had published these patients' stories. Kelly tracked down 100 of these exceptional people and asked them: "Why do *you* think you healed?"

She conducted detailed interviews with these remarkable cancer survivors worldwide, some of whose uplifting stories are recounted in her book. All were attempting to bolster their body's self-healing systems, such as the immune system, although the approaches taken were varied. Some used a combination of conventional and alternative medicine, while others used alternative approaches alone. Among the more than 75 health promoting factors mentioned by these survivors, Kelly deciphered nine common factors which almost all 100 of them had attributed to their healing. These are reported by her, chapter by chapter as follows:

- Radically Changing Your Diet
- Taking Control of Your Health
- Following Your Intuition
- Using Herbs and Supplements
- Releasing Suppressed Emotions
- Increasing Positive Emotions
- Embracing Social Support
- Deepening Your Spiritual Connection
- Having Strong Reasons for Living
- (Exercise)

Kelly's book does many things, one of which is to remind us that the mind and body are not separate. How we feel, the love we receive, our sense of social connection, all translate into chemical and hormonal messages affecting our immune system and our ability to self-heal, even from cancer. While not yet constituting scientific proof, it does give compelling support to the idea that spontaneous remissions are not just random events. It suggests that those people represented by the far end of the bell-shaped curve are long-term survivors for reasons other than mere chance.

Add exercise to this list and you could argue you have '10 Keys' for staying well or enhancing self-healing from any illness. Kelly points out exercise only missed out because many of the people with cancer she interviewed had been too weak to participate in this, but did so as they gained in strength.[35] Each of Kelly's nine keys embody a general principle, so that in terms of specifics what works for one individual may not work for another. What deepens one's sense of inner peace or spiritual connection, for example, will vary between people. Still, *Radical Remission* gives hope, inspiration and some guidance to those with cancer wishing to take a more active role in their healing. Complementing the book, Kelly's website www.radicalremission.com serves as a collection point for freely accessible inspiring cancer stories.

Simply knowing there are people who have completely recovered from advanced cancer is an extraordinary source of hope and inspiration. Of course not everyone has the inclination or lives in circumstances where they can explore Kelly's nine keys. You may decide to focus on one to start with. Giving yourself permission to do things that bring you joy is a good place to start. As we saw, reconnecting with her love of ballroom dancing and gardening strengthened Mrs Smythe's reasons for living, and was a powerful springboard for better health.

You might be inclined to start at the other end of the list where the consensus diet amongst Kelly's hundred survivors was to focus on a wholefood diet, eliminating or minimizing all sugar, dairy, meat and refined foods. They increased vegetable and fruit intake, ate organic produce and drank filtered water.[36] If this dietary key interests you, you might need some professional guidance with it. Whatever you choose to begin with, doing something positive for your self-healing is uplifting and having gained benefit from working on one key, you may be ready to tackle others.

If you're looking to explore a whole lifestyle changing program or simply looking for more information, two useful websites are www.gawler.org and www.ornish.com

Clearly more proactive research is needed to clarify remission rates with and without positive attempts at self-healing. Evidence that people with breast and bowel cancer who exercise live significantly longer than those who don't, is a promising example.[37] Innovative research has also found exercise prior to or immediately following chemotherapy can significantly enhance the cancer killing treatment, decrease side-effects and increase survival times.[38]

Another area of research involves a comprehensive lifestyle program improving outcomes in men with prostate cancer, details of which will be presented in the Lifestyle as Therapy chapters.[39-42] Increased survival times for people with cancer attending psychologically enriching support groups, is another promising area already mentioned.[43,44]

An initial step could be for conventional cancer researchers to add a profiling of all their participating patients, to ascertain the level of involvement in Kelly's nine (10 including exercise) keys. At the end of their research study they could see whether there was any correlation between those who did best and the extent of their participation in active self-care. A caveat here is this type of research requires particular expertise to be done well, so conventional cancer researchers would need to work with experienced psychosocial researchers to obtain a meaningful result.

A further step would be to run lifestyle programs that facilitate these nine keys, like the ones we will explore in the Lifestyle as Therapy chapters. Cancer patients could then be randomly assigned to usual medical care or usual medical care plus lifestyle program. Researchers could then ascertain whether the extra lifestyle program had a significant effect on quality of life and survival. As I've alluded to, the only study I'm aware of that has done this showed positive results for men with early prostate cancer (see Lifestyle as Therapy - Cancer and beyond).[45]

Healing centers adjacent to hospitals provide an opportunity to build upon these types of research. Examples include the Olivia Newton-John Cancer and Wellness Centre in Melbourne, Australia, Chris O'Brien Lifehouse in Sydney and the Cancer Integrative Medicine Program at Rush University Medical Center, Chicago. As we shall see in coming chapters, growing evidence suggests people with a wide range of illnesses, who do something to contribute to their self-healing, experience better health. It appears cancer is no exception and we as doctors can present prognosis with this in mind, leaving the door of hope open, even when Western Medicine has nothing more to offer.

At age 52, Norman Arnold was a successful CEO married with three growing sons. He developed a sharp persistent pain in his lower back and the diagnosis of gallstones was made. Surgery was performed and to the shock of all concerned a large pancreatic cancer was discovered along with metastases in his liver. The pathology report read; 'metastatic adenocarcinoma of the pancreas, with documented nodal metastases and isolated metastatic disease in the liver.' He was told that 95% of cases in this situation, even with treatment, would die within six to eight months.

After a brief period of depression, Norman decided to take a pro-active stance. He recruited people who assisted him in researching alternative and traditional approaches to pancreatic cancer. He changed his lifestyle dramatically taking up a macrobiotic diet (largely vegetables and rice) and attending a support group, where he opened up to others in a 'breakthrough' for him. There he also learnt to practice meditation and visualization (mental imagery). His family was involved and supportive, his children drawing some of the images he was coming up with to defeat his cancer. He had a partial course of chemotherapy and an experimental monoclonal antibody treatment, a treatment which has since been discovered to have no benefit for pancreatic cancer.

An abdominal ultrasound, seven months after diagnosis showed Norman now had a normal pancreas and no evidence of metastatic disease in his liver. Further testing six months later continued to show that all evidence of the tumor was gone. His wife, Gerry Sue recalls the following conversation she had with doctors soon after

Norman's recovery: "One doctor looked at the other and said, 'Oh sure, it's called an instantaneous remission.' And I said, 'Isn't it funny that nobody ever told us that was an option? I mean, when he was so sick, we kept asking is there any hope? Is there anything good that can happen?' No one said, 'Maybe there will be an instantaneous remission.'"[46] Norman is alive today, well into his 80's.[47,48]

Chapter 2

FINDING MY DIRECTION

Follow your bliss.

JOSEPH CAMPBELL

In my second last year of medical school (1983) I was assigned to admit 43-year-old Ruth Collins to a surgical ward. She was to undergo exploratory surgery the following day. A delightful woman who worked as a librarian, Ruth was happily married and a proud mother of four children, all under the age of 12. A seemingly harmless symptom of indigestion had led her to have a gastroscopy which revealed a stomach cancer. The exploratory operation was to determine the extent of the cancer and if possible to remove it.

The following morning, the operating theatre was cool as I stood by Mr JB, a seasoned surgeon, ready to assist him. Mrs Collins was anesthetized and her surgery began. A vertical incision was made into her abdomen and soon after JB was able to place his hand inside her abdominal cavity. He felt around… "Shit!" he said, "she's riddled with it." I felt saddened at the implications for poor Mrs Collins as JB aborted the operation, skillfully sewing the ends of his incision back together as I, less than skillfully, cut the suture at the completion of each knot.

That afternoon an entourage followed JB as he visited each patient in turn on the surgical ward. Included in this group was a charge nurse, surgical registrar, surgical intern and four medical students, of which I was one. When we reached Mrs Collins bed she looked up expectantly. JB sat down on the end of her bed, "the cancer has spread extensively," he said, "there's nothing I could do." With that, he abruptly stood up and left the room, the entourage in trail. As I stumbled after the group I looked back to see Mrs Collin's ashen face. I ducked back into her room, "I'll come back at the end of the day," I said. She nodded her head.

That evening, with all my student duties completed, I sat with Mrs Collins for an hour and a half as she tried to come to terms with having only a short time to live. At times I held her hand, at times she shed a tear. She talked about her children, her husband and pondered about how they would cope without her. At the end of it all she gave me her phone number and invited me to share a meal with her family. I was torn by this offer. On the one hand, my medical education taught me not to get too close to my patients, on the other hand, I liked Mrs Collins, had made a meaningful connection with her and would have liked to have met her family. At the time, I admit I was also afraid of witnessing her demise. In the end I never called her. While I look back at my younger self and respect the decision I made, on some level I still regret it. She was discharged the next day and I never saw or heard of her again.

This experience taught me a great deal. There is no easy way to break bad news; JB said what he had to say. However, I learnt that good surgeons were not necessarily empathic listeners and empathic listeners were not necessarily good surgeons. While I was all thumbs and would never make any sort of a surgeon, I was a good listener. As my career would unfold, it would become ever clearer that my alternative choice at the end of my high school studies of behavioral science and psychology, was an indication as to where my medical practice would go.

Hospital challenges

Halfway through 1986, I awoke with a realization. I was in my second year of hospital residency as a Junior Resident Medical Officer (JRMO) and I had just completed a 110 hour working week for a cardiology (heart disease) unit. At the end of that week, almost delirious with fatigue, I'd collapsed on my bed and slept for 15 hours. When I woke, I peered out of my bedroom window, the world appeared brighter, clearer. Shimmering light reflected on bright green leaves against a backdrop of clear blue sky, birds were squawking at one another. Drinking this all in for the first time in months, or what felt like years, I realized I'd been living in a foggy overworked haze. 'This is crazy,' I thought, 'this is no way to live.. I'm not going to survive in this hospital!' It was time to plan my escape.

I was one of around 30 second-year doctors at the Alfred Hospital in Melbourne. The 30 would be culled to around 13 third year positions. These were highly sought after as a road to medical specialization. My plan was simple: I realized this road was not for me; and after completing the year, I was going to take a year away from hospital environments to reconsider my options.

With this in mind, I became strangely emboldened in relation to my interactions with my superiors, whose behavior, at times, I found less than respectful. No longer in fear of losing a potential third-year position, the second half of my JRMO year proved to be more enjoyable than the first. First up, let me explain that as a resident you work many more hours than you're actually paid for and at least in my day, this was never challenged. So when I entered the office of the brilliant but intimidating cardiology professor, Prof TP, and presented him with a reasonable request for eight hours of overtime payment, the look on his face was of pure bewilderment. I felt like Oliver in Dicken's *Oliver Twist*, asking for more gruel. I handed him the appropriate pink form and speechless for one of the few times that I'd known him, he signed it. I could have legitimately done this more than once, but I felt satisfied and dared not push my luck. Did this crossing of a taboo line influence the following events? I'll never know.

Towards the end of 1986, I was working in the Accident and Emergency Department (A & E) – aka The Emergency Room - during a time when the hospital's nurses were striking over pay and conditions. For this reason the hospital was only admitting true emergencies. It was a Tuesday morning when I was assigned to assess PJ, a 40-year-old man dressed in builder's overalls, who had walked in from a nearby building site complaining of chest pain. The type of chest pain he described was not typical of heart disease and his ECG and blood tests were all normal. Still, men like PJ don't readily seek help for pain, so I was uneasy about discharging him, but felt he was very unlikely to be granted an admission on my clinical assessment so far. So I spoke with the cardiology registrar, two years my senior, Dr CC, whom I had worked with previously whilst on staff with the cardiology unit.

I knew that Tuesday morning was when exercise stress testing was performed in the cardiology department. I described PJ's story to Dr CC and under the circumstances he agreed to add him to the exercise testing list that morning. At that time, a cardiac exercise stress test involved riding a stationary bicycle whilst connected up to heart monitoring leads. Well, I wasn't there, but the commotion that went on when PJ began to exercise and his monitor revealed significant ischemia (lack of oxygen to the heart muscle), led to the fellow being rushed to the Coronary Care Unit (CCU). Dr CC rang me with the news about PJ and warned me that Prof TP was on the war path. All I remember saying was it was better to have happened under medical supervision than back at PJ's building site.

When Prof TP and his entourage, including Dr CC and eight others, entered A & E later that morning, he headed directly towards me. He fixed me with his gaze and began a voluminous tirade admonishing me for my incompetence in front of 30 other staff and patients, a public shaming for what he believed was an unnecessarily risky referral for an exercise test. I tried to make my case, but it was like trying to blow back a cyclone. I will note here that as it turned out, PJ had an emergency coronary angiogram that very day where it was discovered that he had a 95% blockage of a main coronary artery. This was successfully treated with a balloon angioplasty and PJ's heart was not damaged in any way. He went home a lucky and healthier man.

Like most hospital residents, I made mistakes. Once, when exhausted at the end of a harrowing weekend shift, I accidentally gave an order for a medication at 10 times the correct dosage for an eight-year-old child, which could have resulted, but fortunately didn't, in serious harm or death. I was appropriately taken aside the next day by my superiors and the incident was calmly debriefed. The story with PJ was different: I'd consulted with Dr CC and I honestly felt my actions were reasonable given the nurses strike the hospital was operating under. Even if my actions were inappropriate, Prof TP's public shaming of me was unacceptable.

My ears were boiling red for the next half hour and I had to concentrate extra hard on the work at hand. I was allowed to take an early lunch and without a clear strategy, apart from reminding myself I wasn't coming back next year, I marched straight up to the Cardiology Department. I entered the wide corridor at the exact moment Prof TP and his entourage turned into the corridor from the opposite direction. Like something out of a classic Western, we both stopped when there was just a yard between us, his entourage eyeing me incredulously. I began by telling him loudly and clearly how inappropriate I felt his treatment had been of me downstairs. I also reiterated my belief that I'd probably saved PJ's life. Prof TP continued to assert his belief that I should've organized an admission based on the history of chest pain alone. We agreed to disagree and parted ways. I felt relieved that I had spoken up.

I've related this story in lectures I've given to Deakin University School of Medicine students, encouraging them to speak up in the face of bullying or intimidation, if not directly to the intimidator themselves, then at least via the hospital administration. Internalizing a sense of shame can contribute to mental health disorders and even some of the suicides that occur among medical trainees and residents.

This story didn't end there. With only one month to go before the end of that JRMO year I was sitting in the residence quarters, sipping a cup of tea, when I was approached by Dr CC. He took me to one side and said, "Prof TP wants to offer you a third-year position." My eyes widened with surprise before I replied, "I am honored, but I've decided my future lies in community medicine. Please thank Prof TP for his offer." A fellow JRMO overheard this, and punched me in the arm, "Are you mad? I'd kill for an opportunity like that!" I was honest with her and told her my mental health wouldn't survive another year in this hospital. I was sorry she was unable to obtain a position, but it was not my dream; a future in general practice was much more appealing.

Discovery

I began 1987 feeling freer than I had in years. I'd entered medical school at the age of 17 and now eight years later was finally on an extended break. I began the year working part-time as a locum GP (Family Physician) and got back to one of my loves, swimming, building my fitness once again. In April I met up in London with a friend, who was taking a similar break from hospital work, Dr Leon Chapman. Whilst in the UK Leon and I hired a car and travelled through the lush English countryside before embarking on a 21 day bus tour of Europe. We then flew to Israel, where we were both visiting family and parted ways as closer friends. I had arranged to stay on in Jerusalem studying humanities subjects at University, an enjoyable break from medical science. Broadening my knowledge and learning purely for the sake of it, without the pressure of sitting exams, was a real pleasure.

I rented a room in an apartment with two Israeli guys, one of whom, Nissim, was the cartoonist for the Jerusalem Post newspaper, the only English-language newspaper in Israel at the time. Located near the center of modern Jerusalem, like many buildings in this holy city, the apartment building was built of Jerusalem stone, a lovely pale, yellow brown stone quarried from the local area. We were located on the second floor and my room had its own private balcony overlooking a small tree-lined street. One quirky memory of this time is of sitting on my balcony listening to audiocassettes sent to me from Australia with recordings of the latest Australian Rules Football match. I enjoyed my team, Melbourne, making a late, brave, but unsuccessful run for the premiership.

Invariably my uniform was shorts, T-shirt and sandals. Blue skies and temperatures reliably in the high 20s (degrees Celsius) every day for six months, was a luxury I'd never experienced before. With all my belongings in my cool, tiled room and all my transport by foot or by bus, life was simple.

Enduring memories from this time include meandering through the streets of Jerusalem on long walks just soaking up the atmosphere; singing with a local musician; and a joyful friendship with my cousin, Meyer, and a US emergency physician specialist, Howard Levitin. The three of us would shoot baskets (basketball), reflect on the meaning of life, joke around and generally hang out together.

I decided to keep my medical skills from slumbering completely by doing a little work in Israel. I was accepted as a volunteer with the local ambulance service. On my initial observational trip, sitting in the back of the ambulance whilst it raced around the small, curvy streets of Jerusalem, I became increasingly queasy. When the ambulance arrived at the home of a 68-year-old lady having a heart attack, the paramedics raced to her aid whilst I raced for her bathroom, sick from motion sickness. The crew had a good laugh at my expense, transported the lady to the nearest hospital and dropped me off at a bus stop, my ambulance career over. Still, I managed to work as a volunteer in the Accident and Emergency Department at one of the local hospitals. They were grateful for whatever I could offer and I came and went as I pleased.

After many years of a timetabled existence, having space to reflect and relax was delicious. It also brought to the surface deeper yearnings. What's apparent to me now is that I was at this time existentially searching. Back home I had an attractive girlfriend, owned my own apartment and had a promising career. "This is as good as it gets," my girlfriend had said to me. My heart had sunk at this notion; there had to be more.

Despite my freedom, after several months I was homesick and disturbed by the frequently reported skirmishes between Palestinians and Israelis. Then one night Meyer took me along to a meditation group. I was reluctant at first as this was not something I'd ever contemplated, but after several invitations to attend, I finally agreed. I didn't realize I was about to find an answer to my existential angst.

Having visited Israel before and fallen in love with Jerusalem I had wondered whether I would feel more at home living there. Once again I delighted in the extraordinary beauty of this city along with the warm welcome of my extended family, yet despite all this it didn't feel like home. By contrast, within minutes of attending this meditation group, I had a feeling of coming home on the inside that was not dependent on place, religion or belief. With the echo of this came a knowing that all people and living things were somehow connected to this common thread. The more I practiced connecting with this experience, the more I noticed that I carried this feeling with me throughout my day. As a by-product, my tendency to get anxious and stressed was salved and I became happier and more stress resistant. My inner world was awake to the beauty of life, experienced as a love without end upon which all of creation was woven.

So life changing was this experience that I became an enthusiastic pain in the arse, wanting to share it with anyone who would listen. Yet despite my enlightening experiences with meditation, I remained wary of spiritual groups and religions, believing such experiences should be freely available to all, no hooks attached. I was then and am still particularly riled by groups that claim to have the only true path, elevating themselves above others. My understanding now is that this experience of connectedness occurs to some through love, prayer or meditation, to others through ritual, chanting or dance, and others still through communing with nature. Such deeply meaningful, spiritual feelings can be common ground for unifying interactions between people from different backgrounds; those who miss this point by championing their own way as the best or only way, are losing a great opportunity.

So fearless had I become in my blissful state, that I ignored all warnings to avoid the Old City of Jerusalem where an Intifada (Israeli/ Palestinian conflict) was occurring. I chose to go there to visit my meditation teacher, Rachel, the entrance to her house opening onto a narrow cobblestone laneway. Crazy as it may seem, even to me now, at the time the cups of tea and philosophical chats were worth the risk. Besides, back then I felt bullet-proof in my peace-filled armor.

This did not last. When the number nine bus, the bus route I used to take to the University, was firebombed, fortunately with no one inside, I was shaken by the news. My endless Jerusalem summer of innocence had come to an end; desert winds changed direction, the temperature began to fall; it was December and I needed to be home soon to catch the wave that would start my General Practice Training Program. It was time for me to return to Australia.

Chapter 3

MEDICINE,
AN INEXACT SCIENCE

*... medical students are taught that
everything they learn is going to be obsolete
soon after they graduate.*

SAMUEL ARBESMAN, AUTHOR 'THE HALF-LIFE OF FACTS'[1]

One plus one equals two, but medical practice is far from a simple equation. Place a person in a room with 10 others, some of whom are coughing and sneezing with colds, and you can't be certain whether they will catch the cold or not. It may come as a surprise, but this kind of uncertainty can be found throughout medical practice. The mechanism of action of many medications we prescribe is unknown, and often we do not know the cause of the illnesses we are treating. Hence, the treatment plans we use are ever changing. Paradoxically, this uncertainty brings hope, as there are so many promising new areas to research and new discoveries regularly bring forward potential new treatments.

Let's look at the recent history of treating the mental health disorder, schizophrenia, as an example.[2] When the term schizophrenia was first coined in 1910, recommended treatments included injecting sulfur to induce fever, and locking people away in asylums. As time progressed, brain surgery was tried along with electroconvulsive therapy. When barbiturate medication was shown to help, it was used until antipsychotic medication was discovered in the 1950s.

The mental state of psychosis, which is typical in schizophrenia, is described by some as like experiencing a dream whilst still awake, and not being able to distinguish easily between the dream and the real world. In this state of mind, voices can be heard or images seen which seem real to the person with schizophrenia, but are not to others. Antipsychotic medication helps to dampen these experiences. They were considered a big breakthrough, as they allowed even asylum bound schizophrenics to recover enough to return to the community. Unfortunately, medication side-effects remained problematic, leaving many people affected by schizophrenia unable to work and many feeling so miserable that they would stop their tablets.

Chris was 32 and worked as a part-time laborer. He'd suffered from schizophrenia for more than 12 years. In that time he had frequently stopped his medication leaving him with florid psychosis. In this state he was a danger to himself. Hence, he found himself requiring frequent admission to psychiatric hospitals, where his condition would once again be stabilized with antipsychotic medication.

He consulted with me, pleading with me to offer him a treatment other than medication. "The medication dulls my entire experience of life and I hate it," he told me. At that time I knew of no other effective treatments and after empathizing with his predicament, admitted I was disappointed not to have an answer for him, but that I was not the final word on this and that new research was happening all the time.

It's 20 years since I consulted with Chris and change is afoot. Studies have shown that counselling therapies, such as cognitive behavioral therapy, can achieve better long-term outcomes without the need for medication at all.[3,4,5] If I'd suggested this possibility in the mid-1980s in my final medical exams, I would have failed. The point here is that treatment strategies and ideas are in flux, more rapidly than ever before, as new understandings, therapies and research come to light. So people affected by schizophrenia in Chris's situation now have more options.

In contrast to the ever changing face of medicine, professions such as accounting are based in mathematical formulae and allow us to calculate our bank interest with precision. We have come to expect this precision in all fields of life; after all we can land space probes on comets. So if our accountant said the best he could do was to estimate a tax return between $40 and $3000, we would probably take our business elsewhere. Yet the survival range for some cancers can be four months to 20 years. Medicine is not an exact science in the same way as accounting or rocket science, even if it aspires to be.

While the scientific revolution led to the introduction of machinery in so many areas of our lives, medicine began to look at the body as a machine. This brought us invaluable knowledge, as there are certainly aspects that are machinelike, such as our pumping heart, our various pipes and plumbing and biomechanical skeleton, an understanding of which has allowed tremendous medical advances.

While mechanical metaphors and models can be helpful in certain particular ways, they can also be problematic, as people start to believe them as representing all that a human being is. For instance, the expectation this creates is that doctors can be as precise as mechanics in all areas of practice. This is particularly problematic when dealing with the many chronic diseases that afflict our society. Diseases such as heart disease, cancer, asthma, diabetes, multiple sclerosis, Parkinson's disease, rheumatoid arthritis, fibromyalgia, psoriasis, lupus, depression, schizophrenia, dementia and many more, have causes that are poorly understood. They also have symptomatic treatments that are far from precise and often require a deal of trial and error.

Medications we have developed can improve quality of life and be life-saving, but can also be variable in their benefits and have unpredictable side effects, sometimes even fatal ones. Iatrogenic illness, illness that inadvertently occurs as a result of medical treatment, is a huge problem, listed as the third most common cause of death in the U.S.A![6] Medical practice is not the science of mechanics or accountancy. The art of medicine often comes down to weighing up pros and cons and many other factors in treating each individual.

Human beings are not machines

It is interesting that I've rarely heard a person refer to their pet cat, dog or budgie as a machine. Yet as human beings we are often heard to refer to ourselves as such. Our brains are likened to computers, our hearts are likened to pumps and sportsmen can be referred to as 'big units.' As I've alluded to, using the analogy of a machine may be useful in explaining certain things, but there is a danger in thinking of ourselves like this.

As living beings, unlike machines, we defy entropy (decay), at least temporarily. As old cells die they're replaced with new ones; if we are wounded our body self-repairs; and it constantly works to keep things in balance (maintain homeostasis), whether it be the pH of our blood or our core body temperature.

Miss a night's sleep, skip eating and drinking for a day, or simply knock our shin and we're reminded of our fragility. If we scratch our skin deeply enough we'll hurt and bleed. We also sexually reproduce, experience a range of emotions and raise our young (unlike a machine).

The complexity of how our body systems work together is hard to fathom. Subtle interactions between the nervous system (including our five senses), endocrine (hormonal) system, immune system, lymphatic system, circulatory system, lungs, oxygen carrying system, blood production systems, reproductive system, detoxification systems, waste processing systems, kidneys, gastrointestinal system, and musculoskeletal system, keep us alive and functioning every second of the day. All this takes place with exquisite, accurate monitoring of the interactions between us and our environment, without us having to think about it. Each of these systems has had many a textbook written about them and more recently about the ways they work together, yet there is still so much to learn.

On a microscopic level we are made up of trillions of cells. Each cell (picture as a ball if you like) is surrounded by a constantly vibrating cell membrane. This membrane contains the cell contents and interacts with its environment by allowing certain things in and certain things out. The body's cells never sleep, going about the business of maintaining life, whether that be assimilating nutrition, building new proteins or eliminating toxins. It is worth remembering that there is a lot working well in your body to keep you alive, even if you do have an illness.

Within each cell are a number of smaller parts. These are known as organelles, including our energy producing mitochondria, and a nucleus containing the genetic code that is the template for producing all of our body parts. The 23,000 or so genes contained within this template differ slightly in each individual, creating a blueprint as unique as an individual's fingerprint.

On every other level you care to look, human beings are gloriously complex. We have a wide range of cultures and languages, a compulsion to create art and a genius in innovative technology. We are capable of great acts of charity and kindness, but also acts of cruelty and selfishness. We laugh, we cry, we can appreciate beauty or be oblivious to it all together. Our hearts can grow with love or sear with hatred. Our health and well-being suffers without the company of others, but we also need time alone. We need a level of support to feel like we belong, and a sense of meaning and purpose to help us to get up and face our daily lives.

Apart from the obvious, such as clean drinking water, nutritious food, shelter, and sanitation, our health is influenced by many things. This includes: the company we keep, habits we take up, our employment, how happy or otherwise we are, the attitudes we take, how stressed we feel, food choices we make, the type of exercise we do or don't do, and toxic exposures. All these factors and many more, influence the numerous systems of the body that I've referred to above.

While collectively all humans (billions of us) have arisen from a common African ancestor and have common human traits, we are also individual, inexact creatures. We have our particular personalities, socio-cultural contexts and genetic signatures. Life is fluid and dynamic on every level. Our social situation, our stress levels, our attitudes and inspirations, exercise levels and our diet can all alter regularly. As you will discover in future chapters, quite apart from the treatments we may be having, positive lifestyle changes alone can affect the course of a disease within weeks, influencing our body right down to the level of gene expression.

So it can be helpful to remember that Medicine is an inexact science, especially in the realm of predicting prognosis, which is an ever moving thing. Health will never be found through a simple one size fits all prescription alone, as much as we might like it to.

Models of health - reductionism and holism

The way we think about disease determines the way we diagnose and treat it. Looking through history, this has changed over time. For example, the discovery of microbes causing infectious illnesses was a huge breakthrough in our understanding. This discovery went hand in hand with other breakthroughs in science based on *reductionism;* the view that scientific explanations inherently work by analyzing things into smaller components, like the discovery of microbes.[7] It's a view that relies on 'zooming in' if you like, the microscope being emblematic. In contrast, *holism* relies on 'zooming out,' looking at the wide range of influences which might contribute to the development of disease.

In many ways reductionism is easier to understand. You detect an infectious agent, you treat it or vaccinate against it. A single cause leads to a particular treatment for a specific disease. In certain instances treatment is straightforward and uncomplicated. If you have scurvy, you treat with vitamin C; break a leg, you set it straight. A reductionist diagnosis has the great advantage of specificity. It is also an invaluable asset when treating emergencies. It has led to a growth in 'zooming in' pathology tests and imaging techniques which help us to diagnose and treat a wide variety of problems, from genetic defects to traumatic injuries. Not surprisingly then, reductionism has dominated medical education and therefore the way doctors have thought in the last century.

The discovery of microbes and the early success of antibiotic pills in treating infections set up an expectation that all diseases could be diagnosed and treated this easily. It is tempting to think that there is a 'magic bullet' treatment for every illness. This way of thinking is reflected in the public health pronouncements we hear, such as: 'the War against cancer;' 'the Battle against MS;' 'the Fight against obesity.' Reductionism has also led to a use of language that I was guilty of in my medical training days in hospitals, referring to, "the liver disease in bed five;" a dehumanizing way of referring to Mr Jones, a father of four and a mechanic with a wicked sense of humor, who was afflicted with liver disease.

The great strength of reductionism, its ability to provide specific treatments, can also be a great limitation. For if there are no more specific treatments to try, a practitioner who only thinks in this way, will say, as Mrs Smythe experienced (see Chapter 1), "there's nothing more we can do for you," pulling the rug out on hope. In contrast, a practitioner who also thinks holistically, recognizes there are a myriad of ways that could be suggested or facilitated that could enhance a person's self-healing systems, and at the very least, improve the way they feel. Another important limitation of reductionism occurs when someone does not fit any recognized diagnostic category. In this situation they can be too quickly labelled as a malingerer (one who pretends to be unwell). We will explore this further when we look at Chronic Fatigue Syndrome (CFS) in Chapter 15 - Validity and Social Support.

While faith in reductionism solving all our medical ills remains high in some circles, evidence mounts that the majority of the illnesses of Western society are complex in origin and relate to our socio-economic situation and lifestyle choices.[8] Treating and preventing these requires involvement of the holistic way of thinking. The following analogy from Dr Vicki Kotsirilos and her co-authors helps us understand the holistic approach.[9]

The plant analogy

"If given the 'right conditions', the body has an innate capacity to heal. The body is equipped with natural healing mechanisms. A good analogy of this is the sick plant. Most gardeners know that plants can thrive well by providing the 'right conditions', such as the right amount of sunlight, fresh air, nutrient-dense soil, a stable, nurturing environment free of chemicals, and adequate water. Even if a plant appears unwell, changing any of these conditions can aid the recovery of the plant. If we apply this concept to the unwell person, their needs are very similar. Human needs for maintaining and restoring good health include plenty of fresh air, exercise, adequate water, sunlight, good nutritious unprocessed foods, a peaceful environment free of chemicals, excessive noise and light, good quality sleep, contact with nature and people, meaning and joy in our lives, and minimizing psychological stress."

Another way of conceptualizing this is by referring to the Chinese symbols of yin and yang. In this instance, yin represents the nurturing, gentle, patient approach, while yang is the decisive, directive, active approach. They can complement each other in surprising ways. Here is an abstract from research published in the journal, *Science*, back in 1984:

- "Records on recovery after cholecystectomy (gallbladder removal surgery) of patients in a suburban Pennsylvania hospital between 1972 and 1981 were examined to determine whether assignment to a room with a window view of a natural setting might have restorative influences. Twenty-three surgical patients assigned to rooms with windows looking out on a natural scene had shorter postoperative hospital stays, received fewer negative evaluative comments in nurses' notes, and took fewer potent analgesics (painkillers) than 23 matched patients in similar rooms with windows facing a brick building wall."[10]

Here the 'restorative influences' (yin) of a window view of a natural setting, complemented the surgical therapy (yang). Need I say, all the more evidence we are not merely mechanoids.

The more yin holistic model is much better suited to non-emergency and longer term problems and has the advantage of being applicable in any situation, accompanying specific treatments or even when no more specific medical treatments are of value. In many cases, as in the above cholecystectomy research, the combination of reductionist specific treatments with holistic ones works best.

Let's take the example of a diabetic who might require a medication, yet will also benefit from diet, exercise and stress reduction techniques. In many instances, if they take to the holistic treatments with gusto, they may no longer require medication. Similar scenarios can occur with the treatment of high blood pressure or high cholesterol and a raft of other problems. The challenge of the holistic approach is that it requires the patient (us) to take responsibility for making healthy choices. It also requires different skills for health professionals to both inform and facilitate this process.

The truth is both approaches have potential pitfalls if overly favored. Holistic thinkers can get so attached to their approach, that they can overlook a more accurate diagnosis and specific treatments. Reductionist thinkers can get so stuck in their own approach that they keep looking for a single answer pharmaceutical treatment, when multiple factors need to be addressed.

Developing a good marriage between reductionist and holistic thinking is a formidable task. The search for and provision of miracle drugs is a whole lot sexier than say, changing a diet. Their creation involves the intellectual challenge of diving into biochemical and genetic pathways that can lead to the discovery of a pharmaceutical that can be marketed profitably. This attracts research funding. In contrast, the subtle nuances of motivating and facilitating lifestyle change are not of great interest for many medical scientists. Research funding has been harder to come by for these holistic therapies. However, as research does grow, we are coming to appreciate that the very biochemical and genetic pathways we seek to alter with pharmaceuticals, can also be altered by the simple day-to-day choices that we make (see Chapter 4 - Epigenetics). This may not be sexy, but it's empowering. I'm hopeful the potential of these low-cost interventions will increasingly attract the interest and funding of governments battling burgeoning health costs. Not surprisingly, health insurance companies wanting to limit their liabilities encourage healthy lifestyle choices.

Matt first came to consult with me on a Tuesday morning. He had recently returned from a holiday in Bali and was complaining of abdominal pain and diarrhea. Thirty years of age, he worked as a store-man and packer, was single and lived alone. Apart from the fact he was obviously overweight, the first thing that struck me was the stench of alcohol. When I examined him, the most significant finding was an elevated blood pressure of 170/100. I inquired about his drinking patterns. He admitted to having 30 pots of beer every Friday night with his mates after work and that he had hit the booze heavily during his recent vacation. I organized for him to have some blood tests and reviewed him with those results a week later. He agreed to abstain from drinking until then.

He came back looking a little brighter, smelling fresher and he no longer had any stomach problems. His test results showed abnormal liver function tests and significantly elevated cholesterol and the other fat marker, triglycerides. At this stage of my career, I had not learnt the subtle skills of motivational interviewing, where you get a person to reflect on the pros and cons of their unhealthy behavior. Instead I showed him his results and told him if he kept drinking the way he had been, that he would be lucky to reach 50. Fortunately, he didn't charge for the door. In fact, I felt him engage with me for the first time as I explained that all of these abnormalities, along with his elevated blood pressure, could be caused by his heavy drinking. He shared that he had also lost his license for 12 months for drink-driving. Determined to take advantage of the moment, much to the chagrin of my next patient, we went overtime developing a strategy for him to stay off the booze. He came up with the idea of riding a bike to work instead of taking public transport, and skipping the Friday night pub event. We set a short-term goal of two weeks.

Two weeks later he looked a little better again. His blood pressure was now 150/85 and he was enjoying riding to work. We worked on a few more strategies for avoiding temptation and developing new habits, including a few dietary improvements. We stretched the next short-term goal to one-month, which he achieved. I kept reviewing him intermittently for the next six months, at which time we repeated his blood tests. By this visit he had lost 12.5kg (28lbs), his blood pressure was 120/80, his liver function, cholesterol and triglycerides had all returned to normal. He felt happier and healthier and had joined a 10 pin bowling team, where he had made new friends.

Matt's example demonstrates how reductionist and holistic approaches can work together. If a purely reductionist approach was taken, he may have been treated with cholesterol-lowering medication and blood pressure lowering medication, without the time and attention being given to the key issue, namely his behavior. If a purely behavioral approach had been used, we may not have found the key motivational factors of serious disease markers on his blood test results. Instead, the coordinated approach of zooming in to specific diagnostics, together with a zooming out lifestyle overview, gave the time and space required for Matt to pull together pieces of his life and get off a downward, alcohol-fueled spiral. This type of good result for Matt also extends benefits to his nearest and dearest and the wider community, as well as lessening the strain on the health system.

The dance between zooming in and zooming out is not an exact science. The challenge for governments and medical education is providing the incentives and skills for doctors and other health professionals, to learn to dance this dance in a flexible way. It requires adequate provision for longer consultations along with the teaching of communication skills and non-pharmaceutical treatments with a broader emphasis, to complement the application of more specific computer-based protocols. The potential rewards are high, as we will explore in Chapters 6 and 7 - Lifestyle as Therapy, for comprehensive lifestyle therapy does not only prevent disease, but can actually treat it.

The Therapeutic Relationship

Why is it that two doctors, who on the surface are providing the same therapy, will have different outcomes with different patients? There is something in the relationship itself at work here.

A Canadian research study demonstrated the importance of this.[11] It involved 21 family medicine practitioners and 265 people presenting with newly diagnosed headache. The doctors were asked to record their diagnosis and management plan at their first consultation with the patient. Each patient was then interviewed six weeks after the initial consultation and asked an extensive series of questions. They were then sent two questionnaires at six and 12 months after the initial visit.

The doctors classified 56 of the patients as having organic headaches (sinusitis, neck problems, and injury etc) and 209 as having non-organic headaches (tension, migraine etc). Two thirds of the patients indicated that pain and concern about the cause of their headache were major reasons for attending. Having no headaches in the month prior to the 12 month survey and stating that headaches were no longer a problem was defined as a good outcome.

When the researchers correlated the 12 month findings with the data collected at the six-week interview, they discovered some revealing things. Only three factors were statistically significantly ($p< 0.05$) and independently associated with a good outcome. Of these, one factor was clearly the most strongly linked: that was the patient's assessment at six weeks, *that he or she had had the opportunity to discuss his or her problem fully.* Interestingly, this correlation held for both organic and non-organic headaches, (the other two correlating factors were a lack of visual symptoms and an organic diagnosis). Medications, investigations and referrals were notably absent from the list of significant variables.

Another fascinating finding was that the doctor's lesser degrees of liking the patient, at the first visit, was a predictor of poor outcome. Further analysis found that there was a highly significant correlation (p = 0.001) between the patients' perception of full discussion and the physicians liking the patient.

In the discussion of their findings the authors stated the following: "The outcome of the illness is indeed influenced by the doctor-patient interaction, the question arises as to how the effect is produced. The visit of a patient to his or her family doctor, or to a chosen consultant, has all the elements of the 'healing context' within which the so-called placebo effect is thought to occur." (Note: We will explore the placebo effect in Chapter 9 - Meaning.)

Given that headache is one of the most common presenting problems for GP's,[12] the potential benefits of putting a greater emphasis on the therapeutic interaction and less emphasis on drug therapy, are substantial. Of course the benefit of feeling listened to without judgement extends beyond just headaches.

Mother of six, Therese, was no stranger to surgery or to pain. She was born with a condition called Multiple Hereditary Exostoses, and had required multiple surgeries from the age of 3 to remove the non-cancerous bony outgrowths that occur with this condition. In 1991 at the age of 47, following years of back and hip pain, she was diagnosed with hip dysplasia and underwent a hip replacement. Following the operation her back pain worsened and she experienced terrible muscle spasms. She tried a variety of medications, physiotherapists and chiropractors, but received little relief. One of the physios unhelpfully told her she only had the problem because she was too fat!

She heard that Dr S was a GP with a special interest in musculo-skeletal problems and booked in to see him. She describes from the outset a feeling of being listened to, received and empathized with. He did not judge anything she had tried in the past and she felt respected. He treated her with acupuncture, and with forewarning, painful stretching maneuvers. They built trust and rapport and she willingly performed the specific exercises he taught her, including some that helped her self-mobilize (free up) her back. The pain and spasm began to respond and over a 12 month period he lengthened the time between visits until she became independent in managing her back pain. Twenty-three years later she continues to lead an active life, walks 30 to 60 minutes each day and still uses the techniques that Dr S taught her. Recently, she completed an honors degree in Philosophy.

The relationship you have with your doctor is an important part of any healing process. It is enhanced if your doctor displays sincere, accurate empathy, warmth and genuineness, and if you trust her or him.[13] Therese's interaction with Dr S is a testament to this. Other key factors that increase your chances of getting well following a consultation are the confidence with which your doctor prescribes his or her treatment and whether or not you feel adequately informed about what is going on.[14] We'll explore this further in the chapter on Meaning.

Clearly it's worthwhile finding a GP whose competence you trust, who listens well and whom you can get along with.

Trudy's story

When I gave a lecture on 'Counselling in General Practice' to fourth-year Monash medical students, I presented Trudy's story to emphasize the importance of listening.

It was a Friday afternoon at the end of a busy week when I received a phone call. On the other end of the line was a woman I'd never met before pleading with me to see her daughter, Trudy. I was consulting in my role as a GP and asked my receptionist to fit Trudy in at the end of my session. At that time in my life, Friday night dinners were spent at my parents, where my siblings and their partners would gather for a family meal, something I looked forward to. I informed them I would be late and to start without me.

I followed my second last patient into the reception area and looked out at a near empty waiting room. An agitated figure sat hunched in a corner beside a pot plant. "Trudy," I called. She rose at the sound of her name, her tall angular frame bounding ahead of me into my consulting room. As I sat down she emptied half the contents of her handbag onto my desk, spilling forth six prescriptions for various sedatives and tranquilizers. "I've seen six different doctors and all they give me is this! This isn't going to help me!" Her eyes were wild, desperate and she was shaking.

I felt bombarded and out of my depth, but I sat and listened, allowing her to vent. Gradually her story unfolded. Trudy had gotten involved with the wrong sort of crowd in her late teens, becoming a heroin addict and prostitute by her early 20s. An only child, her parents separated when she was five. Her mother remained her most steadfast supporter and the rock upon which this latest attempt to withdraw from illicit drugs and find a new life could rest. At 28, and having been through many drug rehabilitation programs that proved ultimately unsuccessful, Trudy was determined to succeed this time - going cold turkey.

About halfway through hearing her story I experienced a flashback. It was a cold winter's night; tired, nearing the end of a 12 hour shift, I was an intern in the Accident and Emergency Department at the Alfred Hospital in Melbourne, keen to get home. My final patient for the evening was a distressed young lady who had been working as a street prostitute when she was badly beaten by a client. I carefully assessed her, noting many tender areas and bruises and organized for a number of x-rays to exclude fractures. It was 1 a.m. and my shift was at an end when I came to check on her trolley which was in a queue outside of X-RAY. Two trolley-beds lay ahead of her and two behind, like planes awaiting clearance on a runway. As I walked past her I noticed a bruise behind her left ear which I'd not noted before. Forgetting her state of mind and without warning her as to what I was about to do, I moved closer to inspect it. What happened next took only a matter of seconds, but would etch its mark on my memory. Spooked, Trudy lashed out, swinging her right arm; I drew my upper body backwards like a limbo dancer; two orderlies rushed to my aid, her fear further inflamed by their arrival, she climbed out of her trolley, grabbed her clothes and wearing a hospital gown and yelling expletives, bounded out of the building.

My shift was over. Exhausted and feeling like an incompetent fool, I finished the appropriate paperwork and I too left the building. I arrived home, it was empty and dark. I opened the front door, turned on a light, glanced in a mirror and caught the vision of blood red welts across my forehead, where her fingernails had met my skin. Being physically struck by a patient under my care had broken an unspoken protective belief I had around the doctor-patient relationship, and I was shaken; I sobbed.

Now six years later, the same young lady was sitting opposite me, oblivious as to our previous encounter, and a strange feeling settled upon me, a positive omen if you like; I would have another chance to help her.

After clarifying her story, I drew two contiguous side by side spirals on a piece of paper. I pointed to one and said, "this is the chaos spiral where you find yourself now. It's possible to weave out of this and into the peaceful spiral where you can experience a deep sense of connection to your calm self."

Shaking, she looked up at me and said, "Bullshit!"

"You may think so, but that doesn't stop me believing this is where you can get to," I said. "Would you be willing to try a relaxation exercise that might start this process?" Just desperate enough to overcome her suspicions, Trudy agreed to try. She lay down on my examination couch and over the next 20 minutes I talked her through an exercise in which she strongly tensed, then relaxed, various parts of her body. Much to my relief, Trudy calmed down. She returned to her seat where she sat, somewhat stunned by the fact that she was no longer shaking. I pointed out how this demonstrated that she had more control over her withdrawal symptoms than she'd realized and I encouraged her to practice the muscle relaxation exercise at least once, preferably twice, a day. After what turned out to be a 90 minute consultation, we agreed to meet again in a week's time. She walked out of the building.

Over the weeks and months that followed, Trudy managed to stay away from heroin, marijuana and stimulants and was able to wean slowly off diazepam (Valium). We both agreed that her cigarette smoking could wait to be tackled at a later time. While she was doing this drug withdrawal, we worked on a four pronged approach to restoring her health and well-being: relaxation; nutrition; exercise; and fun. Trudy had forgotten how to have fun and I discovered she spent most of the day watching horror videos. I suggested she not only walk her dog more often but play with him as well. I also suggested that she swap the horror movies for comedies. This was instantly beneficial.

I continued to consult with Trudy over a four-year period and in this time I witnessed her transform her life. She moved to a different part of town, initially living with her mother and eventually independently; she helped to inspire some of her 'bad' old friends to get off the drugs too and made new friends; she trained herself in arts and crafts, producing jewelry which she sold at local markets; and she stayed drug-free. She also quit smoking. Interestingly, all my subsequent consultations lasted no longer than 60 minutes. Trudy just needed me to bear witness to her ups and downs and her overall positive progress.

I shared with the medical students that Trudy had told me, some years after our initial meeting, from her point of view there were two keys to our successful interaction: I'd really listened to her at that first consultation; and I'd believed in her. I encouraged my audience to practice listening, an invaluable skill that did not require a degree to acquire. Two students in the lecture were so inspired by Trudy's turnaround and the potential benefits from being a good listener, that they organized a group of fellow fourth-year students, with the assistance of the hospital's Social Work Department, to provide supportive counselling for hospital inpatients. Forty students, one quarter of the year group, signed up for this voluntary out of hours work.

Chapter 4

EPIGENETICS - HOW GENES CHANGE THEIR TUNE

It's not just a matter of playing the genetic cards you're dealt. We have the power to shape our own lives. The reality is a much more optimistic scenario than if it were just a matter of picking the right parents.

JOHN ROWE, PROF OF GERIATRICS AT HARVARD MEDICAL SCHOOL, CHAIRMAN, MACARTHUR FOUNDATION RESEARCH NETWORK ON SUCCESSFUL AGEING.

The leap in understanding from genetics to epigenetics is analogous to the jump from Newtonian to quantum physics.

TORI SOMMER

When Watson and Crick discovered the double helix model of deoxyribonucleic acid (DNA) in 1953, it felt like the secret of life itself had been unraveled. The DNA code was found to contain a variable sequence of four chemical bases: Adenine, Thymine, Cytosine and Guanine, (abbreviated as A, T, C, G). They had found the template for the construction of all living things. They discovered that the two strands of the molecule spiral together with A lined up across from T, while C forms a complimentary pair with G. The molecule unzips itself to allow for replication of the DNA or to allow a smaller molecule, messenger ribonucleic acid (mRNA), to read a section of the DNA (i.e. a gene), and translate this into the production of a protein. It then elegantly zips itself up again. So efficient is this molecule that only rarely do errors in replication, known as mutations, occur.[1] All the information contained within the DNA is compacted into 46 chromosomes (23 pairs) contained within the nucleus of each cell.

While the discovery of genes was in its infancy towards the end of Darwin's time, it would tie in beautifully with his theory of evolution. It gave a mechanism, in the form of random genetic mutations, conferring a life-saving advantage or disadvantage to an organism, allowing for the slow process of evolution by natural selection, 'survival of the fittest.' It was associated with the belief that the genetic code you were born with was unchangeable, 'Darwinian determinism.' In other words, your fate was cast in your DNA, a belief that many of us still hold.

Genomics, a discipline in genetics, is changing our beliefs. It is involved in sequencing and analyzing the function and structure of genomes which are the complete set of DNA within a single cell of an organism.[2] When the Human Genome Project was completed in the year 2000, it had taken over 10 years to sequence 3 billion genetic chemical base codes at a cost of over $2 billion (with New Generation Sequencing it now costs closer to $1000 - and falling!). It had also led to some surprises. Many scientists had predicted the code for producing a human being would contain at least 100,000 genes. In fact the number was closer to 23,000, a similar number of genes to that found within an earthworm's genome. Interestingly those 23,000 genes only took up 2% of the DNA found in a human cell. The remaining 98% was labelled junk, in that it was thought to have no function, although it contained intriguing sequences consistent with our evolutionary past.

For example, our most recent evolutionary relatives, the chimpanzee and bonobo monkey, share 99% of the same genetic code as us.[3]

What has become increasingly apparent is that what distinguishes us from earthworms is not the number of genes we have or just the differences in code, but the way in which these genes are 'played.' If we use an analogy of a musical instrument, we can picture these 23,000 genes as keys on a very large piano, each key being a gene containing thousands of chemical base codes. Until recently, it was thought that we were born with a particular genetic code that couldn't change its tune. A branch of genomics, known as the science of epigenetics, (meaning in Greek, 'around the gene') has shown that this is not the case.[4]

Our genes are in fact in constant flux, being influenced by the environment around them. While the template of codes remains the same, they're either being switched off (down regulated) or switched on (up regulated). Codes are most commonly down regulated by a biochemical process called methylation that covers parts of the code making them unreadable. They are generally up regulated by a biochemical process called histone modification. With this flexibility, it turns out that a single gene can produce a variety of different proteins depending on the environment it finds itself in.[5,6]

Our understanding grew with the discovery that the non-coding or junk DNA, the rest of the piano and pianist if you like, wasn't junk at all. In fact it played important structural roles, such as forming the telomere caps to stop our chromosomes from unravelling, as well as a role in 'playing our genes' by, for example, attracting enzymes into the mix. Hence, this so-called junk, our deep, past genetic history, was somehow involved in influencing our present and future.

The combination of the differences in our genetic code and the complexity of how our genes are played, distinguishes us from the earthworm, chimpanzee and each other. Our tune can subtly and importantly alter all the time. Alterations produced by methylation, for instance, can lead to changes in our tune that can be passed on through several generations. Other changes can be more fleeting. Some days we'll be more in the groove than others, as some keys (genes) are being played more heavily while others are played more softly, subtly nuanced or not at all.

The protein products of the gene along with changes in the chemical milieu within the cell, both of which are influenced by our environment, affect gene expression. Approximately 90% of our genes are engaged in cooperation with signals from the environment in this way.[7]

If there is a conductor in all this, it is in the dance between these interplaying factors. I use environment here in the broadest sense, including our social situation, how we feel, think, the air we breathe, the food we eat, what we drink, the pills we swallow, and the list goes on. This dynamic interplay between our genes and our environment can make us sick or keep us well.

Epigenetics suggests thousands of combinations, sequences, and pattern variations in a single gene are possible (analogous to the thousands of combinations, sequences, and patterns of neural networks that are possible in the brain).[8] With more than 23,000 different genes to look at, scientists are now hoping to map the many millions of possible epigenetic variations that exist in a cooperative effort known as the Human Epigenome Project.[9] The complexity of this endeavor dwarfs the earlier Human Genome Project. While knowing our genetic code (genome) provides us with some useful information about our strengths and weaknesses and some treatments we would be best suited to, knowledge of our epigenome offers huge potential for learning how to 'play our code' so that we can be at our healthiest.

So let's be clear, while our personal genome (genetic blueprint), does not change, the way these genes express themselves, our epigenome, does change. The extent to which this is possible we are only just beginning to appreciate. This discovery is leading us to new understandings not only of health and disease, but also of epigenetic inheritance and evolution itself.

Nutrition and our genes

To make the link between our genes and our environment more tangible, let's spend some time looking at some examples of how basic nutrition interplays with epigenetics. Nutrigenomics is the study of the effects of foods and food constituents on gene expression. It also involves the study of how our individual genetic differences can affect the way we respond to different foods.[10] Here are a few examples of nutrients that alter gene expression:[11,12]

- Glucosinolates -- found in vegetables such as broccoli, cauliflower and brussel sprouts, activate genes responsible for cleansing the body of toxins.
- Genistein -- found in soy, activates a gene whose action increases the level of HDL (good) cholesterol.
- Resveratrol -- found in red wine, stimulates a gene that protects tissues against damage from destructive molecules called free radicals.
- Lycopene -- found in tomato products, slows down the gene involved in prostate cancer.
- Gama-linolenic acid -- found in evening primrose oil, reduces the activity of a gene involved in breast cancer and other malignancies.[13]
- Curcumin -- found in the spice turmeric, suppresses genes associated with inflammation.
- Omega-3-fatty acids -- found in cold water fish, such as

salmon and sardines, and plant foods such as flax seeds, also helps down regulate inflammation genes.

An example of the potential importance of individualized genetic testing directing nutritional advice, involves folate, homocysteine, and the gene called MTHFR (methylene tetrahydrofolate reductase). Homocysteine is produced in the making of certain proteins. When inefficiently metabolized in the body, it can build up to dangerously high levels, increasing the risk of heart disease, life-threatening blood clots and stroke. High levels of homocysteine during pregnancy are also associated with abnormal formation of the nervous system in the developing fetus.

Adequate levels of B vitamins, particularly folate, help to keep homocysteine levels low. The MTHFR enzyme assists in this process. About one in eight people have a gene variation of the MTHFR that makes the enzyme very inefficient. Research has shown that when such individuals have a diet low in folate, their homocysteine levels rise sharply. By increasing their intake of folate these levels can easily be brought down to normal. Genetic testing can detect this need so that vulnerable people can make sure their diet is high in folate rich foods, such as green leafy vegetables.[14]

Genetic testing is still relatively expensive and is not routinely done in medical practice, although this could soon change. Private companies do offer this testing without a doctor's referral. If you choose to take this path, I still advise you to discuss the results with your doctor so that he or she can help bring perspective. Without this some people have been unnecessarily frightened when receiving their genetic test results. Apart from the potential emotional implications of genetic testing, there are also privacy and insurance issues. If you take out a new life insurance policy or adjust an existing one you will have a duty to inform the insurer about any significant genetic test results.[15]

Nutritional genomics promises more personalized medicine and health advice based upon an understanding of our individual nutritional needs, health status and our genome. Nutrigenomics also promises to have impacts on society, from medicine to agriculture, and from dietary choices to social and public policies. Its application is likely to exceed that of even the human genome project. Chronic diseases (and some types of cancer) may be preventable, or at least delayed, by maintaining a balanced, individually suited diet. In addition, knowledge gained from comparing diet/gene interactions in different populations may provide information needed to address the enormous problem of global malnutrition and disease.[16]

Evolution on speed

Before Darwin, the 18th century French scientist, Chevalier de Lamarck, proposed the idea that in adapting to their environment, animals acquired new characteristics which were then passed on to their offspring.[17] Lamarck's theory of evolution, published in 1809, the year Darwin was born, was heavily criticized in France by his peers. While Darwin considered Lamarck's ideas possible, Lamarck and his theory were in fact ridiculed for the best part of 150 years, while Darwin's slower evolutionary model took center stage.[18] Lamarck was blind and penniless when he died and was buried in an unmarked lime pit somewhere in northern France.[19] Belated, appropriate recognition is long overdue. Lamarck's rapid evolutionary process became known as soft inheritance. We now call this epigenetics.

While in awe of Darwin's theory of evolution, I've always wondered whether this theory fully explains the speed with which species adapt to environmental change. Epigenetics relieves my conundrum as it complements it and adds booster juice! At its core it refers to the fact that the tune (genetic expression), being influenced by the environment, can change during a single lifetime, and that this change can be transmitted to generations to come. This has profound implications. Let's look at animal research that demonstrates this:

> Mammals like mice share around 90% of their genes with us, including most of the known disease genes. In this remarkable experiment the simple alteration of diet in a pregnant Agouti mouse was found to alter the offspring from chubby blondes to skinny brunettes. Moreover, the effect of grandma's diet during her pregnancy was passed on for three or more generations until it faded.[20]
>
> The Agouti gene normally produces a yellow pigment, obesity, diabetes and a propensity to develop cancer. If it is switched off by methylation-inducing chemicals in food, it produces a brown pigment and healthier mice. The special diet contained chemicals that had extra methyl donors that encouraged methylation. These included vitamins like folate, B12 and choline, commonly found in many healthy foods such as leafy vegetables, liver, cauliflower, beans, nuts and garlic.
>
> Remember, this reversible inherited change didn't alter the DNA structure but simply its expression. This is the essence of epigenetics and shows how rapid and powerful an effect it can have. [21-24]

Human transgenerational research

Plant and animal studies confirm the immediate heritable effects of environmental change on offspring.[25,26] But what about us?

Several studies of human populations have looked at the effects of famine or plenty on future generations. The Dutch hunger winter for example, occurred from November 1944 to May 1945, when the Dutch in the German occupied Netherlands lived through a severe famine. Rationing allowed for between 500 and 1,000 kcal per day, per person. Rationing stopped in May 1945 when the Dutch were liberated. Detailed health records allowed analysis. A total of 311 people who were born or conceived during this famine, and their healthcare records, were compared with same-sex siblings who were conceived before or born after the famine (also 311 of them). A control group of 349 unrelated people were also studied.[27]

Researchers looked at the insulin-like Growth Factor 2 (IGF2) gene. IGF2 is involved in human growth and development and it can be methylated. They compared how many methyl groups the IGF2 gene had in each of the three groups. More methylation (methyl groups present) meant down regulating the gene, leading to less IGF2. Six decades after being conceived or born during the Dutch hunger winter, famine exposed people had less methylation on their IGF2 gene compared to their unexposed same-sex brother or sister. This suggested the epigenetic inheritance not only occurred, but persisted and led to physical differences.

The differences included: impaired glucose tolerance (a precursor to diabetes), elevated cholesterol, raised blood pressure and higher rates of obesity in adulthood.[28-31] However, these researchers didn't delineate whether these differences were because of epigenetic changes or developmental problems caused by the famine.

Why would being conceived during a famine make you more likely to have metabolic and cardiovascular problems? The researchers postulated it was because our body would try to become as efficient as possible at storing calories, since there wasn't much food around during early development. That would work well, until suddenly you had all the food you needed and more. Once you had too many calories, or even simply enough calories, your body would continue to store them. This would cause you to have metabolic and cardiovascular problems associated with being overweight.

In another study, Swedish scientists looked at the effects on grandchildren if their grandparent went through times of famine or plenty in their childhood. Surprisingly times of plenty in key periods of the grandparent's lives had the biggest impact on the grandchildren. The study was conducted utilizing historical records, including harvests and food prices, in Overkalix, a small, isolated municipality in Northeast Sweden. The study consisted of 303 people, 164 men and 139 women, born in 1890, 1905, or 1920, and their 1,818 parents and grandparents. Only 44 were still alive in 1995 when the follow-up for this study ended.[32]

Environmental effects such as famine or good food supply during the so-called slow growth period (8 to 10 years in girls & 9 to 12 years in boys) prior to puberty, when environmental factors have a larger impact on the body, had most impact on future grandchildren. More recent analysis of this data, suggests it is sudden changes in food availability that may create this epigenetic inheritance.[33]

Grandmothers who when growing up experienced a good food supply during either their fetal/infancy period or between eight and 10 years of age, passed on a significantly higher risk of mortality to granddaughters but not grandsons. Conversely, grandfathers who lived through a time of plenty when they were growing up between the ages of nine and 12, passed on a higher risk of mortality in grandsons but not granddaughters.

Given the times of plenty experienced in the Western world since the Second World War, this study may explain some of the impacts on the health of young people today.

Gastric bypass surgery and children's obesity

Another intriguing study looked at previously severely obese mothers, who had successfully treated this obesity with gastric bypass surgery, and the obesity rates in their children.[34]

Those born after the surgery were 52% *less* likely to be obese compared to their brothers and sisters born while their mother was obese. That siblings shared their mother's new habits with respect to diet, food purchases, and other activities, suggests those who experienced an intrauterine environment in a non-obese mother, received some epigenetic advantage over their previously born siblings. Unlike their siblings, their prevalence of overweight was reduced to current population standards.

Apart from the obvious causes of diet and a sedentary lifestyle, it is now thought that the obesity epidemic confronting western society is, at least in part, being contributed to by obesity itself passing down the generations unhelpful epigenetic metabolic patterns.[35] (Another unexpected contributor to this obesity problem is the bacteria transferred from a mother to her newborn and we will look at this in Chapter 18.)[36]

Developmental Origins of Health and Disease

Epigenetic changes most likely lie behind a recently recognized phenomenon, called the Developmental Origins of Health and Disease (DOHaD).[37,38] The idea is that our experiences in the womb and early childhood can 'program' our future health. It is likely that epigenetics is part of the programming language involved. For instance research in rats demonstrates that a mother's licking and grooming behavior influences subsequent stress levels in their offspring, mediated by an epigenetic change to a gene involved in the stress response. Newborn rat pups whose mothers spend time licking and grooming them grow into calmer adults, whilst pups who receive little maternal attention tend to grow into more anxious adults. Grooming alters the pattern of epigenetic marks, which in turn alters gene activity of the stress regulator gene. Interestingly, when neglected rats were treated with a drug that altered these epigenetic marks, both their anxiety and the accompanying epigenetic changes could be reversed.[39,40]

It is not only rats where parental care can profoundly influence future development, it is relevant to all mammals. This is well recognized in newborn humans where inadequate loving physical contact, like we have seen with rats, also affects stress sensitivity. This can lead to an increase in vulnerability to mental health disorders.[41] Hence protocols in neonatal care units now include, as a vital priority, loving physical contact with newborn premature babies.

Lessons from cloning

Every cell in our body (except the red blood cells) contains all of the genetic information to build an entire body. Yet skin cells only produce skin; liver cells, liver; brain cells, brains and so on. The reason for this is epigenetic. Only the relevant codes are switched on within cells located in the appropriate areas. This differs from stem cells which are undifferentiated and still have the potential to form any body part. Returning a differentiated cell, such as a skin cell, back into its undifferentiated state was the scientific breakthrough that allowed for cloning. Most famously, Dolly the sheep was cloned from a breast tissue cell after 277 unsuccessful attempts. Unfortunately, she developed many degenerative problems and this demonstrated once again how important and difficult it is to mimic epigenetic factors in the healthy development of a living being.[42]

Biotech companies offering cloning of pets have charged customers between $50,000 and $150,000 for this service. Many have stopped offering this due to the high failure rate and complaints from customers that their beloved animals don't look or act exactly the same, despite having the identical genetic code to their previous beloved pet. A belief that cloning would produce identical copies of a living being in every way, simply reflected our misunderstanding of how genetic/epigenetic inheritance really works.[43]

Lessons from Twins

There was a time when geneticists believed there would be a simple genetic answer to most diseases. Studying identical (monozygotic) twins, born with a 100% identical genetic code, the closest thing we have to perfect clones, has illuminated our understanding. Research has been conducted on literally millions of pairs of identical twins and it has been discovered that most diseases and character traits have some level of heritability. But it's complex, not simple. How genetics plays its role is proving to be more challenging to uncover than geneticists initially believed. Single gene mutations causing diseases, like Huntington's disease, are rare.

As leading geneticist and twins researcher, Dr Tim Spector, points out in his very readable book, *Identically Different,* the glaring observation in the identical twins research is not just the similarities that they possess, but the differences.[44] Pointedly, more often than not they *do not* suffer from the same diseases. For instance, if one twin suffers from Rheumatoid Arthritis, a disease with a high level (60-70%) of heritability, there's only a 15% chance that the identical twin will also suffer from it.[45] Clearly it's not just our genes that are involved.

Taking our understanding of these differences further, so that we may learn from them, is a research study that involved 41 identical twin pairs, in which one of the twins developed cancer whilst the other did not. Blood tests looking at DNA methylation sites sought to uncover epigenetic differences between the identical twins. They revealed patterns of difference between the twin who developed cancer and the one who did not. Extraordinarily some of these patterns were present five years prior to the cancer's diagnosis. This research has helped hone in on a part of the epigenome relevant to cancer development and could lead to a simple blood screening test for cancer, well before it can be detected by any other means.[46]

What's become apparent is that rather than a single gene predisposing us to a disease or behavior pattern, many different genes play a role in a complex fashion interacting with their environment. Even eye color, once thought to involve only three genes, has now been shown to involve 10 genes.[47] There are even rare instances of identical twins with differing eye color.[48] As Dr Spector puts it, "we now know that whether you eat garlic or take regular exercise, drink milk or smoke cigarettes is influenced by your genes, regardless of your environment. There are few if any examples of environmental factors without a genetic component, and conversely genes don't work alone and are usually dependent on the cells they live in and their environments. So in a world where hundreds of genes are working together to influence a trait or a disease (along with just as many environmental influences - my words) the old distinction between nature and nurture is simply no longer relevant."[49]

Dr Spector concludes: "The most important lesson that we've learned is that you can change your genes, your destiny and that of your children and grandchildren. It really does matter what you do to your body, and importantly what your grandparents did to theirs many years ago."[50]

How we can change our tune

That nurture can change nature by influencing it down at its fundamental DNA level is the mind expanding revelation of epigenetics. Whilst we need to be respectful of the genetic tune we've been dealt, we also need to realize we have a big say in how that tune is played. We're not just helpless victims of our genes. It opens exciting new possibilities for preventing and treating disease. Scientists and pharmaceutical companies are investigating the possibilities of new medications to alter gene expression. But perhaps the greatest potential exists in the way we live our lives and organize our societies. It's early days in terms of research, but we've already seen how changing nutrition (nutrigenomics) can affect genetic expression. Let's look at some other examples.

Focused relaxation and our genes

Tangible beneficial epigenetic effects can occur quite quickly as evidenced by research on the relaxation response (RR). The relaxation response is a physiological and psychological state opposite to the stress or 'fight-or-flight' response. It was defined by US cardiologist Dr Herbert Benson in the mid-1970s. The RR is elicited when an individual focuses on a word, sound, phrase, repetitive prayer, or movement, and disregards everyday thoughts.[51] These two steps break the train of everyday thinking. Millennia-old mind-body approaches that elicit the RR include: various forms of meditation; different practices of yoga; Tai Chi; Qi Gong; progressive muscle relaxation; contemplative prayer; biofeedback and breathing exercises.[52] Elicitation of the relaxation response has been studied widely and been shown to have wide-ranging health benefits. We will look at these more closely in another chapter. For now our interest is in the research of its effects on epigenetics.

In a landmark study published in 2008, 19 healthy long-term RR practitioners were compared with 19 healthy controls who did not practice any form of RR. There were more than 2000 differences in genetic expression between the two groups. When the 19 controls, who had never practiced RR techniques before, underwent an eight week relaxation response training course, where they practiced eliciting an RR for 20 minutes each day, their genetic expression profiles changed. Importantly, 433 of the previously differently expressed genes were now shared between the two groups. This study provided the first compelling evidence that the relaxation response elicits specific gene expression changes in short-term and long-term practitioners.[53]

In a more recent study, blood samples were taken immediately and 15 minutes after a RR session undertaken by experienced practitioners and novices. The results were summarized as follows: "Relaxation response practice enhanced expression of genes associated with: energy metabolism, mitochondrial function, insulin secretion and telomere maintenance, and reduced expression of genes linked to inflammatory response and stress-related pathways."[54] In other words, particularly beneficial changes in genetic expression were seen in both groups, in particular the long-term practitioners, which could help to explain the health benefits of this practice. If you haven't found one already, it's worth finding an RR style that suits you. (For guidance with this see Appendix 1 and 2.)

Lifestyle change and our genes

In the chapters on Lifestyle as Therapy you will read in more detail the work of Dr Dean Ornish. His research on early prostate cancer has been particularly revealing. Men with early prostate cancer who had been randomly assigned to a lifestyle program, not only had a significantly better outcome over five years, but showed significant epigenetic changes.[55,56] The program included: a low-fat vegan diet; exercise, consisting of a 30 minute walk six times a week; and stress management including yoga, meditation, and group support. Testing of participants revealed that oncogenes, genes that promote cancer, were switched off after just three months on the lifestyle program. This raises the possibility that cancer, such a feared diagnosis, could be influenced not only by medical therapies, but by the lifestyle choices we make. This may well be the beginnings of an explanation as to how spontaneous remissions occur. Could it be that individuals, such as those studied by Kelly Turner[57] (see Chapter 1 - Changing the Odds), switched off their cancer-causing genes?

As epigenetic testing becomes more affordable and accessible we may discover some of the answers to this question, which I suspect may vary between individuals. Comprehensive lifestyle change may hold the key for many, for others an emotional breakthrough or attitudinal shift, a fever, a dietary change or a profound experience during meditation may be the triggers, the research possibilities are tantalizing. For example, if every cancer patient had relevant areas of their epigenome tested and psychological state and lifestyle profiled at the time of diagnosis, those that underwent spontaneous remission could be retested to see if/how their genetic expression had changed. They could then be re-questioned to explore the factors that may have contributed to their unexpected recovery. It might bring us closer to an understanding of this phenomenon, allowing innovative therapies to be developed. The same approach could apply to any number of diseases.

Finding the specific epigenetic triggers, whether they be food, drug, lifestyle, environmental toxin, infection etc., that switch on or off particular diseases, will be the Holy Grail of future research.

We have only touched the tip of the carrot top in terms of investigating this area. Epigenetics may well drive the push towards more individualized research methodologies and health care. It is already profoundly changing the way we think about evolution, health and disease, opening new pathways for hope and healing. What is clearer than ever, is that the choices we make today can profoundly affect ourselves and future generations.

Chapter 5

MEDITATION AS MEDICINE

To be yourself in a world that is constantly trying to make
you something else is the greatest accomplishment.

RALPH WALDO EMERSON

When I organized my 'escape' overseas after reaching my boiling point at the Alfred hospital in 1986, I deliberately left my return open-ended. So when I arrived back in December 1987 the best training positions for 1988 were long gone. This could have proved problematic as I needed to apply for one more year of hospital experience working as a Senior Resident Medical Officer (SRMO) in an approved general practice training position. I spoke with the Family Medicine Program (FMP) training coordinator soon after my return, who'd confirmed the worse, informing me of the few unappealing rotations left unfilled. I would have to take one of these if no other options appeared. Noting my disappointment, she suggested a long shot, that I ring hospitals directly because sometimes residents would pull out of their jobs at the last minute.

I sat and reflected for a while before opening the Yellow Pages and looking up the phone number for Dandenong Hospital. It had a reputation for having a friendly working environment and that would more than compensate for the two-hour daily car travel I would have to do from my bayside suburb, if I found work there. So I called and asked to be put through to the hospital administration. After introductions, the conversation went something like this:

"Are you responding to our advertisement?"

"What advertisement was that?" I asked.

"One of our Senior Resident Medical Officers (SRMO) has pulled out for the year because her mother is gravely ill."

"I'm sorry to hear that. What rotations are you offering?"

"It's an FMP approved position, with three months of Pediatrics, Obstetrics, General Practice, and Accident and Emergency."

These were the perfect job experience options I would have chosen. "How do I apply?"

I faxed my CV and was invited to attend a job interview. The evening after the interview I was offered the job and three weeks later I began my first rotation covering nights in A & E. This was nerve wracking, as I was the most senior doctor on the hospital's frontline at that time of night. Let's just say my newly found practice of meditation came to my rescue, helping me to keep a clear and relaxed mind in the face of some hairy emergencies.

The year rolled along. The work was hard, the hours long, but the promised friendliness delivered, in the form of a respectful camaraderie and cooperation between staff. When I neared the end of an enjoyable three-month general practice term in the nearby suburb of Narre Warren, I received a phone call from the FMP Training Program coordinator. "Would you be interested in presenting to a group of new trainees about the experiences you've been having during your first general practice placement?" she asked.

"I'd be delighted," I said.

"That's a relief, you're the 14th person I've tried!"

On the afternoon before my presentation, I had a space in my patient appointments and sat at my desk jotting down a few pointers that I would refer to that evening. Fortuitously, it was the same afternoon that the roving GP education supervisor had chosen to drop in on me. She enquired as to what I was doing and on discovering the purpose of my jottings, asked me if I enjoyed that sort of thing. I replied that I enjoyed teaching, having worked as a high school math tutor and said that being a Leo, I also enjoyed being on the stage! She then let me know that in two weeks hence, applications would close for a 1989 FMP training rotation that would involve both GP work and being a lecturer attached to the General Practice Teaching Department of Monash University Medical School, where I'd undergone my undergraduate training. If all parties agreed, there would be an option of completing my FMP training with a second year lecturer position in 1990.

My whole being said, "How do I apply?"

The evening presentation went well and I applied to Monash University days later. In filling out the application I also discovered that as a prerequisite for consideration, I needed to have the exact training experience I was receiving at Dandenong Hospital. How lucky I had been.

There were three positions open and seven of us were granted interviews. Whilst waiting to be called in for my interview, the next applicant arrived and we introduced ourselves. He was Dr Craig Hassed. We would both end up with a position but it would be a full 12 months before we would realize that we had a common interest in meditation, stress management and self-care. This happened when the subject was raised at a departmental meeting and both Craig and I spoke up about its importance. We returned to our respective offices after the meeting and then simultaneously poked our heads out into the adjoining corridor, laughed, then got together for a chat.

Soon after this, we teamed up to speak with Prof Neil Carson, the department head, about offering final year medical students an optional meditation session at lunchtime. Neil was an open-minded, creative fellow and agreed, as long as it was well received by the students, which it was.

Not long after these lunchtime sessions began, Prof Carson was at an interdepartmental meeting where the Psychology Department presented some disturbing research about the levels of stress medical students were experiencing. Prof Carson mentioned the meditation sessions we had recently offered to students and much to our surprise, the Psychology Department got in touch with Craig and made available some of its teaching hours for us to provide meditation-based stress management sessions. Craig devised a mindfulness-meditation based stress management program, while I produced a discussion paper collating research regarding mind-body medicine and stress management.[1] Together we taught meditation at both undergraduate and postgraduate levels.

At this time (1991) meditation was not commonly accepted by the mainstream medical establishment and our approach was seen as an innovation. It wasn't long before the news got out and we were being interviewed by various media outlets as to what we were up to. From this publicity I was invited by various high schools to assist VCE students; then nurses, air traffic controllers, careers counsellors and courses for GPs under the auspices of the Royal Australian College of General Practitioners. It was enjoyable and rewarding work.

In my general practice I was also aware that it would be of great benefit to many of my patients if I could teach them how to meditate. I started doing this on an individual basis but soon realized this was inefficient, so I sought and was given permission by the group practice I was working in, to offer evening courses over a six-week period for an hour and a half, one night per week. These were popular and I capped the number of participants at 10. Fascinating to me was that not only were these participants benefiting in terms of managing their anxiety and stress better, but they were also experiencing better physical health. Many were able to reduce their asthma medications, migraines reduced or disappeared, and one lady found she was able to reduce her antiepilepsy medication. This served as fuel for my interest in mind-body medicine and I eagerly read the latest research.

Let's turn to this exploration right now by briefly overviewing stress and its antidote, the relaxation response.

Stress

Stress takes its name from the so-called 'fight, flight or freeze' response, aka the stress response. A little stress can be useful to help us get out of bed and to perform at our best, but when it goes beyond that it can be more harmful than helpful. The stress response is typically activated when we find ourselves under threat or feeling awkward or out of our depth. It can also be triggered by negative thoughts we may not even realize we are having. The key factors here are whether we perceive our ability to cope is being exceeded, whether the demands placed upon us exceed our resources, or whether we lack a sense of control over the demands placed upon us.

In these situations, the sympathetic nervous system and the Hypothalamic Pituitary Adrenal axis (HPA axis) are activated, leading nerves to fire impulses and hormones to be released, including noradrenaline, adrenaline and cortisol. In response muscles tighten, our heart rate and blood pressure increases, we sweat and our breathing becomes rapid and shallow. This can be useful if we need to fight or take evasive action, like jumping out of the way of a bus. In this case the response is switched on and then switched off and no harm is done, assuming we got out of the way of the bus! But when it is regularly switched on by getting fed up sitting in traffic, or worrying about finances, work or home, or replaying an argument in our mind, it can become a problem.

Unchecked, in time stress can become habitual, developing its own momentum, and this can lead to chronic stress. In this situation we can become so used to, and some might say addicted to, its presence, that we live life in its shadow. It tires us, undermines our health and happiness, disturbs our concentration and impacts on our relationships. We can miss out on experiencing the present moment as we worry about things from the past, or things that might be to come.

Chronic stress can also come from deeper unresolved problems in family or work dynamics and lead to mental health disorders, such as anxiety and depression, and physical symptoms, such as headaches, backache, dyspepsia, irritable bowel syndrome and fatigue. It can also lead us to take up unhealthy behaviors, such as excessive alcohol intake, drugs, smoking and violence as ways of coping or dealing with the stress. In addition it aggravates any existing medical conditions. For example, it can have a deleterious effect on the immune system, increase inflammation, worsen diabetes and turn up the volume on pain. Finally, through epigenetic influence it can also be a contributor to the causation of many diseases.[1,2,3]

Stress management

The most obvious place to start in managing stress is to identify any problems that might be causing the stress and address them. Problem-solving alone or with the assistance of a friend or counselor may be enough to resolve the situation. Nonetheless, it is worthwhile developing skills that make us more resilient as well, because the chances are we will continue to be confronted with stressful situations in our lives. One proven preventive and treatment technique is to regularly trigger the relaxation response.

The Relaxation Response

In the late 1960's Harvard University cardiologist, Dr Herbert Benson, became interested in researching the effects of Eastern meditation techniques arriving in the U.S at the time. He even took his equipment to the East to study meditating monks. In time, he researched a variety of meditation and relaxation techniques and he identified a bodily response, mediated by the parasympathetic nervous system, which they all had in common. He called this response the 'relaxation response' and published a book with this title in 1975.[4] During the relaxation response, heart and breathing rates slow, blood pressure lowers, muscles relax and the body receives a deeper restorative rest than at any time during sleep. We are happily relaxed while at the same time clearly awake. Our concentration improves and we function well in this state of restful alertness. Athletes describe this experience as being in the 'zone.' Subsequent research has shown that it can be triggered in a variety of ways. Deep breathing, meditation, progressive muscle relaxation, visualization, repetitive prayer, jogging, tai chi, yoga, knitting... the list goes on. Personal preference plays a part. Knitting may not be for everyone!

Importantly, all of these activities require our active participation and give our minds something to focus upon. In other words, while the stress response is often triggered without us knowing, perhaps paradoxically, the relaxation response requires our conscious attention. Furthermore, Dr Benson's research found that if someone practiced a focused relaxation technique for as little as 10 minutes a day, after just one month their quality of life and ability to cope with stress had all improved. This concurs with my experience of when I ran my groups. Learning how to invoke this response with techniques that can be used anywhere and anytime is a wonderful life skill and I believe an essential one if you are facing chronic disease. For those who might be interested, I've created a self-explanatory audio recording which introduces beginners to meditation and relaxation using the techniques I incorporated into my group work. (The complete text of this can be found in Appendix 1 and 2)

If you need more convincing reasons for looking into this, here is a comprehensive list of the scientific benefits of invoking the relaxation response (from Dr Craig Hassed's discussion paper):[5]

Physiological Benefits of Relaxation and Stress Reduction

- marked decrease in oxygen consumption and metabolic rate well below that achieved in sleep, decrease in respiration rate and minute ventilation associated with greater efficiency and economy, and a lowering of catechol receptor sensitivity.[6,7,8]
- reduction in blood pressure and heart rate.[9]
- reduction in serum cholesterol[10] more than would be accounted for by diet alone, sharp increase in skin resistance (low skin resistance is an accurate marker of stress responses), decrease in blood lactate, associated with anaerobic metabolism which is high in stressful situations.[11]
- changes in EEG patterns associated with the state of restful alertness including an increase in alpha and theta waves and EEG coherence (coordination of EEG waves).[12]
- a reduction in epileptic seizure frequency.[13]
- changes in neurotransmitter profile including high serotonin production as seen in recovery from depression.[14]
- a suggested selective increase in cerebral blood flow.[15]
- reduced TSH and T3 levels.[16]
- improved response time and reflexes.[17]
- improvement in perceptiveness of hearing and other senses.[18]

- improved immune function. For an immune system under-active due to chronic stress, it is stimulated, and for over-active immune systems, such as in auto-immune and inflammatory illnesses, it seems to reduce its over-activity.[19]
- cortisol levels are lowered by the relaxation response preventing increased calcium loss and osteoporosis that is associated with high cortisol levels and depression.[20]
- very beneficial as an adjunct to therapy for a variety of illnesses such as heart disease, cancer, chronic pain,[21] asthma,[22] diabetes[23] and many more.

Psychological Benefits of Stress Reduction

- decreased anxiety.[24,25]
- more optimism, decreased depression as indicated by elevation of serotonin.[26,27]
- greater self-awareness and self-actualisation.[28]
- improved coping capabilities.[29]
- happiness tends to be less conditional. Improved well-being and as an adjunct to psychotherapy.[30]
- reduced reliance upon drugs, prescribed and non-prescribed, or alcohol.[31]
- improved sleep;[32] more restful, less insomnia, and in time less sleep is needed.
- reduced aggression and criminal tendency.[33]
- improved I.Q. and learning capabilities, including the aged and intellectually impaired.
- greater efficiency and output and reduced stress at work.[34]
- better time management and improved concentration and memory.[35,36]

- reduction in personality disorders and ability to change un-desired personality traits.[37]
- stimulus reduction was the most effective known form of treatment for infantile colic.[38]

Having read all these benefits you might be fired up to take up a practice. What to choose? Generally the best technique is the one you practice regularly and persist with and that feels right to you. You may need to experiment. If you're looking for a recommendation to begin your search, then Mindfulness Meditation is a good place to start; it has been widely researched, is taught by some psychologists along with others, need not be affiliated to any group, and like most meditation techniques, provides portable skills that require no equipment. (The guidelines contained within Appendix 1 and 2 may help here.)[39]

Incorporating the relaxation response into your daily life is one effective way of introducing mind-body medicine to improve your health. In the following chapters we'll touch on other examples of how the mind can be worked with to assist physical healing.

Please note that for some people, having a low threshold for stress can be the result of early childhood or later traumas, which, in addition to relaxation response techniques, may benefit from more specific psychotherapy.

Julia's Story

"If there is a doctor of medicine on board, could they please make themselves known to flight staff." This isn't something most doctors like to hear. On a two-hour flight from Melbourne to Brisbane, I waited 30 seconds for other call buttons to ring out; there were none. I pressed the button. A stewardess approached, "I'm a doctor," I told her.

"We've got a lady sitting in the rear of the aircraft who is complaining of chest pain and breathlessness, could you help?" On the way down the aisle she added, "the pilot will need to know if he needs to land the plane."

I accompanied her to the back of the plane, where Julia, whom I estimated to be in her 30s, sat looking anxious and breathless, an oxygen mask attached. Beside her sat her eight-year-old daughter, Amy, gripping protectively onto her mother's arm.

I introduced myself to both of them. I quickly ascertained that the chest pain she was experiencing was sharp in nature and worsened with deep breaths, something a doctor would characterize as pleuritic, meaning it was arising from the outer surface lining of the lung, the pleura, rather than the heart. I had no medical equipment but established her pulse was bounding away at a regular rate of 100 bpm, that she was breathing rapidly and shallowly and that she felt feverish. I removed the oxygen mask in order to assess her more fully. Importantly, her lips and tongue remained a good color, not bluish, which would have indicated a lack of oxygen in her blood. The short duration of the flight along with the fact she had a fever made the more serious diagnosis of a blood clot in her lungs (pulmonary embolus) unlikely, so that provisionally I diagnosed Julia's problem to be an infection, possibly pneumonia. I reassured her of this likelihood and that she would be okay.

I informed the stewardess that the pilot did not need to make an emergency landing and that the flight could safely continue for the remaining hour to Brisbane. I then returned my attention to Julia, who despite my reassurance was still in some distress. I sat beside her and offered to talk her through a simple relaxation technique. She agreed.

To begin with I asked her to place her hands on her belly and to see if she could shift her breathing so that her belly moved more with each breath. We spent a few minutes doing this. I then in-

77

structed her to close her eyes and feel the weight of her body in the chair... "Now listen to all the sounds you can hear, identifying each sound before moving on to the next," I instructed. Her breathing rate began to decrease. "Now I want you to take yourself in your imagination to a place where you feel safe, relaxed, calm. ...What can you see in this place? ...What do you feel under your feet... around your body? ... Are there any fragrances? ... Sounds? ... Now simply allow yourself to rest in this place, there's nothing for you to do ... just simply be there." Julia's breathing became even easier and within minutes she fell asleep.

I continued to sit beside her for the rest of the flight, while Amy involved herself with coloring in books provided by the stewardess. Upon landing, Julia awoke. She was stunned that she had fallen asleep. She felt and looked better and her chest pain was markedly diminished. A wheelchair was brought onto the plane and Julia, with Amy in tow, was taken to the nearest hospital. Before she left I gave her my card so that she could let me know of her progress.

A month later, Julia sent me a delightful thank you card and filled me in on some of her story. The night before her flight she had been in an acrimonious argument with her husband and had barely slept. She had decided to separate from him and was flying to Queensland with her only child Amy, to spend time with her parents. At the hospital, a chest x-ray confirmed that she had pneumonia, from which, after a course of antibiotics, she fully recovered. She was keen to explore meditation and relaxation techniques after being surprised by the benefit she had received in such a high stress circumstance.

Chapter 6

LIFESTYLE AS THERAPY – HEART DISEASE AND BEYOND

Whenever a new discovery is reported in the scientific world, they say first, 'It is probably not true.' Thereafter, when the truth of the new proposition has been demonstrated beyond question, they say, 'Yes, it may be true, but it is not important.' Finally, when sufficient time has elapsed to fully evidence its importance, they say, 'Yes, surely it is important, but it is no longer new.'

MICHEL DE MONTAIGNE (1533-1592)

Improving our lifestyle to help prevent us from experiencing disease, whilst not always practiced, is well accepted in our society. Most of us know that if we stop smoking, eat well, exercise, manage our stress and get a good night's sleep, we will be more likely to remain healthy. Less well promoted is that lifestyle change can actually influence the course of established disease. Modern medicine has tended to downplay this influence and to limit its promotion to a handful of diseases: diabetes, hypertension, heart disease and osteoporosis, being examples of these.

In the last decade recognition that the majority of these chronic diseases can be significantly improved by changing our behavior, has led to the formation of Lifestyle Medicine Associations around the world.[1-4] These associations estimate that 70% of all diseases are lifestyle related. Their ideal is to coordinate a variety of health professionals to impart the motivation and skills required for people to change their lifestyle. Lifestyle Medicine sees itself as a bridge between public health messages, like the Quit Smoking campaign, and one-on-one clinical practice.[5] It represents a shift from seeing your health problem as something to be solved in consultation with an individual doctor, to a consultation with a team of health professionals, who can guide and assist you in taking personal responsibility for managing your health.

To understand how disease might be effectively managed in this way, it is worth taking a step back. In a big picture sense, one way of conceiving this is to realize that the context in which we find ourselves is reflected in the biochemical environment that bathes and literally feeds our body's cells. In other words, our healthy or unhealthy lifestyle choices affect the way our cells work at a microscopic level. In addition, many of our cells die and are replaced many times during our lifetime, providing ongoing opportunity to change the pattern they are expressing. In some regions, such as the lining of our mouth, stomach and nose, the turnover is rapid, occurring in a matter of days. In other areas, like our red blood cells, it takes four months to replace old cells, whilst a liver cell takes about a year.[6] By changing our lifestyle, the nutrient and chemical context that our cells find themselves in is altered, affecting the way they function. In addition, the process involved in the production of new cells also comes under this fresh influence. In these two ways, a body part's cells expressing disease can change to expressing health. Epigenetic research confirms this potential, as we've seen in the Epigenetics chapter.

A model of health?

John Robbins in his excellent book, *Still Healthy at 100*,[7] presents compelling evidence for the ultimate healthy lifestyle. He reviews research on the longest living peoples: Abkhasians of the Caucasus Mountains; Hunzans of northern Pakistan; Vilcabambans of South America and the Okinawans of Japan. Importantly, this research was done before westernization had significantly altered these communities. In each group there was a strong sense of community and the elderly were revered as much as our culture reveres youth today. Extensive daily physical activity was performed at all ages and remarkably, a lack of chronic disease was present. People not only lived well into their 90s or 100s, but did so, for the most part, in excellent physical and mental health. By contrast, here in the West our life expectancy has risen in recent decades, but this has gone hand in hand with an increase in chronic degenerative diseases, making ageing and dying for many, a long and distressing process.

By contrast, elders in these long-lived cultures experienced levels of physical fitness that were superior to those typically found in much younger people in the West. When it came to strength, coordination, flexibility, reaction time, stamina and other ways of assessing fitness, 90-year-olds in these societies very often surpassed 60-year-olds in the modern industrialized world.[8]

It is now increasingly recognized that a lack of exercise, as characterized by a sedentary lifestyle, may lead to accelerated ageing, diseases of the body and brain, and an overall decline in the quality of life.[9] On the other hand, unlike any pill you can take, exercise can help you stay lean and fit as you age, protecting your heart, bone and brain. It makes you stronger, more confident and less susceptible to depression, whilst improving your sleep, mood and memory. It also reduces your risk of cancer and neurodegenerative disease and all the while adds to the quality of your everyday life.[10] Edward Stanley put it succinctly back in 1873, "Those who think they have no time for bodily exercise will sooner or later have to find time for illness."[11]

What about the diet of these long-lived communities? John Robbins sums this up as follows:[12]

- Even though their lifestyle was very active, their caloric intake was comparatively low (around 1900 cal a day) compared to the average Westerner (2650 cal per day). Obesity was not a problem.

- Their diets were all high in good carbohydrates, including plenty of whole grains, vegetables and fruits.

- They ate wholefoods, with very little if any processed or refined foods, sugar, corn syrup, preservatives, artificial flavors or any other chemicals.

- They all depended on fresh foods, eating primarily what was in season and locally grown, rather than relying on canned foods or foods shipped long distances.

- Their diets were all low (though not super-low) in fat, and the fats came from natural sources, including seeds, nuts, and in some cases fish, rather than from processed oil, margarines or saturated animal fats.

- They all derived their protein primarily from plant sources, including beans, peas, whole grains, seeds and nuts. Meat was rarely eaten. The Okinawans included fish and tofu in their diet, while the Abkhasians included a cultured milk drink (matzoni).

This research is corroborated by the largest epidemiological study on diet ever performed, a 20 year study conducted in 65 Chinese counties, known as The China-Cornell-Oxford project. The research was conducted prior to the mass westernization of the Chinese diet.

It involved a comparison of counties that had genetically similar populations, yet had tended, over generations, to live and eat in distinct ways. So while the dietary patterns were consistent within each county, they varied widely between counties, allowing for a clear comparison between styles of eating and health.

What did they find? The study concluded that counties with a high consumption of animal-based foods had higher death rates from "Western" diseases, while the opposite was true for counties that ate more plant foods, with the most plant-based diets having a much lower incidence of chronic diseases, including cancer and heart disease, than the highest animal food based diets.[13]

Dr T Colin Campbell, the Project Director, presents the significance of this research in the bestselling book, *The China Study*.[14] In it he includes evidence from his own laboratory research, which confirmed an earlier report from Indian researchers, that rats fed a diet of 20% animal protein in the form of casein (from dairy), developed cancer when exposed to a cancer causing toxin. In comparison, rats fed a 5% casein diet exposed to a similar toxin did not develop cancer.[15,16,17] When those rats on the 20% casein diet were switched to the 5% diet, their cancer went into reverse. By contrast, 20% protein diets derived from plant-based sources, soybeans and gluten from wheat, were not only not cancer promoting, but reversed cancer. So convinced by the lab findings and Chinese epidemiological results was Dr Campbell, that he and his family changed their diet to being 99% plant-based. You can view a You Tube video of Dr Campbell discussing these results as part of a documentary, *Forks over knives*, at: https://www.youtube. com/watch?v=pGW48HLEv1o

Further support for the benefits of being vegetarian comes from studies of the Adventists, a Christian denomination many of whom are vegetarian and many of these vegan (avoiding dairy and eggs). A review concluded: "Vegetarian diets confer protection against cardiovascular diseases, cardiometabolic risk factors, some cancers and total mortality. Compared to lacto-ovo-vegetarian diets, vegan diets seem to offer additional protection for: obesity, hypertension, type-2 diabetes, and cardiovascular mortality."[18]

All this is not the news someone who enjoys a good steak, like myself, wants to hear. But with this knowledge I began by increasing the whole foods in my diet, reduced animal products and introduced more vegetarian days. I am now on my way to a predominantly wholefood plant-based diet, with some similarities to the Mediterranean diet, which along with vegetables and fruits, emphasizes protein sources in the form of legumes and fish.[19,20,21]

The good news is that for those of us not ready to become vegetarian, large epidemiological research studies spanning five to 26 years suggest that simply increasing the number of vegetables and fruits in your existing diet can decrease your overall mortality risk and chances of developing cancer or heart disease.[22,23,24] By contrast increased consumption of red and processed meat increases death, cancer and heart disease rates.[25]

This reseach suggests vegetables confer more benefit than fruit, with raw vegetables, such as salad, providing the most protection. Seven or more portions of fruit and veggies per day (a variety of each) is optimal, a portion varying from half a cup (eg mashed sweet potato) to two cups (eg lettuce). In order to achieve this one inevitably needs to reduce the volume of animal foods in favor of plant-based foods. Any move in this direction will be of help.

Given the ever growing burden of chronic disease in our Western societies, the question is not only - can we reverse this trend with this knowledge? But can changing one's lifestyle in this manner impact positively on those of us, like myself, with already established chronic disease?

Dr Dean Ornish shows what's possible

Scientific evidence of just how strong the effects of lifestyle change can be, first came to my attention in 1990. The Lancet, a prestigious medical journal, had just published a landmark study from Dr Dean Ornish and his colleagues.[26] I was working at Monash University at the time, when we reviewed the study at our weekly Journal Club.

Dr Ornish had recruited 48 people with significant coronary heart disease (blockages in the 'small pipes,' called coronary arteries, supplying blood to the heart muscle), that had been identified on angiogram x-rays. All 48 had agreed to a repeat coronary angiogram x-ray at the end of 12 months, at which time a comparison would be made and the study ended. These people were randomly placed into one or other of two groups. The first group received the usual medical care, while the second group also received the usual medical care plus an additional lifestyle management program. This program consisted of a low-fat vegetarian diet, group support meetings, exercise and stress management, including yoga and meditation.

At the end of 12 months, 82% of the lifestyle management group showed improvement in their coronary arteries on their repeat angiograms. These x-rays had been independently assessed and compared to their original x-rays. In the group of people who received the usual medical care without specific lifestyle management support, 53% had a worsening of their coronary artery disease (CAD) on x-ray. Not surprisingly the difference between the two groups was statistically significant and this corresponded with symptom improvement. In fact, within a few weeks of commencing the lifestyle program the occurrence of angina chest pain amongst participants began to reduce.

This program was so effective that many of the attendees had to reduce their medication dosage, as they no longer required as much medical assistance. They were also able to perform activities, such as playing golf, which they had lost the capacity to do prior to the program. The study had conclusively shown that lifestyle change alone could reverse coronary artery disease, that is, literally unblock these arteries without cholesterol-lowering drugs or surgery.

A lively discussion ensued at Journal Club, with many thinking the best approach from here on was to ascertain which of the factors was most important in producing this reversal in heart disease. Most people thought it was just the diet. Others argued that given we all agreed that risk factors for heart disease, such as, high blood pressure, smoking and obesity combined to multiply risk, why wouldn't interventions such as stress management, group support and diet synergize in their effects in helping people to recover. When Dr Ornish was asked if it was just the diet, he pointed out that the group support helped people to stick to the diet, while exercise and stress management helped people stay off the smokes as well as reducing their chances of eating poorly. All these factors helped people in some way to maintain their lifestyle change.[27]

As doctors we wish to streamline the approach and identify the key component(s) in the program. This is a valid ideal. However, holistic thinking recognizes people need a lot of assistance to make and maintain behavior change, like changing your diet. As it turns out a three-year follow-up study of the original 48 people found an even bigger difference between the two groups, with the lifestyle therapy group continuing to improve. This led a US health insurance company to fund the full Ornish lifestyle program, with estimated savings of $58,000 per cardiac patient treated this way when compared with heart bypass surgery.[28]

The following story taken from the Ornish study illustrates the potential impact of this approach.[29]

"I'm Werner Hebenstreit, and I'm a business consultant. When I first began this program, I had terrible chest pains, tremendous burning pains with even minimal exertion. It was even a problem for me to cross the street against a traffic light, because I couldn't walk fast enough to make it without getting severe chest pain. Pains, pains, pains. Even taking a shower or shaving caused me to have intense chest pain, although there's practically no physical effort. I was hardly ever without angina pains.

After a few weeks on this program, my chest pains began to decrease. After a few months, I had no more pains whatsoever. Now I walk for an hour with no pain. Or I swim an hour a day, 20 lengths in an Olympic-sized pool -- no chest pains. I just relax and meditate while I swim. I don't even think about having angina pains any more. And I got off many of the medications that I had been taking, with all their blasted side-effects.

Now, my wife and I can hike four to six hours at a time. Last year, we hiked the whole day at the Grand Teton National Park at six thousand feet high and had no pain.

My mental well-being has improved as much as my physical well-being. I enjoy life much more than I did before. I was known, I would say, as a man with a very short fuse. I felt attacked very easily.

I had a tendency to get upset and frustrated about things over which I had no control whatsoever. A newspaper headline could get me into such a bad mood that I couldn't enjoy my breakfast: 'What kind of a politician would do this or that?' Waiting for a late bus got me so full of rage that I decided to write letters to the bus company complaining. And so on.

Then, one day, I recognized it was so stupid to bring up my blood pressure and to get annoyed over things I had no control of. And to illustrate it for myself, I started to write down whenever I got upset in a notebook. On my very 'best' day, I had 33 times where I got angry over occurrences over which I had no control whatsoever.

Now, I don't even carry notebooks around anymore. Whenever I feel frustration coming up, I think of the notebook and I start to smile. I laugh. And I'm much more patient. I take time to analyze, discuss, and evaluate before I shoot off my mouth, which I used to do. My fuse is much longer now. Some days I'm fuseless.

And from a business point of view, I'm much more successful than before my being sick. The program was a godsend for me. It gave me hope. I faced death, and now I'm facing a second chance at life. Before, I was very negative about things. I thought I would have to be an invalid for the rest of my life. Now I am very positive, I'm able to do so many things that were impossible before. Instead of dreading each day, my wife and I look forward to each day. We enjoy each day as it comes.

My angiogram showed that the blockage reversed from 53% to 40% after one year and 13% after four years! I knew how much better I was feeling, but to have scientific evidence proving that -- well, the feeling was just unbelievable.

When I first heard of this program, I thought it would be too late for me to benefit from it. I mean, I'm 77 years old! But, of course, I changed my mind. You're as old as you feel -- and I'm getting younger all the time."

Dr Ornish's pioneering work has inspired other lifestyle programs for managing heart disease, including a similar program run by the Benson-Henry Mind Body Institute (MBMI) - named after cardiologist Dr Herbert Benson who coined the term, the relaxation response (see previous chapter). The MBMI program differs from Ornish in that it involves less intensive follow-up and a less demanding non-vegetarian diet, based on the American Heart Association guidelines; recommending 30% or less calories from fat. Ornish's vegetarian diet recommends 10% or less calories from fat.

Both programs have been taken up by US hospitals, as they have been established to improve health and save costs, with more than 40 American health insurance companies funding part or all of these lifestyle treatments. US health insurer, Medicare, conducted a three-year follow-up of 461 elderly patients who had either an acute myocardial infarction (heart attack), a cardiac procedure within the preceding 12 months or had stable angina. They were assigned to either the MBMI or Ornish lifestyle management programs (LMPs) and compared with 1795 controls, who received standard care with either the usual cardiac rehabilitation or no rehabilitation.

The rates at which patients needed to be admitted to hospital, for both reasons related to and not related to their heart condition, were lower in lifestyle program participants than controls in both the Ornish and MBMI programs and were statistically significant for the MBMI ($p < 0.01$). Program costs of $3,801 and $4,441 per participant for the MBMI and Ornish Programs, respectively, were more than offset by a trend towards reduced health care costs, yielding three-year net savings per participant of about $3,500 in MBMI and $1,000 in Ornish. In MBMI participants, there was also a trend towards lower death rates compared with controls ($p = 0.07$).[30]

The paper concluded that: "Intensive, year-long Lifestyle Management Programs reduced hospitalization rates and suggest reduced Medicare costs in elderly beneficiaries with symptomatic coronary heart disease." If the trend of less health care utilization continues, as one might expect, further savings will be even more apparent in future years, along with a diminished burden on the health system generally. Younger participants would also have less sick days away from work.

Different programs will appeal to different people. It's early days in terms of evaluating these two programs, but in their current form there is some evidence the less stringent MBMI is at least as effective as the Ornish program and less expensive to implement. It has also been shown to be more easily taken up than the Ornish program by people with coronary artery disease (CAD) willing to enroll in a year-long intensive lifestyle intervention.[31]

Dr Esselstyn's dietary research

Another pioneer in lifestyle management is general surgeon and researcher, Dr Caldwell Esselstyn. Dr Esselstyn's research has shown that with intensive dietary counseling and follow-up, patients with coronary artery disease (CAD) can adhere to a vegetarian plant-based wholefood diet. This can reverse their heart disease (demonstrable on coronary angiograms) if their total cholesterol level falls below 150 mg/dL (3.89 mmol/l).[32] Interestingly, this concurs with Dr Campbell's research in China which found that below this level of total cholesterol, CAD fatalities were practically non-existent. It is worth noting that Dr Campbell also found that as total cholesterol decreased from 170 mg/dL (4.40 mmol/l) to 90 mg/dL (2.33 mmol/l), corresponding with a diminished intake of animal food products, the incidence of a whole range of cancers also decreased.[33] This effect is not seen with cholesterol lowering medication alone.[34]

The big question here was could people adhere to such a big shift in their diet? To assess this possibility, Dr Esselstyn recruited 198 consecutive CAD patients who agreed to follow his prescribed plant-based diet, along with their usual medical care. They were asked to eliminate: oil, dairy products (except skim milk and no-fat yogurt), fish, fowl, and meat. They received intensive dietary counselling in which they were taught and encouraged (with biweekly follow-ups) to eat grains, legumes, lentils, vegetables, and fruit. If needed, additional cholesterol-lowering medication was prescribed. The goal was to achieve and maintain a total serum cholesterol of <150 mg/dl (3.89 mmol/l).

The patients were followed up for an average time of 3.7 years, during which severe cardiac events, considered evidence of recurrence of CAD, were noted. An impressive 177 (89%) patients stuck to the diet, amongst whom only one (0.6%) had a recurrence. Amongst the

21 patients who didn't stick with it, 13 (62%) had recurrences. This is encouraging both from the high rate of adherence achieved and the better health these people experienced. For those motivated to do so, intensive support for such a significant dietary change seems well worth it.

The researchers concluded, "This dietary approach to treatment deserves a wider test to see if adherence can be sustained in broader populations. Plant-based nutrition has the potential for a large effect on the CVD (cardiovascular disease) epidemic."[35]

Atrial fibrillation benefits from weight loss

Atrial fibrillation (AF) is a problematic irregular heartbeat, whose incidence is on the rise.[36] It can lead to blood clots in the brain (strokes) and other abnormalities of heart function that can significantly affect quality of life and survival. Obesity is thought to be a major reason for its increasing prevalence. There are various mechanisms by which this occurs, including the enlargement of the left atrial chamber of the heart.[37]

A research study, conducted by Dr Hany Abed and his colleagues at the University of Adelaide, looked at the potential for including weight reduction as part of the treatment of people with AF.[38] One hundred and fifty overweight people with this condition were randomly assigned to either an intervention group, which received the weight loss counseling, or usual medical care (the control group). There were 75 people in both groups and all 150 underwent intensive management of cardio metabolic risk factors. This means that any high blood pressure, elevated blood fats, signs of glucose intolerance or diabetes, sleep apnea, and alcohol and tobacco use was screened for and if necessary, treated in both groups.

In addition to this, the intervention group received a two phase weight management approach. In the first phase, weight loss was produced over eight weeks using a modified very low-calorie diet (800 -- 1200 kcal per day). This was achieved by providing participants with a very low-calorie meal replacement sachet for two of their daily meals. Their third meal of the day consisted of calorie controlled foods with high levels of animal and plant protein and a low glycemic index (GI). There was also a written exercise plan that prescribed low intensity exercise (walking or cycling), starting with 20 minutes three times weekly, before increasing to 45 minutes three times weekly.

The very low-calorie meals were gradually phased out and replaced with low GI meals, increasing exercise and counseling to assist with behavior change, for a period of 13 months. Face-to-face clinic visits were scheduled every three months, sooner if desired, and participants were provided with 24-hour e-mail and telephone support. Every member of the intervention group was also required to maintain a diet, activity, and blood pressure diary.

In contrast, the control group received written and verbal nutrition and exercise advice at their first visit, but no further follow-up regarding this advice. A diary of diet and activity was not requested from them.

Both groups were monitored three monthly for the next 15 months. To check for episodes of AF, a seven-day portable heart (Holter) monitor, which recorded the heart's rhythm, was performed at the beginning of the study and 12 months later. The four chambers of the heart were also viewed and assessed at these times using an echocardiogram (heart ultrasound).

The results were startling, with a dramatic difference between the two groups. For starters, the intervention group lost on average 14.3 kg (31.5 lbs) compared with the control group's average of 3.6 kg (7.9 lbs) weight loss (p<0.001). The intervention group also had a marked reduction in AF symptoms, severity and number of episodes (p<0.01). This was reflected in the Holter monitor recordings, which at 12 months showed the combined length of AF attacks over the seven-day recording period had decreased from 1176 minutes to 491 minutes in the intervention group. In contrast, the control group showed an increase in the duration of AF attacks from 1393 minutes to 1546 minutes.

Interestingly, the structure of the heart, as measured by the echocardiogram, had changed significantly in the intervention group too, with a healthy decrease in left atrial size.

Other positive side-effects noted in the intervention group were a decline in excessive alcohol consumption, a decrease in blood pressure and requirement for antihypertensive medication, a decrease in LDL-cholesterol and triglycerides, a decrease in glucose and insulin levels, and a decrease in C-reactive protein (CRP), a marker of inflammation in the body. Improvement in those people also suffering from obstructive sleep apnea, in itself a known risk factor for AF, was also noted.

The researchers concluded that their lifestyle and risk factor management program was feasible to deliver, effective, associated with little chance of side-effects and resulted in a substantial reduction in suffering from atrial fibrillation. I would add to this that it is likely to be cost-effective, given the reduction in medication usage requirements and the other health benefits noted above.

In the next chapter we'll look beyond heart disease to further explore the potential of lifestyle as a treatment.

Further Resources

www.ornish.com

www.dresselstyn.com

www.nutririonstudies.org

Ornish D. Dr. Dean Ornish's program for reversing heart disease : the only system scientifically proven to reverse heart disease without drugs or surgery. Ballantine, New York 1991.

Campbell TC, Campbell TM II. The China Study. Benbella books Inc., Dallas 2006.

Chapter 7

LIFESTYLE AS THERAPY – CANCER AND BEYOND

*Until you really feel good,
you don't realize how bad you felt.*

BOB L, PARTICIPANT IN THE ORNISH LIFESTYLE PROGRAM.

In the previous chapter, we investigated how lifestyle change is being researched as a treatment for existing heart disease. What about cancer and other diseases? Could lifestyle alone influence the progress of these illnesses too?

You might recall from Chapter 1 there is evidence that people with breast and bowel cancer who exercise live significantly longer than those who don't.[1] Research has also found exercise prior to or immediately following chemotherapy can significantly enhance this cancer killing treatment, decrease side-effects and increase survival times.[2]

In this chapter we'll look at some detailed research that gives us a clue as to how these positive influences might be coming about.

Prostate Cancer Responds to Lifestyle

After demonstrating the potential of lifestyle change to reverse heart disease, Dr Dean Ornish focused his efforts on testing his lifestyle program against another illness, prostate cancer.[3] This was the first published study to assess whether comprehensive lifestyle change can affect cancer progression. Early prostate cancer is ideal for studying lifestyle intervention, because nowadays it is acceptable medical practice to wait and see whether the cancer progresses before proceeding to more aggressive treatments.

Ten years before Dr Ornish first published this research on prostate cancer, I was consulted by 65 year old John with his wife Alice. A stocky fellow with a pleasant smile, John seemed troubled. He shared with me that he had been diagnosed with prostate cancer four months previously, having a Prostate Specific Antigen (PSA) - a cancer marker - blood test reading of eight. His general practitioner of the past 20 years had referred him to an urologist who confirmed the diagnosis of prostate cancer with a biopsy. He then recommended immediate surgical treatment. John wasn't keen on this and to the surprise of his urologist he declined treatment.

Instead, he and his wife attended a ten-day residential retreat at the Gawler Foundation, hoping to learn strategies that might manage his cancer differently. The retreat introduced them both to an approach almost identical to the one used by Dr Ornish in his lifestyle management program. John had recently retired and his wife and he were able to commit to this major change in their lifestyle.

His GP told them they were crazy to take this approach and refused to support him doing it. He was consulting with me in the hope that I would monitor his PSA levels whilst he attempted to reverse the early cancer.

Back then surveillance of early prostate cancer was not considered appropriate management as it is today, and of course Dr Ornish's research was not available to me, so I must admit, I was a little nervous about taking John on. Nonetheless, I had met people with cancer who had significantly improved their health by attending the Gawler Foundation, so I agreed to do so on the condition that if his PSA levels were rising he would consult once again with his urologist. John agreed to this and both he and his wife were visibly relieved to have some medical support. We checked in monthly for the next six months as they took on a vegetarian diet with gusto and practiced three one-hour meditation sessions each day. They both felt healthier than they had done in years and over the six month period, John's PSA level gradually fell to zero. I suggested he return to his urologist to get a final all clear. When I last saw them, they had big smiles and were planning a caravan trip around Australia.

Dr Ornish's study involved 92 men diagnosed with early prostate cancer. Each of these men had chosen a surveillance approach rather than immediate treatment, and they were randomly assigned to either Dr Ornish's comprehensive lifestyle program or to the control group that maintained their usual lifestyle. The lifestyle intervention program was very similar to the one previously employed for heart disease, namely, low-fat vegan diet, exercise, consisting of a 30 minute walk six times a week, and stress management including yoga, meditation, and group support. Two blood test markers were used to monitor progress, namely, prostate specific antigen (PSA), a marker of disease severity and LNCaP, a marker of the body's defense against prostate cancer.

At 12 months follow-up, of the 43 men assigned to the Ornish lifestyle program, none had gone on to require further conventional treatment. In contrast six of the 49 men in the control group required conventional treatment due to rising PSA levels or magnetic resonance imaging (MRI) studies indicating progression of disease. The average PSA level dropped 4% in the treatment group and rose 6% in the control group. LNCaP testing found that on average, the blood of the intervention group inhibited prostate cancer cells eight times more than the control group. All these findings were statistically significant ($p<0.05$). Interestingly those men who got stuck into the lifestyle therapy the most, had the better results, there being a direct relationship to the improvement in prostate health and how much lifestyle change was made.

Since then, a two year follow-up found that just two (5%) of the men from the lifestyle program had required conventional aggressive treatment, while 13 (27%) men from the control group had gone on to need more aggressive treatment.[4]

Several years later, Dr Ornish designed a separate study to see if an understanding of the mechanisms of how lifestyle change brought about this result could be found. Thirty men with early prostate cancer, who chose surveillance rather than immediate conventional treatment, were studied. All 30 men had biopsies of their prostate before and after three months of intensive lifestyle intervention. In the biopsy tissue samples significant alterations in gene expression following lifestyle therapy were found, with known cancer-causing genes (oncogenes) being down-regulated, while known health promoting genes were up-regulated. The differences between the genetic expression patterns before and after lifestyle therapy were statistically significant, suggesting a fundamental genetic mechanism for bringing about improvement in prostate health.[5]

A further five-year follow-up study looked at another aspect of how the DNA in the cells of participants was affected. Recall that a cell's genetic material, DNA, is located in intertwined chromosomes, which in turn are found in a central nucleus within each cell. At the end of each chromosome is a small 'cap,' called a telomere. This 'cap' prevents the chromosomes from unraveling when the cell divides. A telomere of diminished size is associated with ageing and disease. So in the case of telomeres, size does matter.

When blood samples, taken from 10 lifestyle program participants and 25 control group participants, were compared with their original sample taken five years previously, major differences were found. Once again the lifestyle participants trumped the control group with an average increase in telomere length. In contrast the control group showed a decrease in length. The difference between the groups was statistically significant. Closer scrutiny also found that those participants who adhered more closely to the lifestyle program had proportionally greater increases in telomere length.[6]

Multiple Sclerosis shows promise

In 1999, at the age of 45, George Jelinek, a Professor of Emergency Medicine and family man, was diagnosed with Multiple Sclerosis (MS). His mother had died 18 years earlier, severely disabled by the same disease. As editor of a medical journal and an academic emergency physician at the University of Western Australia, he was well qualified to search the medical literature for ways in which he might overcome his disease. He found answers and shares these in his book, *Taking Control of Multiple Sclerosis*.[7] Let me highlight some of the research that George uncovered.

Population (epidemiological) studies suggest having a diet high in saturated fat, dairy products and a lack of sunlight exposure, with subsequent low vitamin D levels, all increase the risk of developing MS.[8] The saturated fat link is particularly interesting because of a study conducted by Prof Roy Swank. In 1949 Dr Swank recruited 150 people with MS and placed them all on a low (less than 20 g per day) saturated fat diet. What's remarkable about this study is that Dr Swank followed these people's progress for 34 years! His results were published in the *Lancet* in 1990[9] and *Nutrition* in 1991.[10]

In a nutshell, approximately half (72) of the people maintained the low-fat diet and their progress was markedly more positive than those that didn't. For example, good dieters who were relatively well with MS when they began the study, were still physically active 34 years later. By comparison, poor dieters with similar levels of disability prior to commencing the research study, on average ended up wheelchair, bedbound or deceased 34 years later. Regardless of how progressed the MS was at the beginning of the study, for those who stayed on the low-fat diet their illness had only progressed marginally. In contrast, the illness of those unable to stick to the diet had progressed markedly and 58 were dead at the 34 year point (compared with13 deaths among the good dieters). The difference between the two groups was highly statistically significant (p < 0.005).

As you can correctly deduce from all this, the solutions George found from his exploration of the scientific literature largely related to lifestyle change. George instituted these changes in his life and to date has not had a relapse of MS since his diagnosis in 1999. Determined to teach and scientifically investigate the effectiveness of these strategies with other people with MS, he runs intensive lifestyle training programs for groups.

Recently he published a five-year follow-up study.[11] In this research there were 274 MS participants who completed detailed questionnaires covering areas including quality of life, physical and mental health. Each participant attended an intensive five-day lifestyle training retreat. The lifestyle program involved a low-fat plant-based diet, exercise, adequate sunlight exposure, vitamin D and omega-3 supplementation, and meditation and stress management. Follow-up questionnaires were completed after one and five years. After 12 months, quality of life measures improved by a median 11.31%, while at five years this had risen to 19.58%. The median rating physical health improved by 18.6% in 12 months and showed a 17.8% improvement at five years. Mental health median improvements were 11.8% at one year, rising to 22.8% after five years. The study lacked a control group, but had nonetheless shown very promising possibilities for a disease that is generally regarded as unrelentingly progressive, especially as the benefits of the treatment seemed to build over the five years following just a single point of intervention over five days. Further larger studies are currently underway.

A Low-tech Vision

It seems that while healthcare budgets are exploding all over the world, a low-tech solution may be at hand. Clinics and hospitals of the future could contain Lifestyle Medicine Units (LMU's), with as much funding and facilities as surgical units. They could be staffed by highly trained professionals in the areas of dietary advice and food preparation, exercise therapy, health coaching, group support facilitation, meditation, and stress management.

I had breakfast with Susie, a dear friend whom I had not seen for some time. It was the day after her son's wedding and we were enjoying a cooked meal in a hotel restaurant. Susie was clearly obese and I tried not to judge her as she ate her hash-browns, bacon and eggs. At one point the conversation moved away from the wedding and Susie confided that three months prior she had experienced severe chest pain and was rushed to hospital. A diagnosis of unstable angina (a serious lack of oxygen to the heart muscle — a potential indicator of an imminent heart attack) was made and following a coronary angiogram, stents were put in place to open up the blockages in her coronary arteries. Susie, in her late 40s, seemed in denial about the seriousness of this. When I gently asked if anyone at the hospital had advised her of any lifestyle changes that might help her condition, I was shocked to hear not, but that she was told it was highly likely that she would need coronary bypass surgery soon. As an addendum she mentioned someone at her health insurance company had said something about lifestyle. "Maybe I'll do a little bit of swimming," she said.

Changing lifestyle is not easy for most people and having a team of skilled facilitators to support people along this road would be an invaluable addition to any hospital or clinic. Outcome studies, such as those I've just presented by Drs Ornish, Esselstyn, Abed and Jelinek, confirm just what can be done with adequate skilled support. Further similar research could be performed by LMU's looking at other diseases, along with more reductionist research. This could help streamline and define the different nuances of lifestyle change required to best manage each particular disease. Certainly the most common diseases such as heart disease, diabetes, obesity and cancer, could be managed in this way, in conjunction with existing therapies.

Twenty-five years ago I became enthused by Dr Ornish's low-tech vision for improving healthcare. I was soon to discover this vision was not every medico's cup of tea when Dr Daniel Lewis, a friend and a rheumatologist (joint disease specialist), invited me to present to a group of his fellow rheumatologists at their annual recreational conference. Apart from introducing the group to meditation, I also presented the Ornish study on heart disease. I suggested that a similar lifestyle program might benefit their patients with arthritis and could be researched. Let me just say that with the exception of Dr Lewis, the response was underwhelming. Some thought, quite reasonably, that their patients were unlikely to take up the type of intensive lifestyle change Dr Ornish was suggesting. My response was that Dr Ornish had demonstrated how willing seriously unwell people are to making changes that might help them, especially if it is recommended by their doctor, backed up by a team of lifestyle change professionals and funded because it saves the health system money. There was palpable disinterest in exploring the possibility further. Fortunately, times are changing, as the formation of Lifestyle Medicine Associations attest.[12-15]

A Teachable Moment

The beauty of Lifestyle Medicine is that it does not require high cost equipment. It can easily be adapted for both inpatients and outpatients, along with doctors consulting rooms and Community Health Centre settings. Every patient admitted to hospital could be considered for a Lifestyle Medicine referral at some stage during admission or soon after discharge. Why so? It is an ideal time, not in small part because as a hospital inpatient you're a captive audience in your bed! More importantly, when you're vulnerable you're open to change. In behavioral psychology terms, it's a 'teachable moment.' These moments can change the lives of people in such wonderful ways and at the same time break the cycle of expensive medical care, a win-win for all. Matt's story in Chapter 3 - Medicine an Inexact Science, is a good example of this.

You may have picked up that I've been on this barrow for some time! Back in the 90's I came up with a proposal for a Patient Education and Health Promotion (PEHP) trolley. The trolley was to be located on hospital wards, so that not only would nursing staff take their drug trolley around to each patient, they would also take the PEHP trolley around at some other time of the day, with the question, "have you had a 'PEHP' talk today?" The trolley was also to be accessible as a mobile educational aid, with handouts, audio and video, a mini whiteboard etc, for other health professionals and family members of patients to use. Nowadays it could also be offered online as most patients bring a laptop or tablet to hospital.

Two separate hospital wards at different major hospitals in Melbourne were recruited to trial the idea. The nursing staff were quite excited about it, seeing it as an opportunity to shift the focus from a disease treatment orientation, allowing a positive health promotion interaction with their patients. I also hoped by its presence that it would change the conversation around the ward. The research proposal was shortlisted for funding, but alas, fell at the final hurdle. Life took me in a different direction and I was unable to follow through with it further. Still, it would stand alone as a valuable resource, could be adapted for an inpatient television network and would tie in well with a Lifestyle Medicine Unit. It's an idea freely offered to anyone who's interested in running with it.

Let me conclude this chapter with a reflection on the positive side effects that Lifestyle Medicine could introduce into our health system:

- Teach people that they can have an impact on their health without relying on the healthcare system alone.
- Impact positively on many diseases at once.
- Make our hospitals and community health settings places where people can not only be treated for their presenting illness, but also leave with new skills that can help them to stay out of doctors' clinics and hospitals in future.
- Help create new healthy role models from people previously facing serious illness. They could impact their families and communities with lifestyle management skills that could inspire others to lead a healthier life.
- Reduce the financial and over-stretch burdens on the health system.
- Improve the health of the workforce, thus boosting the economy generally.
- Save the health budget a bucket load of money.
- Learning to take responsibility for one's health can have positive flow on effects to other areas of life.

What are we waiting for? Let's do it!

Further Resources

www.gawler.org

Jelinek G. Taking Contrrol of Multiple Sclerosis. Hyland House, Flemington 2005.

Hassed C, The Essence of Health: The Seven Pillars of Wellbeing. Ebury Press 2008.

Chapter 8

MIND-BODY WEAVING

This is the reason why the cure of so many diseases is unknown to the physicians of Hellas; they are ignorant of the whole. This is the great error of our day in treatment of the human body, that physicians separate the mind from the body.

HIPPOCRATES (460 BC – 375 BC)

In many traditional cultures the understanding of what it takes to be healthy is regarded as a seamless weave of mind and body. In Western culture, we are only just beginning to integrate this understanding.

There is evidence in Western civilization that the consideration of the mind and body as divided entities began in Ancient Greece. While Hippocrates believed mental illness would be reflected in biological abnormalities in the brain, Plato and Aristotle believed that this was not the case and that mental illness could only really be cured through adopting a healthier philosophy.[1]

In the 17th century this division became a chasm when French philosopher René Descartes famously outlined a path for medical science to travel, the (corpus) body being in the realm of science, and the (ame) mind, which included the soul, belonging to the realm of religion. This so-called Cartesian split[2] freed science from the shackles of religious ritual, control and superstition, allowing it to bound ahead in extraordinary ways. This provided the intellectual foundation stones upon which today's modern medicine was built. However, it had some unforeseen downsides.

For many doctors and medical researchers inexplicable healing effects that seem to involve the mind, rather than provoking curiosity and inquiry, have been dismissed as just 'the placebo effect,' perhaps subconsciously still being treated as unsuitable for the realm of scientific exploration. This dismissal can translate into inadequate attention being given to the subtler aspects of clinical practice, leaving unwell people feeling like they are being treated more like robots than human beings. Yet we are rediscovering that when these aspects are integrated skillfully, new healing possibilities can unfold.

Imagery

"If a feeling becomes strong enough, it might become an image. This image can be of help for the mind."

TS ELIOT

Ian Gawler, a remarkable cancer survivor who has helped thousands of people affected by cancer over more than 30 years, shares the following experience about the use of imagery in his book, *The Mind That Changes Everything*:[3]

"Ellie was a young girl who was battling with an almost overwhelming brain cancer. When we first met, her mother had been told that Ellie was not responding to treatment, nothing more could be done for her and she only had weeks to live. On request, Ellie completed a series of drawings with me that proved to be both insightful and therapeutic.

When Ellie drew her bedroom, it seemed to me to contain an image that powerfully represented the cancer. Amongst her bedroom furniture she drew her dressing table with a large mirror above it. Here Ellie placed the only discordant image in her drawing - she scribbled heavily, angrily, wildly all over the mirror. When it came to depicting the outside of the house, Ellie had drawn a happy garden and a clothesline. So we put these images together and created a healing sequence.

Ellie was instructed to close her eyes, to relax a little and then to imagine the house and the clothesline. In her mind she then created what in one sense was a fantasy; however, the instruction was to imagine she actually was in this fantasy. Ellie began by moving to the back of the house. There she collected a bucket, filled it with water and took a cleaning rag off the clothesline. Next she walked into the house, up into her bedroom (which she had drawn on the first floor) and proceeded to wash off the mirror. The cloth became quite dirty, and she rinsed it in the bucket until the mirror was clean. Then she returned outside, flushed the dirty water down the gully trap, rinsed the cloth and hung it on the line.

Now Ellie had begun this in early December of the year we first met. At that time she was blind in one eye and her mother had been told by the specialists there was little hope of her living to Christmas. Early in the New Year not only was Ellie feeling much better but her sight was back to normal!

Then late in January a new development. Ellie's mother rang me, very disturbed, saying that having been in the routine of diligently practicing imagery morning and evening every day, suddenly Ellie had stopped, saying she did not want to do it anymore. It seemed to her unnecessary and a waste of time. Ellie's mother was quite anxious, but I told her that often as people's physical condition changed, the imagery also could change. As recommended she returned to her doctors and thorough tests found all the cancer had disappeared. Ellie had made a remarkable recovery! Was

she just lucky? Was the time of starting the imagery just a coinci-
dence? Maybe. But none of us closely associated with her at the
time thought so."

To work with people in this way requires an individualization
of approach that involves engaging with subconscious aspects of the
mind. Ian adopts a Buddhist conception when describing this: the
mind broadly having two aspects, the thinking mind and the nature of
mind. The former, containing the conscious and unconscious minds,
can be enlisted in the healing process through techniques such as the
active visualization performed by Ellie.

The term 'nature of mind' is used to describe the profound part
of us that is stable and enduring and is capable of being aware of our
thoughts. This aspect is at the core of our being, an ever flowing river so
often unnoticed and yet available as a constant source of inner strength
and confidence. It is experienced in the deepest stillness or silence of
meditation. Connecting with this aspect of ourselves, coming home to
home base if you like, can also be profoundly healing,[4] as evidenced in
part by the benefits of the relaxation response (Chapter 5).

Which technique to use, the more active visualization type or a more
passive silent meditation? Much more research is needed both to determine
the benefits and to clarify the method best suited to each individual. Ian
recommends incorporating both techniques in healing, but obviously
some people will be more suited to some methods than others.

It is worth noting that our health experts of the mind, psychologists
and psychiatrists, utilize imagery in a variety of ways to assist their
patients in easing psychological distress.[5] However, it is interesting to
consider that the lingering influence of the Cartesian split means that
they do not commonly use, or are referred to, for this therapy for a
physical problem like Ellie's cancer. Should we consider it strange that
the mind's help can be enlisted to treat physical problems? Or have we
simply been taught to believe this is strange?

Attitudes are changing. Sports psychology has led the way in the utilization of imagery in a proactive, positive sense. Research confirms that imaginal practice of sports skills consistently enhances performance and skill development. In addition it is known that top sports people use imagery more than lower-level performers.[6] Legendary golfer Jack Nicklaus describes it this way:

"I never hit a shot, even in practice, without having a very sharp, in focus picture of it in my head. It's like a color movie. First, I 'see' the ball where I want it to finish, nice and white and sitting up high on the bright-green grass. Then the scene quickly changes, and I 'see' the ball going there: its path, trajectory, and shape, even its behavior on landing. Then there's sort of a fadeout, and the next scene shows me making the kind of swing that will turn the previous images into reality. Only at the end of this short, private, Hollywood spectacular do I select a club and step up to the ball."[7]

Many scientific studies on mental rehearsal prove that when you concentrate on a particular region of the body, your thoughts stimulate the region in the brain that governs that part. If you keep doing it, physical changes in the brain will then follow.[8] One could confidently predict that Jack's neural circuits for every aspect of the art and craft of golf would be highly developed. This is not surprising given our understandings about neuroplasticity; neurones that frequently fire together, wire together, creating new physical circuits.

This was demonstrated beautifully in a Harvard University study. The research subjects had never before played the piano. Half of them were taught to mentally practice a simple, five-finger piano exercise for two hours a day for five days. The other piano novices were taught and physically practiced the same activity for the same amount of time. When before and after brain scans were examined, regions of the brain that controlled finger movements had increased dramatically and equally in both groups.[9] As far as the brain was concerned, the imagined training activity was real enough for it to respond. It did so by developing the corresponding neurological pathways that were created for the real practitioners, thereby creating new brain maps from thought alone.

Given the nervous system communicates with the rest of the body, one would expect that thought exercises would not only influence the structure of the brain, but the whole body itself. This has been confirmed in a number of studies which have demonstrated that repeated imagining of lifting weights to increase muscle strength, without actually lifting anything, does in fact do so, and that these gains in muscle strength can be maintained for three months after the mental weight lifting stops.[10,11,12] In one study those who imagined lifting heavier weights activated their muscles more than those who imagined lifting lighter weights.[13]

Our Virtual Body

Another area that points to the power of imagery is body image; the image we hold of ourselves in our mind, a virtual image if you like. In a healthy person this image is in sync with their actual body, unless they have just had a numbing injection such as a dental one, in which case their virtual image will temporarily insist that their lip is enlarged against all physical evidence to the contrary. More serious longer term distortions, for example with people affected with anorexia nervosa, can cause a person looking into a mirror at an emaciated frame to insist that they are overweight.

Distorted images can also be used in a positive way. Researchers stumbled upon the fact that if a person affected by painful arthritis looked at a real-time distorted image of their hand, made to look stretched or stumpy, much in the way that funny mirrors would do at an amusement park, then their pain could be rapidly relieved (halved) and movement improved in 85% of those tested. Interestingly, different types of distortions worked best for different people.[14] How this works remains a mystery.

Mind styles

Deciding which mind-body technique best enhances physical healing in any particular person is a subject of research in the area of hypnosis. The psychiatrist, Dr Herbert Spiegel and his wife Dr Marcia Greenleaf (PhD), have had extensive experience in treating people using hypnosis.[15] When a person enters into a trance their mind is particularly open to suggestions and this can be usefully employed to help them (clinical hypnosis). Dr Spiegel developed a rapidly administered 10 question survey, initially named the Apollonian-Odyssean-Dionysian Cluster Survey,[16] now called the Mind Styles Questionnaire.[17] It reflects how hypnotizable somebody is and correlates this with particular personality characteristics. Their research has determined how best to manage a person based upon their mind's style of operating.

Dr Spiegel determined that at one extreme, the *Apollonian*, named after the Greek god Apollo who was guided more by reason than emotion, shows less flexibility in responding to new stimuli and tests at the low end of hypnotizability with the Hypnotic Induction Profile (HIP). Apollonian's give priority to their 'brain-minds' rather than their 'heart-minds.' They prefer to be in charge; they judge things critically at the time of presentation; they are above average in taking responsibility for their actions; they prefer to figure things out rather than dream them up and they are prone to taking a lot of notes. In treating people like this, time needs to be given to explaining 'why' particular strategies are being suggested, so they can understand the rationale and go with the process rather than fight or control it.

At the other extreme is the *Dionysian*, named after the Greek god, Dionysus, known for unrestrained and undisciplined spontaneous behavior. Dionysian's test high for hypnotizability on the HIP and have a strong tendency to be guided by emotion rather than logic. They have a marked ability for becoming totally absorbed in an activity. They easily suspend critical judgment and they are most likely to comply with others impositions. Of all the mind styles, they are the most sensitive to the environment they find themselves in and the most vulnerable to persuasion. People with this tendency respond well if given clear instructions on 'what' treatment strategies are going to be used, with less emphasis on the 'why,' as too much information of this kind will tend to create anxiety.[18,19]

In the middle, the *Odyssean*, named after Homer's mythical man, Odysseus, who wandered far and wide to find his way home. Testing in the mid-range on the HIP, the psychologically healthy Odyssean is a balancer and mediator. Fifty percent of the population belong to this grouping and do best with a mixture of 'why and what' information.

It might be useful for you to reflect on whether you are a 'why' or a 'what' personality, or 'a like to dance between the two' sort of person when it comes to facing your own ill-health.

How significant is this understanding in clinical situations? Well it is known that hospital settings with continuous background noise and activity unwittingly encourage spontaneous trance (hypnotic) states, making a patient receptive to suggestions, whether they be negative or positive. Hence, communication from all hospital personnel to patients becomes crucial.

Research data from the Albert Einstein College of Medicine suggests that people who are highly hypnotizable (Dionysian) are so sensitive to the suggestive influence of the noisy and confusing atmosphere of the Intensive Care Unit (ICU), that they have significantly longer periods of unstable blood pressure compared to those in the mid-range and low end of hypnotisability.[20] In addition, many medical patients suffer from a *nocebo* effect, a negative placebo effect if you like, when statements from hospital personnel and family members make dire predictions for the effects of treatment.[21]

In emergency situations this is particularly crucial. It may be a person suffering from horrific burns, an accident victim being rescued at the scene or a person coming out of anesthesia in the ICU. It has been shown that helping the patient focus attention away from fear and pain with suggestions for safety, comfort, healing, and recovery, can make a significant difference in outcome. Such phrases as: "Everything you need for your recovery is here for you," "These are soft plastic tubes made to fit your body, bringing you everything you need for your comfort and healing," have been demonstrated to decrease morbidity and mortality in the Emergency Room, at the scene of an accident, and in the ICU. This approach not only enhances healing and recovery, but also raises the morale of the health workers involved.[22, 23, 24]

In appreciating the importance of the mind-body connection in all areas of medicine, the potential for innovation and research into working with the mind to promote healing is mind-boggling. For those interested in the science, let us review chronologically some of the key research that has been helping us to appreciate this knowledge.

Reconnecting Mind and Body – Research Milestones

1865	French physiologist, Claude Bernard, described the concept of homeostasis, the body's ability to maintain a finely tuned equilibrium in many areas of its function, self-monitoring and regulating its internal environment in response to changes in the external environment. Examples include maintaining body temperature and pH (acid-base balance). Harvard physiology professor, Walter Cannon, went on to popularly coin the term 'homeostasis' in his 1932 book, *The Wisdom of the Body*.[25]
1911	Walter Cannon also first introduced the concept of the 'fight or flight' response when it was published in the *Mechanical Factors of Digestion* in 1911.[26] Cannon's work with animals showed that emotions such as anxiety, distress or rage caused the stomach to stop moving.[27]
1932	University of Montréal researcher Hans Selye demonstrated stress effects on animals. Despite exposure to acute physical or mental stress animals adapted and healed. However, if exposure to stressors was unremitting they would eventually weaken the immune system, killing the animal. Post-mortem examinations revealed enlargement of the adrenal gland, gastric (stomach) ulcerations and atrophy (deterioration) of the thymus, spleen and other lymphoid (immune system) tissue. These were physical changes caused by stress. Selye was also the first to recognize the important role of the endocrine (hormone) system in the stress response via the Hypothalamic-Pituitary Adrenal (HPA) axis.[28]
1975	US cardiologist, Dr Herbert Benson, published a book called *The Relaxation Response*.[29] In it he outlined research which had uncovered a counter balancing response to the fight or flight (stress) response, that he named the relaxation

response. Whereas the stress response involved the activation of the sympathetic nervous system, the relaxation response activated the parasympathetic nervous system, which some people have called the 'rest and digest' response.

1975	Scientists Robert Ader and Nicholas Cohen demonstrated classic conditioning of the immune system. In experiments with mice at the University of Rochester they defined a link between the mind (psycho), the nervous system (neuro) and the immune system, coining the term 'psychoneuroimmunology.' While studying taste aversion in mice, they discovered that the immune system can be conditioned in the same way as Pavlov's dogs. If you recall these dogs eventually learned to salivate in response to a bell, even when food no longer accompanied it. In the mice study, mice prone to the autoimmune disease, Lupus, were offered a saccharin flavored drink at the same time as they were injected with a potent immune-suppressing drug to treat their disease. Once the association was learned, the taste alone (with no injection at all) reduced inflammation and symptoms of Lupus almost as much as the drug alone. The experiment demonstrated the nervous system could influence the immune system.[30] Scientists formerly believed that each of these physical systems functioned independently.
1981	Indiana University of Medicine scientist, David Felten, found nerves connected to blood vessels and cells of the immune system in the thymus and spleen, ending at clusters of immune function-regulating lymphocytes (white blood cells), macrophages and mast cells. This provided further physical evidence that the nervous system was communicating directly with the immune system.[31] Combining their work, Ader, Cohen and Felten published the book *Psychoneuroimmunology* in 1981, in which they proposed

	that the brain and immune system worked together to keep the body healthy.[32]
1989	Pharmacologist, Candice Pert at Georgetown University, demonstrated that cell wall receptors for neuropeptide chemicals, like serotonin and dopamine, released by the brain and nervous system, were located on the surface of immune cells.[33] Furthermore it was discovered that immune cells produce and release similar neuropeptide chemicals, indicating evidence of a two-way conversation, which could explain how emotions influence our immune system. It also could imply that given these chemicals represent emotions and are being produced throughout the body, that the mind is not confined to the brain. A 'gut feeling,' for instance, may be exactly that.
1990	A study published in the New England Journal of Medicine confirmed the impacts stress can have on the immune system. Amazingly, 394 volunteers were found who agreed to having one of five different cold viruses injected into their nostrils, after having completed a detailed assessment of their physical and psychological state. Independent of other immune depleting risk factors, how psychologically stressed the person felt was a strong predictor of actually catching the cold. [34] This relationship held for all five viruses, providing evidence for something that most of us have observed to be true, we are more susceptible to viral illnesses when we are run down by stress.
2000	The Nobel Prize in Physiology or Medicine was awarded to Eric Kandel for demonstrating that as learning occurs, the connections among nerve cells increase. Known as 'neuroplasticity,' this discovery overturned a 400 year old mainstream view of the brain; that it could not change.

In 2007, psychiatrist Dr Norman Doidge made this knowledge available to a wide audience in his excellent book, *The Brain That Changes Itself*.[35] In it he described through ground-breaking research and patient stories, just how significant this discovery was. In my medical education I was taught that the brain was incapable of producing new pathways or cells after childhood. We now know that it can do this at any age, giving great hope to those suffering from brain damage or disease. For instance, if one area of the brain is damaged, another undamaged area can learn to take up its function by growing new connections, changing its physical structure. So you can teach an 'old dog new tricks,' the key being that the lesson is repeated again and again. It has also been demonstrated that the brain's physical structure can change simply in response to meditation or counselling therapies, such as psychotherapy.[36]

2009	Neurosurgeon and scientist Kevin Tracey and Ulf Anderson reported their discovery of the neuro-inflammatory reflex, a mechanism by which the brain directly regulates inflammation throughout the body.[37] By electrically stimulating the vagus nerve they were able to treat a man with disabling rheumatoid arthritis. In other words activation of the vagus nerve decreased inflammation through its communication with the immune system. The vagus nerve arises in the brainstem at the base of the brain and is an essential part of the parasympathetic (rest and digest) nervous system, which is responsible for calming organs after they experience activity or stress. Via thousands of tiny branches, it carries messages to and from all the organs residing: in the chest, such as the heart and lungs, and in the abdomen, such as the stomach, spleen and liver. Having good vagal tone is an

	indicator of good health. It is indicated by heart rate variability, whereby the level of activation of the nerve varies with both the in breath and the out breath. Exercise, positive emotions, social connectedness and meditation have all been shown to improve vagal tone.[38-41]
	Since Tracey and Anderson's discovery, a pilot study involving 20 people affected with rheumatoid arthritis has been conducted. In this study patients had a vagal nerve pacemaker inserted into their chest with a wire running up to their neck, where it attached to the vagus nerve. Results have been promising with 16 people feeling significantly better, with this being mirrored by improved reductions in inflammatory markers on their blood tests. Many were able to reduce or cease their anti-inflammatory medications.[42,43] It is hoped this method or other ways of improving vagal tone may be useful in treating the myriad of other autoimmune inflammatory conditions, where medication can be problematic or inadequate. Other conditions in which vagal nerve stimulation treatment is being explored include: asthma, inflammatory bowel disease, Chronic Fatigue Syndrome, diabetes and obesity.[44]
2015	The embracing of the phenomenon called 'epigenetics' (see earlier chapter), in which the internal environment surrounding our cells influences the genes that switch on or off and therefore which proteins are produced within our body, has added another dimension to our understanding of how our mental state can influence our physical health. For this internal environment is not only influenced by external factors, such as: diet, exercise, medications or supplements, but also by our thoughts and feelings. All these things can rapidly alter the chemical milieu surrounding cells, thus affecting

genetic expression. Combined with the insight into the need for repetition to induce neuroplasticity, as Ellie's story attests, positive psychological inputs consistently internalized could play a fundamental role in healing or ameliorating disease.

It is one thing believing in the power of the mind. It is another thing altogether to discover that we have found ways in which thoughts and feelings can translate through immunological, neuroplastic and epigenetic effects to literal physical changes in the body. With this evidence, even the most Apollonian of thinkers has good reason to explore how to use their mind to assist them in healing their body.

Chapter 9

MEANING

He who has a why to live can bear with almost any how.

NIETZSCHE

... everything can be taken from a man but one thing: the last of the human freedoms - to choose one's attitude in any given set of circumstances, to choose one's own way.

VIKTOR FRANKL

Saying "yes" to life in the face of personal suffering may be our greatest challenge. Let me share the story of one man whose friendship and example has helped me to walk this road.

Born into a working-class family, Ron could remember sitting in the back of his father's milkman's cart as they wound their way through the streets of Sydney, refilling empty bottles in the early hours of the morning.

Ron loved his dad but was destined to escape his neighborhood, performing well enough at a select state high school to enter university. His studies led him to the behavioral sciences and eventually he became an organizational psychologist. Ron was bright, ambitious and a highly skilled people manager, so much so, that in 1982 at the age of 42, he had become managing director of the international management consulting firm, the Hay Group. He was at the peak of his powers, when without warning, he experienced severe chest pain. His wife, Di, drove him to hospital whereupon his heart stopped beating. Accident and Emergency (A&E) staff managed to revive him and he was rushed to an operating theatre for an urgent coronary bypass procedure. Di was told he would be lucky to survive the night. Ron survived, but unfortunately most of his heart's function was lost. Six months later another bypass operation was attempted, with minimal success; a bleak prognosis lay before him.

Happily married to Di, his second wife, and with three loving daughters from his first marriage, Ron was not ready to depart without a fight. He was also a man of faith and an active member of the Anglican Church. Another thing in his favor was that he believed in modern medicine and medical innovation and that if he hung in there long enough, a new therapy would be developed that could help him.

After getting through the initial survival stage, Ron and Di had to face the disorientation of the loss of their previously busy lives. In order to care for Ron, Di, who ran her own staff recruitment consultancy, had to modify her working hours. Out of necessity, their priorities changed. As often happens in these situations, some of their old friends stayed away, which was hurtful. But new friends were found, including their next-door neighbors, who would become a strong source of support in the years to come.

When I first met Ron, he had already defied the medical odds by more than 20 years and had survived a further coronary bypass surgery, another cardiac rehabilitation program and half a dozen coronary stent procedures, any one of which could have ended his life. It's hard to fathom the courage, tenacity and determination he mustered to face procedure after procedure for a chance at a little bit more life. Ron, with Di's unfailing support, faced this time and time again so admirably, his desire for life seemingly infusing him with an anti-death factor.

He had been right about the value of hanging in there. Over time, he benefited from improved cardiac medications and technologies, such as a defibrillating pacemaker and a CPAP machine, the latter to assist him with a problem he developed with poor breathing patterns at night, sleep apnea.

In between crises, he did return to some part-time work at the Hay Group. It proved to be a hard reality check, being more than he could manage and a difficult step in acknowledging his limitations. In time, Ron accepted this, set up his own company and succeeded in providing some private psychology consultancy work from home. Yet all the time the specter of cardiac events, in the form of abnormal heart rhythm episodes and chest pain, hung close. He and Di were no strangers to ambulance travel, emergency rooms and coronary care units. Despite this, they would travel to their holiday house on the Great Ocean Road, take their beloved golden retrievers to the beach and face up to the occasional blood-pressure-raising ambulance journey, along the winding roads out from their remote home.

Ron had a passion for social justice and he played a pivotal role in bringing two disparate church charities together under the one arm, which became known as Anglicare, Australia's largest church charity. He saw this as one of his life's greatest achievements. It wasn't long after this that he found he was unable to continue working as a psychologist, and they sold their Melbourne home and moved to their Ocean Road house. There, Ron volunteered his skills to the local hospital board, Health Foundation charity and Anglican Church. He also started the Apollo Bay Discussion Group, inviting interesting speakers once a month to present and answer questions over a meal at the local pub. This injected welcome stimulation into the intellectual life of the community, and it continues to this day.

Whenever I met Ron, he always had an interesting book on the go, inevitably about psychology, theology or philosophy and I enjoyed and welcomed our discussions about such things. He also subscribed to the latest psychology journals. When visiting his home, Radio National was often playing in the background whilst he was reading or tinkering with something. His keen interest in current affairs along with his sense of humor and conversation was always interesting. He thought deeply about life. As he put it succinctly, "the less I'm able to do in the physical world, the more of my life happens behind my eyes."

One of Ron's biggest battles was with the 'black dog' of depression, and he railed against this and the increasing fatiguing debility his illness was inflicting upon him. His diminishing heart function meant less blood flow to his brain and failing kidneys, affecting his precious ability to concentrate and to think. Apart from professional assistance, he tackled this by finding joy in what was meaningful to him: his loving family (now including grandchildren); his contribution to others; his friendships; and remaining intellectually engaged and involved as much as he was able.

When I asked Ron his secret to longevity, given the poor prognosis he had been given so many years ago, he said, "never giving up hope and swapping my specialist every 10 years, because the younger ones are more up-to-date with the latest treatments." Ron trusted his doctors and took any new medication they recommended with enthusiasm, swallowing up to 30 plus pills each day. It was clear to me that his belief in the effectiveness of medical interventions enhanced their benefit. But beyond this was his bloody-minded determination, his ability to adapt to his changing circumstances and the meaning he absorbed from the nurturing aspects of his life, which kept him fighting to stick around.

Ron lost his battle in the end, as we all must eventually do. But he had lived to the age of 75, contributed greatly to his community and to those that knew him, and fittingly died with all his family surrounding him.

At Ron's funeral the tones of Monty Python's, 'Always Look on the Bright Side of Life' (Ron's choice), echoed around us as we filed from the church.

Navigating suffering

As Ron's story demonstrates and my own experience confirms, serious and chronic illness can throw our world into chaos. Unable to participate in life as we once knew it, we must find new ways to get through each day. Initially, most of our focus will be on treating the disease and reducing its impact upon us, and if this leads us to having a better sense of personal control over how we can manage symptoms, like pain, then acceptance of our situation can be reached more readily. Even so, acceptance can take a considerable amount of time, because more able-bodied memories remain.

While the quest for better health can be meaningful in itself, other questions inevitably surface, such as: How will I survive financially? How can I contribute to my family? Will I work again? How can I feel useful? If I'm unable to work, who am I? My experience is that a significant period of grief over the loss of one's health, previous abilities and position in society follows.

Apart from the hope for improvement or recovery, another source of hope, as research confirms, is that if we can get through this phase, the longer we have the illness for, then the more likely we're going to be able to adapt to its presence and find new meaning in our lives.[1] For instance, relationships may deepen, new or voluntary work may give us a sense of purpose, and we may come to savor the glitter of sunshine again, perhaps even more than we did before.

As the Existentialist movement suggests, "to live is to suffer, to survive is to find meaning in the suffering."[2]

Clarifying our journey

In the 1980s psychologist James Pennebaker began a series of fascinating experiments. Typically, college students were randomly assigned to one of two 15 minute writing tasks, for four consecutive days. One group, the control group, was told to write about everyday, ordinary phenomena. The other group was told to write about their very deepest thoughts and feelings regarding the most traumatic experience of their lives. The second group of students found the exercise enjoyable and psychologically beneficial. What was unexpected was that these students also needed to attend the student health clinic far less in the months following this exercise. Their physical health had improved as well.[3]

This experiment has been repeated many times in different places around the world with similar results. In another variation of this study, medical students were given the same written assignment, just before they were to receive hepatitis B vaccination injections. When followed up, the students who wrote about their emotions were found to have a much higher antibody response to the vaccination than the control group, when blood tests were taken 4 and 6 months later.[4] In other words, their immune system was functioning better and they were now better protected against the hepatitis B virus than their control group colleagues.

Other researchers have looked at means other than writing to achieve the disclosure of difficult feelings. For example, Holocaust survivors were asked to talk for an hour or two about their personal experiences during the Second World War (talks were videotaped). Their health was followed up for 14 months following this. Analysis of the videotapes found that the degree to which survivors opened up during the interview was found to be positively correlated with long-term health benefits after the interview.[5]

It is helpful to realize that finding a way to express the deeper aspects of our lives, even for just 15 minutes a day for four days as Pennebaker's students did, can be beneficial both psychologically and physically. Like a jigsaw puzzle, the more pieces that fit into place, the more satisfying and whole we feel and our health seems to mirror that satisfaction. Of course some pieces can be hard to find or even to hold on our own, so just as Ron discovered, we may need a friend, counsellor or psychotherapist to help us to make sense of and/or clarify our story.

Placebo, the Meaning Response

"The healing process has been relegated to the position of a disturbing effect, summed up under the name 'placebo,' equated to some kind of noise in the system."

DR NORMAN SARTORIUS, WORLD HEALTH ORGANIZATION

While finding meaning can help to bolster our health and give us reasons to live, it can also play a more subtle, unconscious role in our everyday health, in the form of the placebo effect.

How is it that inactive substances, like sugar pills, or fake treatments of any description can have a healing effect? Welcome to the world of the placebo, an inactive medication or treatment whose effect is not well understood, but demonstrates that our culture and beliefs influence our biology.

Placebo is derived from Latin and means 'to please.' Daniel Moerman, who has studied and published widely on the placebo effect for more than 25 years, prefers the term, 'meaning response' to placebo response. He believes this is a more accurate representation which allows the effect to be considered within the larger pool of what brings meaning to our lives, and more easily discussed as a contributing factor in the effectiveness of all treatments, not just inactive ones.[6] He suggests a way to help us understand this effect is to tease out three ways in which healing occurs:

- Autologous healing - the body's own innate self-healing ability.
- Specific treatments - such as drugs, surgery or complementary therapies.
- Meaning.

For example, if we cut our finger the majority of the wound's healing is done without any conscious effort, i.e. by autologous healing. It may be hastened if we clean the wound and use a Band-Aid (a specific treatment). For a child, it might be helped further if their mother kisses it better (meaning).

The placebo effect is encompassed by the third category, meaning, and therefore cannot be understood without understanding the broader webs of significance in which a doctor-patient encounter takes place. Let me provide you with evidence of this (remember the placebo is a chemically inactive treatment in these examples):

- people who take their placebos diligently do better than those who take them only occasionally.[7,8]
- placebo injections work better than placebo pills in the US, but not in Europe.[9,10]
- brand name placebos relieve pain better than generic placebos.[11]
- blue placebos are better sedatives than red ones[12] – except for Italian men, for whom the opposite is true.[13,14] This is thought to be because, whereas Italian women associ-

ate blue with the Virgin Mary, Italian men associate blue (azure) with the color of their national soccer team, the Azzurri, whose team slogan, "losing is not an option," is not a notion conducive to a nice nap![15]

- Germans with ulcers respond to placebos at a rate twice that of people in the rest of the world. In fact, the placebo healing rate for ulcers in Germany is almost three times that of the Netherlands or Denmark. In studies of blood-pressure drugs rather than ulcer drugs, the situation reverses itself. In blood-pressure studies, the Germans have the lowest placebo response rate in the world. No one has an adequate explanation for this, although in Germany, unlike other countries, doctors treat low blood pressure as well as high blood pressure, so perhaps Germans are more concerned about having their blood pressure lowered, so subconsciously resist the effect of the medication.[16,17]

Clearly the placebo response varies between nations, evidence that healing is being influenced by different cultures and beliefs. This is more easily encompassed by calling it the meaning response. If phenomena such as this puzzle us, Moerman suggests it is because we have grown too accustomed to the machinery model of medicine. According to the machinery model, placebos should not work at all. If we fill our car engine with water instead of oil, we know the result, but if we inject water instead of morphine into somebody suffering severe pain, it might do the job. As Moerman says, it is as if someone had designed a joke spanner that looks real but won't turn a nut, and secretly slipped it into a mechanic's toolbox. But when the mechanic uses it, the joke spanner works just fine.[18] As I've emphasized earlier, human beings are not machines. We've explored some of the pathways that might explain some of these findings in the chapter entitled Mind-Body Weaving.

The Birth of the Randomized Controlled Trial

Harvard educated American surgeon, Henry Beecher, was serving in World War II when he ran out of morphine, which was in short supply. At the time he was about to operate on a badly wounded soldier. He was afraid that without a painkiller, the soldier might go into fatal cardiovascular shock. What happened next astounded him. One of the nurses filled a syringe with saline (salty water) and gave the soldier a shot, just as if she were injecting him with morphine. The soldier calmed down straight away. He reacted as though he'd actually received the drug. Beecher went ahead with the surgery, cutting into the soldiers flesh, repairing what was necessary inside him back up, all without anesthesia. The soldier felt little pain and did not go into shock.[19]

After that stunning success, whenever the field hospital ran out of morphine, Beecher did the same thing again; injected saline, just as if he were injecting morphine. The experience convinced him of the power of placebos and upon return to the US after the war, he began to study the phenomenon.

In 1955 Beecher published a landmark paper which looked at 15 other research papers. Entitled *The Powerful Placebo* and published in the *Journal of the American Medical Association*, it discussed the huge significance of placebos and called for a new model of medical research that would randomly assign subjects to receive either active medications or placebos, so that the powerful placebo effect wouldn't distort results.[20] Thus the randomized controlled trial (RCT) was born. So now, the most respected research, whether in conventional or complementary medicine, includes a placebo treatment, as well as a "real" treatment, in order to compare the two.

It is worth noting that RCTs are only necessary because placebos (disguised inactive treatments), do work to a significant extent. While the main focus of developing an RCT was to distinguish which active treatment actually added further benefit, beyond its placebo benefit, exploring ways in which the placebo aspect might work and be enhanced, has been a far less popular scientific endeavor. What is clear is that while the placebo itself is inert, the act of receiving and/or taking a placebo is not inert.

This effect was illustrated clearly by functional Magnetic Resonance Imaging (fMRI) of patients' brains when they received either an antidepressant tablet, or an identical looking sugar pill. It showed the brain activation of those who received the active chemical to be almost identical to that of those who received the sugar pill.[21] This finding is supported by reviews of published research data, which suggest that the level of placebo effect of antidepressants is 60 to 80%; that is, only 20 to 40% of the benefit can be attributed to the chemical. Other reviews that included published and unpublished research were even more dramatic, suggesting that antidepressants were no better than placebo for mild to moderate depression and only marginally better than placebo for severe depression.[22,23]

One might have thought that this placebo activation pathway in the brain would be common to other placebos, but sugar pills disguised as pain killers have been shown to activate different brain pathways related to the reduction of pain.[24] These pathways cause the specific release of appropriate neurochemicals, such as serotonin to elevate mood or endorphins to relieve pain. The body was effectively cooperating with the instructions the mind was giving it, by selecting and releasing appropriate specific chemicals from its 'internal pharmacy.' The selection depended upon what the person believed the placebo was being directed towards relieving.

Earlier research in 1996 had demonstrated the release of endorphins, the body's internal painkilling opiate, in response to a placebo. Fabrizio Benedetti and his colleagues designed an elegant experiment in which 223 research subjects had pain induced by a tight blood pressure cuff, whilst an IV line was available on their free arm to inject medication into. They were instructed to report when their pain level had reached 7 out of 10, at which time they were given an intravenous injection of inactive saline in full view whilst being told the following: "I'm going to give you a painkiller. Your pain will subside after some minutes. Be calm and comfortable and report your pain sensation during the next minutes."[25]

Over the next hour, following the placebo injection, the majority of participants reported increasing pain, reaching a rating of 10. However, 60 were strong placebo responders and their pain levels dropped to a rating of 5. These 60 were then secretly given either a further injection of saline or the opiate antagonist drug, Naloxone. Naloxone is commonly used to reverse the effects of a heroin overdose by competing with opiates (like heroin, morphine, codeine and endorphins) for the receptors on the surface of brain cells, thus reducing the opiate effect. When the placebo responders who'd received Naloxone began to complain of increasing pain once again, whereas those who'd received a further saline injection did not, this was proof that their internal opiates (endorphins), induced by the placebo, were now being competed with by Naloxone.[26] Solid evidence that placebos could trigger real biological effects, a fact now backed up by fMRI brain imaging.

Interestingly, fMRI brain scans also show the activation of different pathways again when recovery from depression occurs through counseling with cognitive therapies as opposed to antidepressant medication. In future, when treating difficult cases of depression, it may be possible to use these patients' brain scans to determine whether they will respond best to drug or cognitive therapies.[27,28,29]

Influencing Placebo

While it might be easy to assume that people who respond to placebos are somehow more gullible or have particular personality characteristics, extensive research has found this is not the case. As counterintuitive as it may seem, the characteristics and qualities of individual patients makes no significant impact on the placebo response rates.[30] More recently there has been research suggesting genetic markers may help to define placebo responders, but it is early days.[31]

What we do know makes a significant impact is the effect of the doctors themselves. Studies have shown that the same treatment given by two different doctors, one adopting a neutral stance and the other an enthusiastic, warm confident one, significantly influence the effectiveness of whatever is being administered, placebo or otherwise.[32] Take the case of antianginal medication, for treating the ischemic (lack of oxygen) heart condition, angina. When double-blind RCTs were initially introduced, a number of medications that had been used to treat angina for some years, were put to the test again. In the initial trials, before the RCT, doctors were enthusiastic about the new medication they were prescribing and their patients experienced a 70 to 90% alleviation of their symptoms. When the same drug was re-trialed using the RCT methodology, the doctors administering it, unsure whether it might be a placebo, presented it more skeptically than in the original trials. They had a 30 to 40% success rate, no better than the placebo.[33] The active drug had not changed and yet the results were vastly different.

This pattern of initial trials yielding better results with newer medications is not uncommon. Take the example of Tagamet (cimetidine) an anti-peptic ulcer drug. Moerman reviewed 117 trials. Initial trials consistently yielded a 72% success rate, as proven on endoscopy (i.e the healed stomach ulcers being viewed through a flexible camera). When it was superseded by a supposedly better medication, Zantac (ranitidine), further trials involving Tagamet found its effectiveness dropped to 64%, as the enthusiasm of the doctors prescribing it waned.[34]

Another study which demonstrated the influence of the person administering medication on the patient receiving it, involved the injection of painkilling medication. No placebos were used in this trial. The only difference was that some patients got their painkiller secretly administered through an intravenous (IV) line, while other patients got the same kind of IV medication openly, from an injection by a doctor or nurse who told them, "it was a powerful painkiller increasing their pain tolerance." All patients were encouraged to ask for more pain relieving medication until the pain they reported was half the level of what it was to begin with. Patients who were reassured that they were getting the medication, required substantially less of it than those who didn't know when it was being injected. This study confirmed the power of the placebo (meaning) effect even when the same real medication and no placebos were being used.[35]

What to conclude from all this? Given the effectiveness of all "real" treatments includes a placebo (meaning) response component, and given this response tends to have a honeymoon period of greatest success when the treatment is new on the market, then it would appear to be wise for the doctor and the patient to enhance any treatment with enthusiasm, by finding reasons to be positive about whatever is being administered. Daniel Moerman does it this way:

> "...when I have a headache, or some aches or pains in my back or leg, I shake two ibuprofen (eg Nurofen) tablets into my hand, I look at them carefully, and I say, 'Guys, you are the best, the most powerful and trouble-free drugs in the world.' Or something like that. Then, with a large glass of water ('Water is good too,' I think carefully to myself), down the hatch."[36]

So as you take your medication, placebo or favorite home remedy for that matter, remember you can enhance its effectiveness by saying to yourself something like, "this is providing a boost to my immune system that will help me overcome this illness." Positively cooperating with whatever treatment we take or agree to receive, is a valuable lesson the meaning response can teach us.

How powerful can this be? Consider the testimony of a 76-year-old World War II veteran who was one of 10 men in a study involving knee surgery.[37] Although he didn't know until somewhat later, he had been one of five in the study to have sham surgery on his knee to treat his arthritis. He had been mildly anesthetized and given three stab wounds in the knee, to mimic the visible results of arthroscopic surgery. So effectively nothing was done to his knee apart from these cuts. Despite this, he had an outstanding result. Listen to the patient's description and comments about his surgeon, Dr Bruce Moseley:

> "I was very impressed with him, especially when I heard he was the team doctor for the Houston Rockets... So, sure, I went ahead and signed up for this new thing he was doing... The surgery was two years ago and the knee never has bothered me since. Just like my other knee now. I give a whole lot of credit to Dr Moseley. Whenever I see him on TV during a basketball game, I call the wife in and say, 'Hey, there's the doctor that fixed my knee.'"[38]

Prescribing placebos

Should a doctor be able to prescribe a placebo? Of late, the standard answer has been that because it is deceptive, no, it would be unethical to do so. Most of us, quite rightly, wish to be informed about what we are taking. Yet turning all this on its head is preliminary research conducted by Harvard University medical professor Ted Kaptchuk and his colleagues that suggests that even when a patient knows they are receiving a placebo, it can still be effective.[39,40,41] It seems that generations of conditioning to expect a pill to deliver healing benefits, especially when it is given by a trusted authority, is so hardwired in us, that the very act of taking a pill, even in the full knowledge it has no active ingredients, is received as a reassuring signal by the body to invoke its healing mechanisms. So no deception is required.

Given this, how could placebos be prescribed? Firstly they would be reserved for patients with non-specific complaints and viral illnesses unsuited to medical interventions, conditions where one can afford to wait and see what does or does not develop. All a doctor would need to do is to incorporate the statement the researchers used, for example: "An option I can offer you is to prescribe placebo pills made of an inert substance, like sugar pills, that have been shown in clinical studies to produce significant improvement in (your condition) through mind-body self-healing processes,[42] activating your body's internal pharmacy without the risk of unwanted side effects." Informed placebo prescribing; no deception.

How big an issue is this? A survey of hospital internists and rheumatologists in the United States found that 50% of the medication they prescribed was given to the patient as what is known as an 'impure' placebo.[43] In other words, they thought it best to prescribe something rather than nothing at all, even though they knew the medication was not indicated. In this instance, because the prevailing culture does not encourage prescribing of a harmless placebo, the patient is given an often expensive and potentially dangerous medication as a placebo instead. Many other studies confirm this finding.[44] In other words placebo prescribing still exists, it has just morphed into a more dangerous active form, albeit a culturally acceptable form for both doctor and patient.

The same thing occurs in general practice where antibiotics are too often prescribed for viral illnesses patients would recover from in time, without the need for medicine. In this common scenario, the doctor knows antibiotics are only effective against bacteria and ineffective against viruses, yet both he or she and the patient feel more comfortable involving a pill in the relationship. Unfortunately, the chemical in the pill is useless in this instance. It just increases the potential for harmful side-effects for the sick person, as well as the development of dangerous antibiotic resistant bacteria in the community and costs us all in terms of the health budget. It does, however, have a reassuring placebo effect, that is, believing it will help creates a level of effectiveness. Much better to get this level of reassurance by understanding that with appropriate rest, fluids and nutrition the virus would be overcome by the body anyway. But failing this, it would be preferable to prescribe an inexpensive, harmless placebo. In this situation if you must fire (i.e. prescribe), better to fire 'blanks' than live ammunition, otherwise, a much more dangerous type of deception than the one originally being avoided takes place.

This is a serious problem. In the US, amongst hospitalized patients alone, there are over 100,000 deaths annually due to adverse drug reactions.[45,46] As the survey of hospital internists and rheumatologists suggests,[47] a sizeable number of these would have been from medication prescribed to act purely as a placebo. These deaths, side-effect induced suffering and billions of dollars could all be saved, simply by reintroducing the skillful prescribing of harmless placebos.[48]

Currently I'm aware of a placebo called Obecalp (placebo spelt backwards) which is available over-the-counter in some US pharmacies,[49] but there is a huge market for a pharmaceutical company to introduce a placebo that doctors could widely prescribe. It would be completely safe, so no expensive pretesting would be necessary, making it easy for the company to get into the marketplace. Marketing could include educating the doctor in appropriate prescribing indications and communication.

The main problem we'd face in bringing this about would be changing the culture of prescribing. When faced with a patient they have nothing specific to offer help for, I suspect most doctors, with good intentions, are more comfortable prescribing an essentially useless medication as a placebo, than a completely inactive pill (unaware of the devastating global statistics they could be contributing to in the process). In order to reintroduce the prescribing of harmless placebos, I believe we need to bring to the forefront the "first do no harm" maxim and to re-embrace the understanding of the powerful effects of the mind on the body, and in this instance the capacity of placebos to stimulate the body's internal pharmacy.

The following two examples from my medical training days are a reminder that it wasn't that long ago when the conscious use of placebos was an acknowledged part of the practice of medicine. We may need to do it a little differently these days, but there is much to learn from these examples:

Sir Edward Hughes was a brilliant surgeon who also championed the introduction of compulsory seatbelt legislation. In 1984, my final year of medical training, I was privileged to experience a tutorial with him. In this session he emphasized one of the keys to improving a patient's recovery from surgery. "You must prescribe a liquid vitamin tonic," he said. "It must be red in color. You are to instruct the patient to take exactly five mls (0.17oz) exactly 10 minutes before breakfast and five mls exactly 10 minutes before dinner." He looked each of us in the eye and told us, "you must give specific, confident instructions."

During the same year, I also spent two weeks of work experience with Dr Broughton, a consummate, caring country GP. He was 78 and was greatly respected in the town where he worked. Many had been his patients since he had delivered them as babies. At one point an elderly farmer mentioned how much he missed those purple pills Dr B used to give him for his back pain. After the gentlemen left, I asked Dr Broughton about those purple pills. He shared with me that he used to keep a bottle of purple-coated sugar pills in his cupboard. He said it had been a most useful medication for a whole range of conditions. It was in fact a placebo. My observation of Dr Broughton and the esteem with which he was held would have enhanced the effect of his purple pills. He lamented the fact that for medico-legal reasons he could no longer use placebos for his patients. Now that informed placebo prescribing has been proven to be effective, it would overcome this barrier.

Chapter 10

HUMOR THAT HEALS

The arrival of a good clown exercises more beneficial influence upon the health of a town than of twenty asses laden with drugs.

DR THOMAS SYDENHAM (1624 – 1689)

In the mid-1990s I was fortunate enough to be involved in helping to organize two presentations given by Dr Patch Adams. You might recall that Robin Williams played Patch Adams in the movie of this title. Unlike Robin, the real-life Patch was 6'7" (200 cm) tall, with a wonderfully upright posture and a greying ponytail that almost reached his behind. He had an intense presence that exuded compassion.

He commenced his lecture at Monash Medical Centre Clayton imploring us to enjoy the benefits of wearing our underpants on our head, which he proceeded to do. He then pulled his large clown bloomers all the way up, covering himself from head to foot, telling us how much he enjoyed doing this whilst standing completely still at bus stops. He observed that some people would completely ignore his presence, as if he were a signpost, which he was tall enough to be!

Patch then went on to briefly review the many scientific benefits of laughter (see later on in this chapter) before sharing stories of his travels and experience as a clown in a poor Eastern European hospital setting.

In one moving story, he described hearing the chilling screams of a child coming from a treatment room. He made his way over there, observing a boy with significant burns suffering terribly as a doctor cleaned out his wounds, a procedure that would normally be performed under anesthetic. Patch entered the room in full clown outfit and placed his face within an inch of the child's. The child stopped screaming, entranced by the strange face before him, remaining transfixed and silent for the next 20 minutes whilst the procedure was completed.

After his lecture, Patch donned this very same clown outfit and joined a ward round on the children's wing. The gregarious passionate lecturer come comedian, was now a shy, fragile, introverted clown, his face painted and a bulbous red nose attached. He engaged gently and playfully with the youngsters, before he reached the private room of a 15-year-old girl, Lisa, who had been admitted with Anorexia Nervosa. On the advice of the pediatrician, the rest of us in the entourage remained in the corridor, whilst Patch approached her, wordless and slightly hunched. Subtle exchanges of body language followed until he received her permission to sit on the end of her bed. The delicate encounter continued to unfold over the next 30 minutes. During this time I learnt of Lisa's story from the pediatrician standing beside me. Lisa, he told me, had been in hospital for five days and the interaction we were witnessing before us, was the first time she had opened up to anyone since she had been admitted. When Patch re-entered the corridor he briefly acknowledged the seriousness of this girl's plight and told us of her agreement to keep in touch with him; the two had exchanged contact details.

The ward round had been set up at least in part as a photo opportunity, yet Patch, whilst happy to agree to help with the hospital's publicity, had no qualms about leaving the rest of us waiting while he maintained his priority of patient care first and foremost. His free not for profit hospital, the Gesundheit Institute, founded in 1971, remains an inspired vision of healthcare, with care being its primary motivation.[1]

Laughing illness better

In 1976 the New England Journal of Medicine published a fascinating case report.[2] It referred to Norman Cousins (June 24, 1915 – November 30, 1990), who was an American political journalist, author, professor, and world peace advocate. In 1964 he had been diagnosed with a form of fulminant widespread arthritis, known as Ankylosing Spondylitis. He was admitted to hospital barely able to move without severe pain, his jaw almost locked. His doctor, also a personal friend, suggested he only had a 1 in 500 chance of surviving. Norman was proactive and decided the busyness and negativity of the hospital environment was not going to improve his chances of recovery. So with his doctor's support, he checked himself out of hospital and into a hotel room, where he hired a movie projector and comedy movies. Having done his own research, which indicated the medications he was being given would be depleting his body's vitamin C, he got his doctor to agree to adding high doses of vitamin C intravenously to his treatment regime. He combined this with a positive attitude, love, faith and hope. The inflammation in his body was measured by a blood test, the Erythrocyte Sedimentation Rate (ESR), which was elevated, but was lowered by at least five points after either a period of sustained laughter or a dose of intravenous vitamin C.

His laughter was induced by Marx Brothers and Candid Camera films. "I made the joyous discovery that ten minutes of genuine belly laughter had an anesthetic effect and would give me at least two hours of pain-free sleep," he reported. "When the pain-killing effect of the laughter wore off, we would switch on the motion picture projector again and not infrequently, it would lead to another pain-free interval."

He was able to cease all medications while he continued laughter and vitamin C therapy and one week later walked unaided from the hotel. A fortnight later he returned to work. His bestselling book, *Anatomy of an Illness*, is well worth a read.[3]

Investigating humor

*"Studying humor is like dissecting a frog -
you may know a lot but end up with a dead frog."*

MARK TWAIN

While I can appreciate Mark Twain's sentiment, I am also gratified and amused that scientists take humor seriously enough to research it! Below is a list of some of their discoveries.

- A lack of ability to appreciate humor can relate to right frontal lobe dysfunction in the brain, which may be present in some people with autism.[4]
- There is good evidence that humor helps to reverse the effects of stress both psychologically and physiologically. Stress has been observed to be much less likely to translate into anxiety and all its range of physical symptoms if a person uses humor a lot to break the tension.[5]
- Japanese research has found that diabetic patients improved both their immune system function and glucose control after watching a one-hour comedy video compared to those who attended a one-hour diabetes education lecture. Thirty-nine health promoting genes were positively activated by the comedy.[6]

A list of some of the health benefits of laughter follows:

Therapeutic effects of laughter (from Hassed)[7]

Psychological

- Moderates stress and buffers physical effects of stress[8]
- Improves mood, coping with sadness[9,10] and loss[11]
- Adjunct to psychotherapy[12]
- Reduces anxiety and improves performance[13] and teamwork[14]
- Enhances education[15] and occupational therapy[16]
- Coping with terminal illness,[17] hospitalization and major medical procedures[18]
- Positively associated with creativity,[19] generativity,[20] emotional stability, extraversion,[21] optimism and self-esteem, and negatively with distress and depression[22]

Physiological

- Longevity
- Reduces pain and improves pain threshold[23,24,25]
- Enhances relaxation response[26]
- Reduces stress hormones, e.g. cortisol[27]
- Improves immunity - Stimulates IgA,[28] increases blood leukocytes,[29] reduces stress hormones[30] and buffers against the immunosuppressive effects of stress[31,32,33]
- Improves blood and lymph flow, increases oxygenation, lowers blood pressure and exercises muscles[34]

A Wee Story

In my capacity as a lecturer for final year medical students, I would run tutorials for groups of 40 students at a time. The clock had just ticked on 2:00 p.m. and I could see the students waiting for my arrival in the tutorial room. It had been a busy day and I ducked into the toilet next to the tute room for a quick pee. Paying insufficient attention to my business at the urinal, I looked down to see a stream of urine trickling down my left trouser leg. I quickly corrected the flow direction but it was too late. To add to the effect, it was springtime and I had chosen a light beige trouser to wear that day.

What to do? My mind raced; was there a sports bag in my car with a change of clothes? No; was there someone who could take my place? No; could I just leave the building, do a runner? Boy did I want to, but no, I was too responsible for that.

So I decided to play dumb. I entered the room and started my presentation just as I would normally do. I thought I was getting away with it until a student in the front row kept fixing my gaze. She looked down at my pants leg, then up at my face, at least 15 times. I have no memory of what I was teaching that day, but I have a vivid memory of the look on that student's face!

That evening, I heard from my mother that my sister, who was 20 weeks pregnant, had started bleeding. Dianne and her then husband, Michael, had been seeing a fertility specialist having failed to achieve a pregnancy beyond 12 weeks in the previous six years.

Her specialist advised her to rest quietly and that he would perform an ultrasound the following day. She decided to spend the night at my parent's house. I arrived quite late to visit, but she was not asleep. I sat on the end of the bed. "I'm losing my baby," she said, crying.

Not knowing quite what to say, I sat quietly for a while, then related my day's experience. Well, when I got to the part about the student looking down at my trouser leg then up at my face, my sister laughed so hard, that the tears rolled down her face. She was doubled over so uncontrollably with laughter, I was sure she was going to lose her pregnancy there and then. As it turned out, soon after she fell asleep and when she woke eight hours later, the bleeding had stopped.

There were no further complications during the rest of her pregnancy and at the time of writing this story her only child, Andrew, is studying at University.

Humor makes top 6

In 2004 Christopher Peterson and Martin Seligman, founder of the field of positive psychology, came out with *Character Strengths and Virtues: A Handbook and Classification*.[35] This volume was a significant contribution to psychology, a sort of antidote to psychiatry's *Diagnostic and Statistical Manual's* (DSM) focus on mental illness, and an important reminder to psychologists that humans aren't only full of illness, but also have a lot of character strengths they can draw upon.[36]

The main tenet of the field of positive psychology is that the path to well-being lies in nurturing your highest strengths. The book laid out the following 24 character strengths grouped within six categories:

- Transcendence: appreciation of beauty and excellence; spirituality; gratitude; hope; humor.
- Temperance: forgiveness and mercy; humility and modesty; prudence; self-regulation.
- Justice: citizenship; fairness; leadership.
- Humanity: love; kindness; social intelligence.
- Courage: bravery; persistence; integrity; vitality.
- Wisdom: creativity; curiosity; open-mindedness; love of learning; perspective.

More recently Martin Seligman in his book *Flourish*, presented another way of looking at well-being through five categories, known as PERMA: Positive emotions; Engagement; positive Relationships; Meaning; and Accomplishment.[37]

Researchers tested this theory by studying 517 people with an age range of 18 to 71 years (average age 36 years). They found each of the PERMA categories to be important and interdependent, in that if one category was raised the others would rise also. When analysis turned to the 24 character strengths, each of these was also found to be important to our well-being, with the top stand-alone strength contributing to well-being being gratitude, the love of learning a close second.[38]

I've personally found the positive psychology recommended practice of reflecting at the end of each day on three things to feel gratitude for, to be invaluable, bringing perspective, even on difficult days. It can be the memory of the simplest thing; a smile from a shop assistant, a meal enjoyed, sharing a joke with a friend, or remembering the sight of a magpie doing something ridiculous. As I practice savoring these moments, it reminds me to savor them more often in the moment they are actually happening as well.

Other highly ranking character strengths not far behind gratitude and love of learning were: love, honesty, hope and our good friend, humor.[39]

Humor in the face of adversity

I first met Margot Maurice, a woman of indomitable spirit, in 1995. At one time billed as Australia's Marilyn Monroe, Margot had been a successful performer on stage, radio and television. Later she had become a journalist and newspaper editor. This all changed in 1974 when at age 41 she was almost killed in a horrific car accident.

A car traveling the wrong way along a freeway exit ramp collected her vehicle head on. Rushed into hospital by ambulance, rapidly losing blood, Margot was wheeled towards an operating theatre. At the same time a clerk was rushing beside her pen and paper in hand asking, "What is your religion?"

Despite being in shock, Margot could still appreciate the ridiculousness of the situation and replied, "Zoroastrian!" leaving the bewildered clerk in her wake.

Margot then overheard one of the surgeons commenting on the trouble they were having controlling her blood loss. Using self-hypnosis, she assisted them by slowing her heart rate and breathing. Much later on her surgeon confirmed the benefit this had given him and had enquired as to how she had done this. Margot was well-versed in mindful breathing and meditation well before it became popular.

Margot recovered from multiple injuries over three years involving many hospitalizations for surgery.

A classically trained jazz pianist, as she recovered Margot forged a new career developing her own method of music therapy for children with intellectual disabilities. At the age of 51 she was highly driven, working an 80 to 90 hour week operating two music schools, when her inner guidance told her to get her heart checked. Margot had always been very intuitive, but was feeling well, so it was only when her inner voice persisted with its message that she took heed.

When she saw her GP no problem was found. Months later, however, after developing several viral illnesses, she became increasingly short of breath. Further tests saw her urgently referred to Sydney cardiologist, Dr Choon Lee. In her autobiography, *Six Months to Live*,[40] she retells her experience:

"You have cardiomyopathy," Dr Lee concluded. "That's the condition for which we do heart transplants, but you're out of the age group for which transplants are being done at present. As your heart is only about 25% of normal strength I wouldn't expect you to live any longer than 6 months."

"The condition will improve," Margot said hopefully.

"Cardiomyopathy doesn't improve. The best we can hope for is that it stabilizes, then you may get a few months more." (In 1984 this was the case. Medical treatment offers a much better prognosis today.)

Further tests at Westmead Hospital confirmed a Dilated Cardiomyopathy (DCM) with an ejection fraction of less than 25%. "Only about one in 25 people with cardiomyopathy last longer than five years," a doctor told her.

"Well maybe I can be that one," replied Margot.

Margot was always one to focus on the positive and was horrified by the prognosis. She told her loving partner, John Gallagher, her daughter Vanda and the rest of her family and closest friends that she was going to beat it. Knowing Margot, they all believed and supported her. The fact that Margot chose to trust herself instead of the accepted prognosis she was given by her doctors, is a testament to her character. She backed this belief up with actions; this is what she did:

- Admitted to herself that she had been trapped by becoming a successful businesswoman –"the monster I'd created had started to devour me." Working hours were reduced to 15 per week, which was all she had the strength for. With John's help they sold one of the two music schools.
- She recommitted to her spiritual meditation.
- They moved to a home in a less mountainous area. The new home had a swimming pool that allowed Margot to start her own water exercise program when well enough.
- She returned to the healthy eating patterns she had known prior to running the music schools.
- Made sure she was in bed by 10pm.

The prescribed medications caused headaches but, with Dr Lee's telephone guidance she persisted with them. When she returned to see him three months later he found her ejection fraction had increased to 30%. He was elated, "This is most unusual. It doesn't usually improve. So, just keep on doing whatever you're doing."

Margot was delighted and certain that a combination of meditation, tender loving care by John and family, plus the prescribed medication had collectively aided her improvement. She commenced her daily water exercises and at her next review, Dr Lee reduced her medication. Too soon it seems, as 48 hours later she was rushed to hospital with her first episode of Atrial Fibrillation (AF) – a rapid irregular heartbeat. Stabilized, her medication was increased again.

At times Margot would have no energy for weeks at a time, but as her strength improved she increased her working hours up to 25 per week. Her ejection fraction was now 35% and Dr Lee revised his prognosis to Margot living into her mid-60s.

By 1990 Margot and John decided to sell their business and home and travel around Australia. Around this time two of Margot's friends independently told her about Coenzyme Q10 (CoQ10), a 'miracle substance' assisting heart disease patients in Germany and Japan. When Margot and John reached Perth they decided to settle there. She commenced taking CoQ10 in the form of a cultured Kombucha mushroom drink. Soon she was feeling much stronger and they shifted further south to Busselton and then Dunsborough. Her doctor agreed to wean her off all medication; however, once again a further episode of AF ensued. Unwell with palpitations and shortness of breath, on arrival at Busselton Hospital Margot recalls:

I asked the nurse to move the heart monitor so that I could see what was going on.

"Why do you want to see the monitor?" she asked me.

"If I die I want to be the first to know." Margot soon recovered.

From her unit in Dunsborough Margot pursued a job as a spiritual counselor, published a New Age magazine and with others established a New Age Expo. At age 67 she was employed as an editor and journalist for a local paper. At the same time her cardiologist had told her she would in time need open heart surgery to replace a weakened heart valve.

Desiring to be closer to family they moved to the Gold Coast in 2000. AF attacks and breathlessness were worsening and cardiac surgery was arranged. Preoperative assessments revealed that two valves needed replacing. Interestingly, Margot's ejection fraction was now 58%.

The travails of open heart surgery, intensive care and gradual rehabilitation are well described in her book.[41] Margot's AF persisted post-surgery and she was placed on the blood thinning medication, Warfarin. On this treatment you need to be careful to avoid taking other substances, like vitamin C and aspirin. Margot was therefore unsure about taking CoQ10. The following conversation between Margot and her Gold Coast cardiologist is illustrative of the polarization issue discussed in the Complementary Medicine (CM) chapter:

"How about CoQ10?" asked Margot.

"Well, there's no evidence that it does any good," he said.

"Oh yes there is," she said. "There have been 10 years of research at the Baker Institute in Melbourne using double blind tests and attaining very good results."

"Well you obviously know more about it than I and if you're happy taking it, it won't do any harm."

(While it is important to share any information about CM you may be taking with your doctor, as these can interact with medications, it may be worth questioning if a doctor has defaulted to the negative position on CM, as it is possible he or she has not researched the CM in question. The patient shouldn't assume the doctor has this knowledge. Fortunately, Margot had done her own research and was not fazed by the negative pronouncement.)

Margot had now lived long enough to benefit from newer medications. Stabilized again on these pills, CoQ10 and other supplements, she felt as good as she had in years. Taking a swim each day in her Gold Coast apartment's pool, she focused her energy on her writing, authoring or co-authoring with John, five books including her autobiography.[42] She crossed her 80th birthday milestone in 2013, by which time the function of her heart had begun to deteriorate once more.

On a recent visit to the Prince Charles Hospital several doctors asked her to what she attributed her long survival. She told them: "determination, following my intuition, sense of humor, positive attitude, maintaining my exercises and good eating habits." Apparently they all made notes of these pearls of hard-won wisdom.

Unfortunately for us all Margot's heart rhythm and function has become increasingly unstable and medicine has run out of reasonable options to offer her. In response to the poor heart function her kidneys are also failing, leaving her increasingly fatigued. Yet she continues to write when she is able and draw on her life experience, wisdom and indefatigable sense of humor. Let me finish by sharing with you a section of an email Margot sent me. She writes this after a particularly harrowing period of days spent in the Coronary Care Unit of the Gold Coast University Hospital, where she endured severe chest pain and unpleasant medical procedures before her heart came back into the right (sinus) rhythm.

"I told the nurse not to panic when the rhythm changes & only wake me up if I flat-lined. She thought (that) was very funny. I explained that as I had donated my body to the university it would be easy for them to just put me on a gurney; give it a good push and it would land over at the university. Two nurses both said I had black humor, but they thought it was great that I'd donated my body to the Uni. I told them it was the ultimate recycling as I wouldn't be needing it anyway. It's hard for people to understand my attitude to death, but when they know I have been preparing now for 30 years, they start to see that I won't be surprised when it eventually happens. Now whether I had a heart attack that time, I don't know, but I do know the heart was stressed and I wouldn't want that too often or for too long. I am planning to be here for my 90th birthday in 2022, but I also accept that if the powers that be need me somewhere else to organize something for them, then so be it. Maybe the ablation will be a big help (it has since been done successfully and has helped). Each time I have faced death (the accident in '74) I am told, 'Go back you have more work to do'. So it's out of my hands and I won't be sitting around waiting when I have things to do."

Chapter 11

COMPLEMENTARY MEDICINE (CM)

Healing is not a competition.

DR HUNTER 'PATCH' ADAMS

The World Health Organization (WHO) estimates that approximately 60% of the medicine practiced worldwide is traditional medicine.[1] Traditional Chinese Medicine (TCM) is practiced in many Asian countries, Ayurvedic medicine in India, Unani medicine in the Middle East, Pakistan and India, while Kampo medicine is used in Japan. Like these forms of medicine, conventional or Western medicine, the predominant medicine practiced in developed countries, has been influenced by cultural factors.[2]

Many traditional forms of medicine have been used for centuries, some for thousands of years, and have a long history of use in their societies and cultures. Such traditional forms are well entrenched in their healthcare systems, often alongside Western medicine. There may be little scientific evidence for these therapies, but the absence of such evidence does not mean that their treatments do not work.[3] There is also some inherent safety considering they've been used for a long time, in some cases over 2000 years.[4] These therapies make up some of what we call complementary and/or alternative medicine (CM), but clearly other cultures would consider them mainstream rather than alternative. What does this mean for us in our modern multi-cultural, internet savvy world? We have more health promoting choices than ever before. On the one hand this array of choice can bring hope, on the other it can be overwhelming and at worse, dangerous.

Complementary and alternative medicine, as defined by the United States National Centre for Complementary and Alternative Medicine (NCCAM), is a group of diverse medical and health care systems, practices, and products that are not presently considered to be part of conventional medicine.[5] NCCAM classifies natural, complementary and alternative medicine into five categories:

1. Alternative Medical Systems -- these are built upon complete systems theory and practice such as homeopathic and naturopathic medicine, Traditional Chinese Medicine and Ayurveda (from India).
2. Mind-body interventions -- these include counseling, patient support groups, meditation, prayer, spiritual healing, and therapies that use creative outlets such as art, music or dance.
3. Biologically-based therapies -- these include the use of herbs, spices, foods, vitamins, minerals and dietary supplements.
4. Manipulative and body-based methods -- these include chiropractic or osteopathic manipulation, massage, yoga, Qigong and Tai Chi.
5. Energy therapies -- these involve the use of energy fields. They are of two types:
    a. Biofield therapies such as Qigong, Reiki and Therapeutic Touch.
    b. Bioenergetic therapies involving the use of pulsed electromagnetic fields, such as pulsed fields, mag-

netic fields, or alternating current fields and/or alternating and direct current fields.

Worldwide reports demonstrate that a large proportion of the public are using CM and its popularity is increasing. For example, in Australia up to 70% of the population are using CM.[6] In the United States up to 62% of adults use it.[7]

To try or not to try

"Don't waste money on unproven treatments" is a common sense statement I've heard from fellow doctors and others. Of course many treatments remain unproven because priority funding is not given to assessing them. We'll touch more on this in the next chapter.

Given the relative lack of proof, why are so many people choosing to use CMs? For many people it provides a more meaningful explanation for their suffering.[8] Let me give you a stereotypical example:

> Julie has a sore throat. She sees her doctor who spends six minutes with her, looks in her throat and ears and diagnoses a probable viral illness. The doctor prescribes rest, fluids and paracetamol. Dissatisfied, Julie attends a naturopath. He spends 45 minutes with her and discovers recent stresses, including a one-week visit from her mother-in-law and increased work pressures, and suggests that these have weakened her immune defenses, allowing this viral illness to occur. He helps her to realize she needs some down time and prescribes an immune boosting, stress relieving tonic. Julie leaves feeling heard and satisfied.

Giving people more time to make meaning of their condition in relation to what is happening in their lives, is an important difference here. Another is the fact that modern medicine places more emphasis on the strength of the external treatment to eliminate disease or manage symptoms, rather than building up the strength of a person's defenses. Pointing out social or lifestyle factors, a mineral deficiency or mental and emotional factors that may have led to a disease, can provide a working anchor from which people can make sense of and tackle ill health. It is easy to see why by comparison, conventional medicine's common explanation of a probable viral illness unluckily acquired, lacks something.

Other reasons people choose CM include:

- a cultural and/or philosophical choice, being consistent with values and beliefs about life.
- a wish to take a less aggressive, gentler, holistic approach.
- to feel more of a sense of control over one's treatment.
- to feel better, having responded poorly to conventional medicine.
- Having suffered an adverse reaction to their treatment i.e. drugs or surgery.
- to support the body's self-healing systems whilst undergoing conventional treatment.
- there are no longer any orthodox approaches available to assist the problem.

For the final point, the question is this, if you're landed with a serious illness, do you risk trying an unproven treatment that may make some sense to you physiologically or instinctively, or wait for research which may never happen? It's easy to make a logical assessment when you're not affected. I experienced the truth of this when a medical colleague, who'd been unimpressed with CM and a staunch supporter of evidence-based medicine (EBM), sadly developed an untreatable cancer. To the surprise of some, he tried a number of unproven complementary treatments which gave him some hope and comfort, but did not save his life.

Let's face it, wishful thinking or not, there's a tantalizing possibility of potential cures in unproven treatments, even more so if we hear a testimonial story of recovery using this or that therapy. And more so again if there is even a skerrick of research suggesting a benefit for a particular CM. Now I'm going to say something that many of my fellow medical colleagues will disagree with. If the CM being chosen brings a person hope without too great a financial cost or detrimental effect on their health, then I believe it should be supported. That's right, supported, not poo pooed or just tolerated. It may well be a placebo, but as we discussed in Chapter 9 - Meaning, the placebo effect has mysterious potential benefits, so why should we as doctors try to dent this possibility? Hope fuels life. If some CMs are providing this fuel by playing the role of placebos, is this a problem?

I believe the answer to this is usually no, but sometimes yes. As patients and 'CM users' we can feel reluctant to reveal this use to our doctor. On the other side of the desk, medical practitioners underestimate the extent to which CM is used by their patients[9,10] This can unfortunately mean that serious interactions, such as those between certain drugs and herbs, are missed. The message here is if you're not comfortable sharing this information with your doctor, at the very least check with your pharmacist.

Surveys indicate that 80% of people are happy with their GPs,[11] but if you are in the 20% that isn't, it might be worth trying someone else, especially if you wish them to monitor your health while you use CM alongside orthodox treatments. In my view it's best to have a medical opinion in addition to the opinions of complementary therapist(s) being consulted, as a medical practitioner has superior training in detecting or excluding serious disease. This can be a particularly important issue if a CM practitioner overstates their scope of practice. Once you have a good relationship with your GP make sure you share the various CM treatments you are attempting, in addition to those prescribed by your doctor.

> Sandra was a 52-year-old delicatessen owner, who worked long hours and presented to her GP with shoulder pain. She mentioned that she had taken some magnesium tablets which seemed to help. He scoffed, "that wouldn't help you." Sandra made a mental note not to mention in future, any natural therapies she might be taking.

Supplementing nutrition?

While it is beyond my expertise and the scope of this book to review all five categories of CM, I would like to say a few words about supplements in general.

Some nutritionists are of the opinion that due to diminished soil quality, the nutritional content of most fruit and vegetables we eat has decreased over the last 50 years. Supporting this assertion are the findings of a careful survey in the UK from the Marine Research Centre and Ministry of Agriculture. They compared 27 vegetables, 20 fruits and ten meats over 50 years. They showed average falls of 48% in calcium and 27% in iron content, with similar or greater losses for other minerals like copper or magnesium.[12,13]

So does this mean we should all be taking vitamin and mineral supplements? The answer is not so simple. Taking more is not necessarily better. In addition, vitamins and minerals contained in food are supported and integrated by other compounds within the food. Let's take the example of an apple.

In his revealing book, *Whole - Rethinking the Science of Nutrition*,[14] Professor T Colin Campbell highlights a landmark research study published in the journal, *Nature*. In this article, researchers reported their analysis of the composition of 100g (half a cup) of apple.[15] They discovered that this amount of apple produced an antioxidant effect equivalent to 1500 mg of pure vitamin C. However, when they looked at how much vitamin C was actually present in the apple sample, it amounted to just 5.7 mg. It turns out there are hundreds if not thousands of other chemicals, some of whom were contributing to this vitamin C-like effect.[16] It is mind expanding to think of how all these chemicals may be interacting and working together, influencing thousands of biochemical reactions within our bodies, leading to the variety of benefits we subsequently receive from a simple bite of apple.

In an understated way, as is often the language of scientists, the researchers concluded, "that natural antioxidants from fresh fruit could be more effective than a dietary supplement (of vitamin C)."[17]

Could supplements harm us?

An apple is but one example of the complexity of components that make up the food we eat. Our ability to extract the benefits and nutrients from food has been adapted over thousands of years. So perhaps we shouldn't be surprised that isolating vitamins and minerals into tablets to be consumed may not have the benefits we expect:

> A review of 78 trials involving over 296,000 people showed that taking an antioxidant vitamin pill will not reduce deaths, and in fact may actually - as in the case of beta-carotene, vitamin A and E - slightly increase your chance of dying.[18] One of the 78 trials reviewed was known

as the Beta-Carotene and Retinol Efficacy Trial (CARET). It demonstrates the difficulties of making assumptions in this area. Involving over 18,000 smokers, beta-carotene and vitamin A supplements were tested in the hope that they would reduce cancer risk. This study was done because evidence had accumulated that eating more fruits and vegetables led to lower rates of lung cancer. Fruits and vegetables are rich in beta-carotene (a violet to yellow plant pigment that acts as an antioxidant and can be converted to vitamin A by enzymes in the intestinal wall and liver) and retinol (an alcohol chemical form of vitamin A), and thereby increase blood beta-carotene concentrations. To everyone's surprise, the trial had to be stopped early because the group taking the supplements developed *more* lung cancers than the untreated group![19,20] It appears that raising beta-carotene levels by eating fruits and vegetables well and truly trumps taking it as a supplement. Not surprisingly the U.S. Preventive Services Task Force recommends against the use of β-carotene or vitamin E supplements for the prevention of cardiovascular disease or cancer.[21]

The message from all this would seem to me to be obvious. Focus on increasing fruit and vegetables to obtain the nutrients we need. A regular multivitamin may do us more harm than good.

Can supplements help us?

There are also some promising areas of research in relation to vitamin supplements. For instance, research demonstrates that nutraceuticals (nutritional as opposed to pharmaceuticals) can be used effectively for deficiency states, such as B12 for vegans,[22] iron for heavy menstruation (menorrhagia),[23] vitamin D for those unable to obtain it naturally,[24] and folate and other vitamins for the increased needs of pregnancy.[25] Nutraceuticals can also be used therapeutically: fish oils as anti-inflammatories,[26] magnesium for fibromyalgia[27] and zinc[28] and vitamin C for the common cold.[29]

I'll finish this section with some more detailed examples of promising areas of research. A study that followed more than 3500 adults aged 65 years or older over a 12 year period concluded that those who had higher intakes of vitamins B6 and B12, which included bolstering by supplementation, were less likely to experience depression.[30] Another promising example involved a case-control study of 288 autistic children in California. It showed the use of prenatal vitamins around the time of conception, defined as the three months prior to conception to the first month of pregnancy, was associated with a reduction in the risk of having children with autism. They found an overall 40% reduced risk if mothers took vitamins.[31] Given the devastating impact that autism can have on families, this result needs to be confirmed or refuted by controlled trials as soon as possible.

The case for buying organic

There is a lot more research required to clarify when vitamins and minerals are best taken or not taken. In the meantime the safest thing to do is to eat as many good quality vegetables and fruits as you can. But do we need to buy organic vegetables and fruit? When all the research is tabulated, the experts tell us there is not enough difference in nutritional value, from an individual health point of view, to be of concern,[32] although some organic farms may show marked increases in nutritional value.[33] That said, research does confirm that you decrease your exposure to pesticides by eating organic foods ahead of conventional ones,[34] and that this is the most pressing reason people give for choosing organic produce.[35] Pesticides have been shown to build up in the bodies of children eating conventional food and subsequently being eliminated from the bodies of these same children when they're placed on an exclusively organic diet.[36] The American Academy of Pediatrics acknowledged the potential advantage of organic foods, especially in very young children.[37] Parents obviously agree with this, as sales of organic baby food are one of the fastest-growing organic food items.[38]

My own view is, regardless of nutritional value, I wouldn't be so keen to eat a piece of fruit I'd just sprayed with a pesticide, even after I'd washed it. Unfortunately, when we buy non-organic produce this is most likely what we are receiving. I also find organic produce more flavorsome, especially the tomatoes. So my suggestion would be; the fresher the better, home-grown if possible, then organic produce if affordable and then non-organic, which is still good for you.

There are many other reasons for choosing to buy organic, if you can afford to. It's a more environmentally friendly and sustainable way of farming. Organic farming builds soil, pulling carbon dioxide out of the atmosphere (natural carbon sequestration) in the process.[39] It also benefits soil quality long-term by maintaining the biodiversity of the beneficial soil bugs, and avoids polluting our waterways with chemical fertilizers and pesticides. In addition, a review of over 100 research papers over a 30 year period has shown consistently that organic farms have 34% more plant, insect and animal species on average than non-organic farms, with around 50% more species of pollinating bees, making them crucial oases for our diminishing bee populations and others.[40]

Research also indicates that despite the intensive use of chemical fertilizers and pesticides, conventional agriculture only yields 25% more produce than organic agriculture.[41] Proponents for organics suggest that this shortfall could easily be made up if the same amount of effort and investment was put into large-scale organic farming.[42] In other words, we may not really need to rely upon current conventional farming practices to feed the world. As the scale of organic farming increased, soils would improve along with yields and the price of produce would decrease. Food for reflection.

Hormesis

"What does not kill me, makes me stronger."

FREDERICH NIETZSCHE

Pharmacologists, toxicologists and biochemists are now confirming what traditional healers learnt before them: plant chemicals, produced to protect the plant from insects and often toxic when consumed by us at high levels, can be beneficial when eaten in small amounts.[43] Like healthy levels of exercise,[44] calorie restriction (e.g. fasting)[45-47] or cold exposure,[48] plant chemicals put a mild strain on the body inducing its own production of antioxidants and growth factors. This response involves a slight overcompensation, preparing the body for future strains, strengthening it in the process. This positive effect is known as hormesis.

The key with hormesis is that the stressor or strain (hormetin) is challenging but not overwhelming.

Coffee (caffeine), tea (catechins), turmeric (curcumin), broccoli (sulforaphane), garlic (allicin), hot peppers (capsaicin), grapes (resveratrol), apple skins (ursolic acid) and Brazil nuts (selenium), to name just a few, all contain chemicals which induce hormetic effects. This is almost certainly one of the reasons why eating whole foods is so beneficial to the body, whereas isolated supplements may not be. It is also an area of research which has enormous potential for the development of new pharmaceuticals. Galantamine, for instance, a chemical produced by snowdrop and snowflake flowers and now a prescribed drug for Alzheimer's disease, is thought to work via hormetic effects.[49]

The Future of CMs

As the evidence base increases for the benefit of certain CMs and the lack of benefit for other CMs, all medical practitioners will have a legal obligation to inform patients of the efficacy of relevant complementary therapies as treatment options, and to simultaneously be aware of the potential for adverse events and interactions that CMs might have.[50] This means the education of doctors will need to be broadened in an unbiased manner.

In future some of these CMs may receive subsidies through the Pharmaceutical Benefits Scheme (PBS - in Australia), just as many pharmaceuticals do now, at which time they may no longer be considered CMs, but mainstream medicines. This will be especially so if a CM is found to be as/or more effective than a pharmaceutical, as well as being a lower-cost option.

The following two examples illustrate both the potential and the challenges of introducing complementary medicine.

My wife and I struck up a friendship with Dawn and her husband Len when we were part of a community choir. At 70 years of age, Dawn was a dynamic lady running her own crafts stand at a local market. Invited for dinner one night, she confided in me as a doctor-friend that her medical specialists had only given her two years to live. This was because she had high blood pressure (210/105) which was proving impossible to lower with medication. Her daugh-ter-in-law, a prominent female physician, had made sure she had seen the best cardiologists. Dawn had resigned herself to her fate.

Normally I don't make it my business to interfere with other people's medical management, but I felt compelled to share some informa-tion with Dawn and visited her at her market stall the following weekend. I had recently read of some interesting research about Coenzyme Q10 (CoQ10) and its ability to lower blood pressure. I shared this with her. She was interested, but fearful, as it turned out her daughter-in-law was vehemently anti natural therapies. Still, Dawn decided that the opportunity to see her grandchildren grow-ing up was worth risking the wrath of her daughter-in-law. She attended a local naturopath from whom she purchased a bottle of CoQ10 and took it for a fortnight prior to seeing her cardiologist. Remarkably, her blood pressure had dropped to 145/90. I must admit when I saw her again several months later I expected her to be grateful for the tip I'd given, but I received a mixed reaction. The daughter-in-law was somehow unimpressed with all this and Dawn was clearly affected by her coldness towards her. "If only it could've been a drug," she said to me.

Before looking more closely at Dawn's story, just a little background about CoQ10. Coenzyme Q10 is also known as ubiquinone, a natural substance found in all plant and animal cells. It was first identified in 1957 and it plays an important role in energy production. Heart muscle cells have the highest concentration of mitochondria, a cells 'energy factory' in the body and therefore require a good supply of CoQ10 to function well. Good sources of CoQ10 include meat, fish, soy and vegetable oils. CoQ10 is also an antioxidant.[51]

In Dawn's situation, it is known that CoQ10 depletion can occur with the use of certain cardiac medications, such as cholesterol-lowering statins,[52] and this is thought to contribute to high blood pressure. While research suggests that CoQ10 supplementation may lower blood pressure by around 15mmHg (systolic) and 10mmHg (diastolic),[53] in Dawn's case it was much greater than this, suggesting long-term depletion. It is troubling that she was given such a poor prognosis from her cardiologist, who one can only assume was unaware or unwilling to entertain treatments outside of their sphere of practice. This said, I have come across people whose cardiologists recognize this research and have placed them on CoQ10 along with medication. I'm also aware that Prof Frank Rosenfeldt, at the Cardiac Surgical Research Unit at the Alfred Hospital in Melbourne, has investigated the benefits of CoQ10 for over a decade.[54] Trials involving 450 people, who were soon to undergo cardiac surgery, looked at the effects of providing known beneficial cardiac nutrients or a placebo, two months prior to and for one month after their operation. The combination of nutrients included CoQ10, magnesium orotate, selenium, lipoic acid and Omega 3 fatty acids. The results have been promising, including decreased complications, with less damage to the heart and earlier discharge from hospital, leading to more than a $3000 health cost saving per person receiving the combination of nutrients.[55,56]

Dawn's story illustrates the polarization that occurs at times between mainstream medicine and CM proponents. It seems there is a blind spot on both sides. On one side we have vocal medical proponents angry at unsubstantiated claims made by 'snake oil salesmen.' On the other side we have vocal natural therapy proponents who see medicine dominated by multinational pharmaceutical companies pushing chemicals for every ill. One refuses to entertain the use of any natural therapy, while the other refuses to take any pharmaceutical. Both are actually identifying some of the serious problems within each system. Yet, as imperfect as these systems might be, they both have a lot to offer. The development of Integrative Medicine (a relatively new system in Western medicine that integrates conventional and complementary medicine) is an attempt to work with the best of both approaches, focusing on more evidence based CM, but it too is a work in progress.

In a situation like Dawn's, even if the research is not rock solid yet, it would be worth trying an evidence based low risk treatment like CoQ10. There is more to gain than to lose from this. That her daughter-in-law could not open herself to this possibility even after it had proven helpful, beggars belief. Then again, there may have been more to it; power struggles within mother-in-law, daughter-in-law relationships are not unknown!

This next story presents the other side of the CM coin.

June was a divorcee in her 50's and the mother of three married daughters, one of whom was a close friend of mine. I met June on several occasions and she let me know exactly what she thought of the medical profession, whom she avoided like smelly socks. She was into everything alternative and appeared to be in pretty good health. When her daughter, my friend, died suddenly in a car accident, June turned to alternate ways of dealing with her grief.

One of her other daughters, Marie, rang me one Sunday distressed. She told me that June had taken up with a particular spiritual group who believed they could increase their 'vibration' to such an extent that they no longer needed to eat or drink. June had been on a 10 day fast, gradually decreasing the amount of water she was taking. When Marie visited her, she found her mother partially clothed, talking gibberish. As June did not have a GP, Marie had rung me.

On arrival at June's house her two remaining daughters greeted me with anxious faces. June was indeed hallucinating and although she recognized me, she was uncooperative. I explained to her daughters that their mother needed an urgent full assessment in hospital and for this to happen I would need to organize for a psychiatric team to commit her. This would mean they would keep her in hospital for a minimum of 10 days. They agreed without hesitation.

In A&E (the Emergency Room) June was found to be severely dehydrated. Blood tests revealed that she was in acute renal (kidney) failure. Fortunately, over the next day intravenous fluids returned her kidneys to normal functioning. I visited her and found her sitting upright in bed on a medical ward. The staff informed me that she had not spoken a word to them. They interpreted this to be part of her psychiatric condition. Knowing June's attitude to anything medical, I was not so sure. I entered her room and her eyes acknowledged me. I leaned towards her and whispered in her ear, "If you don't start talking to these people they are going to keep you in here for a very long time."

Her eyes widened as she turned towards me, "Really!"

I nodded my head.

From this point on she became a model patient, spending her requisite 10 days on a psychiatric ward and developing a new found respect for medical people, knowing they had saved her life.

In the next chapter we'll look more closely at Evidence-based Medicine (EBM) and its relationship to CM.

Further Resources

C Norman Shealy, The Illustrated Encyclopedia of Healing Remedies. Element Books Ltd 1998.

http://naturaldatabase.therapeuticresearch.com/home.aspx?cs=&s=ND (accessed February 2016)

http://www.uptodate.com/contents/complementary-and-alternative-medicine-treatments-cam-for-cancer-beyond-the-basics (accessed February 2016) https://www.aima.net.au/ (accessed February 2016)

https://www.acnem.org/ (accessed February 2016)

Chapter 12

THE COMPLEMENTARY CATCH

They call it the art of medicine (AOM), and it's a lot less black-and-white than law, ironically ... science is the underlying guiding principle, but then there's such subtlety that overarches everything you do, you have to know how to appreciate that it is never black and white.

DR BERNADETTE WILKS, ANESTHETIST AND
PAST PRESIDENT DOCTORS IN TRAINING SUBDIVISION
AUSTRALIAN MEDICAL ASSOCIATION VICTORIA.

It has been suggested that an intervention by a health practitioner can be said to 'work' in three distinct but often overlapping ways:[1]

1. It produces a clinically observable change in a set of symptoms. For example, you came in with a wheezy cough and the cough settled after treatment.
2. It produces a change in a set of symptoms that is scientifically demonstrated to be a function of the treatment. For example, a randomized controlled trial (RCT) confirms that an asthma treatment puffer, with active ingredient, relieves asthma cough more effectively than an inactive placebo puffer. This important research helps us to decide which

interventions work beyond their placebo benefit and which do not.

3. It changes your relationship to your affliction so that you feel more comfortable, suffer less pain and are able to manage your normal daily life. For example, after years of caring interactions with their GP, a long-term smoker with emphysema learns to accept the limitations the illness places on his daily life. While still hoping for better treatments, he has learnt to find some joy and purpose despite his limitations.

Let's explore how these three ways of 'working' tie in with the Art of Medicine (AOM) and Evidence Based Medicine (EBM).

The idea of EBM gained momentum in the 1990s with the increasing recognition that large areas of medical practice were still based upon experience and expert opinion, rather than scientific evidence in the form of randomized controlled trials (RCTs). Out of the three points I've made above, the second is most suited to EBM, with the third being most suited to AOM. Nonetheless, nowadays to be taken seriously in healthcare you need to at least claim to have an evidence-based approach. This is leading to much better informed medical practice in certain areas, but is leaving the skills and the benefits of the third way of 'working' in danger of being under recognized. Undervaluing the less easily measured aspects of healthcare is a potential consequence of EBM.

The more subtle skills, often referred to as the Art of Medicine, recognize and take into consideration factors apart from (and including) evidence of effectiveness. These are some of the factors which may influence decision-making: side-effect risks versus benefits; quality of life with or without treatment; costs, effort required; inclination and motivation; support systems in place; access to treatment facilities; and individual preferences. Any of these factors may or may not come into play for a given circumstance, but clearly doctors need adequate training in both AOM and EBM, in order to have the skills to help a patient move towards a treatment plan that best suits their individual situation.

How big an issue is this? Given the plethora of chronic diseases that we can help but cannot cure, one can only conclude it's highly significant. In these many instances, taking into account the nuances that make up each individual will be a big part of coming up with the most appropriate treatment plan for that person. Interestingly, the accepted definition of EBM by Prof David Sackett and colleagues published in 1996, took all this into account.

> "(EBM) is the conscientious and judicious use of current best evidence from clinical care research in the management of individual patients. The practice of Evidence Based Medicine means integrating individual clinical expertise with the best available external clinical evidence from systematic research. By individual clinical expertise we mean the proficiency and judgement that individual clinicians acquire through clinical experience and clinical practice. Increased expertise is reflected in many ways, but especially in more effective and efficient diagnosis, and in the more thoughtful identification and compassionate use of individual patients' predicaments, rights and preferences in making decisions about their care."[2]

This ideal of EBM, which includes the art of medicine, can be easily lost in a computer-based health system, where both accessing information and inputting patient data can dominate a consultation. The very words, 'Evidence Based,' can conjure up lab coats and statistics in one's mind, leaving the holistic sensibility, reflected in the final sentence of the definition above, as no more than a footnote.

In place of this original 1996 definition, today's understanding of EBM effectively leaves out AOM and refers largely to the hierarchical levels of evidence model as defined by the National Health and Medical Research Council (NHMRC):[3]

- Level I Systematic review or meta-analysis of rigorous randomized controlled trials (RCTs).
- Level II At least one randomized controlled trial (RCT).
- Level III Non-randomized controlled trials.
- Level IV Descriptive studies or accepted medical opinion.

To rebalance the ledger, we need a more side-by-side model. In this model, "... more thoughtful identification and compassionate use of individual patient's predicaments, rights and preferences in making decisions about their care," would have its importance upheld, by being considered adjacent to EBM under the title of Art of Medicine.

AOM involves the skills of listening, careful observation, taking a thorough history that includes psychosocial circumstances, and learning how to integrate all this into a management plan. To fully and most appropriately apply EBM as presented in the hierarchy above, requires AOM skills.

Finding EBM

Locating EBM research is possible for anyone with access to the web. Finding Level I evidence, for example, has been assisted by the formation of an independent, non-profit group known as the Cochrane Collaboration. With 31,000 volunteers, the group compiles published randomized controlled trial (RCT) research on the effectiveness of particular treatments. A positive Cochrane review is considered the gold standard of proof. For example, the Cochrane Library has produced a systematic review summary of the effectiveness of cholesterol lowering drugs known as Statins.[4] It has also produced a report supporting the use of the herb, St John's Wort, for depression.[5] In many countries outside the United States, access to this type of summary is freely available at *www.thecochranelibrary.com*. This is a useful resource for both clinicians and patients, providing some guidance where research is available. PubMed (*http://www.ncbi.nlm.nih.gov/pubmed*) is another free way of accessing individual and systematic reviews of research.

Importantly, in this tiered system of evidence, Level I and Level II are considered the most compelling. Research involving pharmaceuticals is well suited to the RCTs required by these levels. Non-pharmaceutical treatments, such as acupuncture, massage, counseling and lifestyle change, don't easily fit into this type of methodology. The upside of this is that doctors can prescribe with more confidence in the evidence base that supports their prescription. The downside is that it can skew their treatment emphasis towards pharmaceuticals, as these usually have Level I evidence whereas non-pharmaceuticals rarely do.

As I've alluded to, in practice it's often not as simple as the linear hierarchy suggests. Often the patient's circumstances and wishes need to be considered above and beyond the research. For example, I have witnessed dying patients faced with terminal cancer make three very different, but reasonable, choices:

- Some chose chemotherapy, which RCTs suggested could prolong life around three months longer than no treatment.
- Some chose palliative therapy alone, to avoid suffering the side-effects of chemotherapy, preferring a shorter but better quality of life over their final months.
- Some chose to try unproven therapies without or with less side-effects, not wishing to experience the side-effects of

chemotherapy, but still wanting to maintain some hope of prolonging their life.

Such choices reflect individual beliefs, life experience, social situations and preferences. A humane, understanding doctor patient relationship, helps people to navigate their path in many situations like this, where evidence and research has a limited role to play. AOM makes room for and teases out these important considerations. If you're a patient facing complex choices, I would advise giving yourself enough time to consider your options, making a longer or further appointment if necessary.

This can mean, as will be emphasized in the example at the end of this chapter, sometimes treatments with Level III or IV evidence trump the Level I evidence treatments as the therapy of choice.

How reliable is the research?

"When money talks, the truth is silent."

ABKHASISAN PROVERB

A health system that involves wealthy pharmaceutical companies has the advantage of stimulating new research and development, and the disadvantage of directing research money predominantly into profit making products, such as drug therapies. This means that priority funding decisions are not always based on need or promising science but rather profit-making potential.

It is also worth noting that RCTs require access to a large number of patients with a particular problem, like high cholesterol. This often involves recruitment of people through university-linked hospitals or doctors' surgeries. Such trials are expensive. To bring a new pharmaceutical onto the market, researched and developed, has been calculated to cost in excess of 2.5 billion dollars.[6,7] Others suggest this is conflated with the true average cost closer to $70 million.[8] Either way, most of the trials being conducted on pharmaceuticals are funded by the companies creating them. Many useful, life-saving and effective drugs have been found in this way, but it is not hard to see why a conflict of interest could occur here. Having invested many millions or billions of dollars, could one accept negative trial results?

Unfortunately, researchers have uncovered serious irregularities in a number of practices in the way some pharmaceutical companies have reported their research.[9] In addition to this, scientific journals have been found to be five times more likely to publish positive ('good news') trial results than negative ones.[10] Hence, even if the Cochrane Collaboration performed a systematic review, they would not have access to the negative trial results that were never published. This casts a shadow on the very reliability of the core research used for EBM.

Take the example of cholesterol lowering statin medications to illustrate this. A recent Cochrane review collated 18 published scientific papers and found statins to be overwhelmingly beneficial in preventing cardiovascular disease.[11] How confident can we be that withheld negative research and publication bias hasn't skewed the assessment? Doubts have emerged about the veracity of Cochrane's conclusion for this very reason.[12] In addition statins do not appear to improve overall mortality rates in people being treated for elevated cholesterol who are otherwise at low risk from cardiovascular disease.[13] It appears, if you are in this category, that statins may well reduce your risk of dying early from cardiovascular disease, but paradoxically increase your risk of dying early from something else instead.

While most patients will tolerate statins, in agreeing to take a long-term medication like this, it is worth being aware of its significant side-effect risks. An analysis by the United States Food and Drug Administration led it to issue warnings regarding an increased risk of diabetes and decreased cognition with statin drugs, along with other side-effects that could require the discontinuation of the medication.[14]

Another vivid example relates to the anti-viral drug, Tamiflu, and further confirms reliability of research concerns. The drug, the product of pharmaceutical giant Roche, had been given a positive review by Cochrane in 2008 as a treatment for influenza (flu) that could prevent the life-threatening complication of pneumonia. On the basis of this, governments around the world had the confidence to spend billions of dollars stockpiling the medication so as to be prepared for a flu pandemic. When just such a pandemic threatened in 2009 the Australian and UK governments requested an updated review on Tamiflu's effectiveness by Cochrane. Around this time a Japanese pediatrician, Dr Keiji Hayashi, left a communication on the Cochrane website pointing out the limitations of the data upon which the 2008 review had been made. Dr Tom Jefferson, who had headed up the initial review, found Dr Hayashi's concerns to be justified, admitted the limitations of the initial review and requested all of the missing data from Roche. Roche, who had no legal obligation to provide this information, did not cooperate.[15]

Independent scientists from the British Medical Journal joined Cochrane in agitating for the release of the hidden data. Finally in 2014, five years after the initial request, Roche handed over the information. At this time research results from a similar drug, Relenza, a product of GlaxoSmithKline, were also obtained. The Cochrane scientists, who'd previously given Tamiflu a positive review, re-analyzed the complete set of data and did a backflip, concluding that neither Tamiflu nor Relenza was effective in reducing complications or the need for hospitalization.[16] Had there been a flu pandemic, the billions of dollars of stockpiled medication would not have done the job it was purchased for.

One can only imagine that there are many other instances where if Cochrane had all of the data, both positive and negative, that their conclusions may change. Hence, without transparency of results reporting, all clinical research and the voluntary work of the Cochrane Collaboration and others are diminished in value.

If EBM is to continue as a foundation stone of healthcare, then the major flaws of withholding negative results and publication bias need to be addressed. With this in mind a group with widespread support, known as AllTrials (*www.alltrials.net*), is advocating for an openly available clinical research registry. They're calling on governments, regulators and research bodies to implement measures to achieve this. As they point out, as things stand, huge volumes of research are being lost, jeopardizing good medical decision-making.[17]

While most researchers are diligent and act with integrity, even if AllTrials succeeds, vigilance will still be required. The story of Celebrex and Vioxx (anti-inflammatory Cox 2 inhibitors) involving results fabrication and the unreported risk of heart attacks, was a salient reminder of just how far some people will stretch the test tube to come up with the results they desire.[18] In response to this debacle, stricter regulations on research reporting were introduced in 2005. Sadly, I still believe that a 'reliability risk' for any research cannot ever be discounted whenever human beings, money and position are at stake.

For those of you looking for extra guidance on choosing medication, diagnostic tests or procedures, *choosingwisely.org.au* is a useful website.

The Catch Up

As EBM gains momentum there is an increasing demand for Complementary Medicine (CM) to prove its worth via research. The problem here is the difficulty or indeed the impossibility for many complementary therapies to attract research dollars. The fact that a natural substance cannot be patented whereas a chemical pharmaceutical can, has been one of the drivers of modern medical research and product development. Simply put, products that are not patentable are less financially desirable to investigate.[19] Even nutritional supplement companies willing to invest in research have a problem gaining access to patients and experienced researchers through universities and hospitals.

Health practitioners prescribing natural substances are left to rely upon traditional usage, often founded on many years of experience, functional research, where, for example, a vitamin or herb is shown to improve immune function, and at best, small clinical trials. If the basic tiers of the evidence model are held up to be sacrosanct, as they are tending to be, then the lack of substantial clinical research to back up the benefits of natural therapies leaves them vulnerable to being dismissed outright. It's not that they may not work; it's just that more clinical research is needed to confirm this, because functional research may not translate into actual benefits for the patient.

It is worth remembering that a vast number of pharmaceuticals were derived from natural plants and/or synthesized plant derivatives. For example, codeine and morphine were derived from poppies, and aspirin (salicylic acid) occurred naturally in the bark of willow trees. Scientists were attracted to the potential of these plants by relying upon their history of many - often hundreds and up to thousands of years - of practical use. I believe it would be a travesty to discredit this experience and a loss of great therapeutic potential, if we became so adherent to the EBM tiers of evidence model, that we prematurely eliminated the use of natural substances, citing lack of clinical research evidence. What is actually needed is more clinical research rather than pronouncements; guilty of being unhelpful without a proper trial!

So in our quest for more and more therapeutic certainty we need to watch that we don't create a funnel that only allows treatments through based on multi-centered RCTs. Let's be clear: this would narrow our treatment options to an exclusive club, those treatments that are suitably tested with RCTs and those with the money and influence to get through the rigors of a model of proof, namely randomized controlled trials, that was only created in the last 60 years.

Let's look at homeopathy as an example of the challenges facing CM research.

Homeopathy

Homeopathy has been a regular villain of conventional thinkers. The lack of plausibility for how it actually works has been put forward as a reason for this.[20] Founded by Dr Samuel Hahnemann, homeopathy is a 200 year old form of CM. The discipline is underpinned by the principle of similitude ('like cures like'): substances that cause symptoms in a healthy person have the ability to treat an ill person with the same symptoms, when administered in tiny homeopathic potencies.

For example, chopping up an onion causes runny eyes and nose in a healthy person. A homeopathic remedy made from diluted, boiled onion water, can be prescribed for someone suffering from a cold with symptoms of runny eyes and nose. This principle is not confined to homeopathy. As discussed earlier, hormesis, as it is applied in toxicology, recognizes that very small doses of certain toxins can strengthen the body.[21]

Specifically, homeopathic remedies are repeatedly diluted and agitated in a process known as 'potentization' or 'dynamization'. Whilst the majority of prescriptions contain small amounts of a diluted substance, some prescriptions go beyond this to a level of ultra-molecular dilutions, where it is unlikely that any molecules of the original substance remain. This is the most controversial aspect of homeopathy. By definition, such dilutions cannot have any classical pharmacological action, since this involves pharmacological molecular keys fitting into the locks (receptors) located on the surface of body cells, triggering chemical reactions within the cell.[22] In these ultra-molecular dilutions there are no molecules left to act as keys.

You might think the discussion should end here, but confounding this logic is the fact that these ultra-molecular dilutions have been consistently shown to be biologically active in repeated scientific experiments. Let's look at the example of allergy. Allergens, such as dust and pollen, trigger the release of a chemical known as histamine from immune cells, called basophils. Histamine is an irritant/inflammatory chemical and causes the itchy eyes and throat, running nose and sneezing we all know as hay fever. It can also cause asthma. One approach to this problem, taken by conventional/allopathic medicine, is to prescribe antihistamines to block the effects of this irritating chemical. Homeopathy on the other hand, using the principle of similitude, prescribes ultra-molecular dilutions of histamine, a dilution so great that no molecules of histamine remain in the remedy.

Seventeen separate studies looking at the human basophil degranulation test, have confirmed that a homeopathic ultra-molecular dilution of histamine, inhibits the release of histamine by basophils when exposed to an allergic trigger. The peak of this beneficial effect was consistently found at the same high level of dilution (16c /10 -32M), a dilution where no molecule of histamine would remain. Testing a similar chemical to histamine, known as histadine, in the same way, showed no active effects.[23,24] Ultra-molecular dilutions of aspirin, similarly have been found to have some of the anticlotting effects that occur when taking an aspirin tablet.[25] How is this possible? Some postulate that in the homeopathic preparation process some vibrational memory of the original chemical remains in the shape of a subtle alteration in the molecular structure of the water it is diluted in, giving it therapeutic power.[26] Whether it is this or some other mechanism, we do not know.

Many doctors are unaware of this research and those that are aware, because they find the explanations so unbelievable, conclude that it must be shonky. On the other hand, if these results are true and we can discover a mechanism by which these biological effects are imparted, it could open up whole new areas of therapy. My own view is that if we can accept the use of pharmaceuticals whose mechanism of action remains unknown, as is commonly the case, then we should accept homeopathics shown to be clinically effective, regardless of how they may or may not work.

So what does the research show in this regard? Scientific reviews of the clinical effectiveness of homeopathy, published in prestigious journals up until the year 2000, tended to be favorable, concluding that it worked for certain conditions, such as hay fever and childhood diarrhea, whilst admitting incomprehension as to how this could be so.[27,28,29] More recent reviews have concluded that it does not work.[30,31,32] It has been argued that this change of opinion has more to do with the reviewers disbelief in the plausibility of homeopathic effects (plausibility bias), than the availability of more recent quality research data.[33]

In Australia a 2014 review commissioned by the National Health and Medical Research Council (NHMRC) concluded there is no evidence for its effectiveness, but also said:

"There is a paucity of good quality studies of sufficient size that examine the effectiveness of homeopathy as a treatment for any clinical condition in humans."[34]

If this is so, I would suggest what's required is more research, for until this paucity is addressed, we can't be definitive as to whether it works or doesn't work. Whatever the truth may be, homeopathy is a cheap and safe CM, not highly profitable, with a poor reputation amongst most allopathic doctors, and would therefore find it challenging to attract the research dollars to fully assess its worth.

Researching CM

For many CMs independent research grants are the only avenue available for researchers. In Australia independent funds for CM research were provided for the first time in 2008. In the USA the National Centre for Complementary and Alternative Medicine (NCCAM) was established in 1991 and this has led to an increase in CM research.

The other major issue for CM research is the fact that many therapies are practiced holistically, being individualized for each patient. For example, two patients, both with asthma, may be treated with different acupuncture points depending on their Traditional Chinese Medicine pulse diagnosis. It is also difficult to produce a placebo acupuncture treatment or a lifestyle or counseling treatment for that matter. So RCTs are difficult to perform on these and on more complex interventions generally. The RCT works well for single substance interventions like pharmaceuticals or nutritional supplements, where placebos can be used to compare the results. Hence, more complex research design is required for many CMs.

Finally, even when useful evidence is available for various CMs, it's not always easy for doctors to become aware of this or to have it reported in an unbiased way.

So here are seven things I believe we need in place for CM to catch up on allopathic medicine's research database:

1. Bridge the funding gap. Both the natural therapy industry and independent funding bodies need to continue to increase their research funds allocation.
2. Green-flag promising pilot-study CM research for priority future funding of larger trials. This would ideally be done by an independent panel of research experts, clinicians and members of the public (i.e. educated consumers). Conflicts of interest would need to be declared.
3. Access to universities, hospitals and research oriented clinics. Increasing this exposure is essential both for utilizing the research expertise and patients for research trials. This would be facilitated by more cooperation between natural therapy and allopathic training schools.
4. Looking beyond the RCT. Acknowledgement and respect for different research methodologies that are required to assess particular CMs unsuited to RCTs.
5. Broadening the education base of both natural therapy and allopathic health students to increase understanding of each other's approach.
6. Mainstream medical journals to include a dedicated section for unbiased reporting of promising CM research.
7. Remembering that clinical research is for the benefit of unwell people or people trying to stay well. From a sick person's point of view, it's not a competition between one treatment or another; it's simply a desire to be helped by the therapies that will best suit them.

Let's bring some of these issues alive with an example that involved myself:

In November 2010 I experienced my first Ulcerative Colitis (UC) attack, with fever, abdominal pain and almost continuous diarrhea for weeks on end. UC and Crohn's disease are both forms of a very unpleasant disorder, known as Inflammatory Bowel Disease (IBD), which commonly cycles between periods of activity and inactivity. By April 2012 I had had four hospital admissions and many near admissions with this disease, had lost 20 kg (44lbs) and almost my life. The medication I was reliant upon to stop these attacks was the corticosteroid, prednisolone. Following each attack I needed to complete a course of this life-saving drug over two months. Unfortunately, I reacted very badly to this medication, becoming unusually aggressive and suicidally depressed, not a happy combination. Prednisolone also has other side-effects, such as osteoporosis, a problem I already had. Having endless courses of this drug was a tortuous prospect, and the hope that complementary medicine could provide a way out from this was like oxygen for me.

So when I was well enough I searched. I tried promising supplements, including aloe vera juice, colostrum, fish oils, probiotics and glutamine; but while soothing, they failed to stop acute attacks. I was becoming disheartened, when my enquiry led me to discover a research paper published in 2007 assessing a supplement (also a Mediterranean food product) known as mastic gum.[35] An extract from an evergreen shrub (Pistacia lentiscus var. Chia – Anacardiaccae), this source of mastic gum grows widely throughout the Mediterranean region and especially on the Greek island of Chios. Documented use of the resin/gum dates back to Ancient Greece, more than 2000 years ago, where it was used to treat gastrointestinal problems. Modern day research has also shown it to be effective in peptic ulcer disease.[36]

The small 2007 colitis study involved 10 people suffering from active Crohn's disease. After one month of treatment all 10 patients were much improved, with seven of them being in remission. It corresponded with reductions, demonstrated by blood testing, in their inflammatory markers, namely, C-reactive protein (CRP) and tumor necrosis factor alpha (TNF-alpha). The only reported side-effect was constipation, something a colitis sufferer can only dream of!

This promising pilot study (Level III evidence) was never followed up with the larger studies the researchers felt were warranted. Remember, of course, a natural substance like mastic gum cannot be patented, and therefore is unlikely to attract any substantial private research funding. Nonetheless, given my severe reaction to prednisolone, my first-hand experience of how difficult it can be to stop an acute colitis attack, even with prednisolone, and despite the small nature of the research study, I felt it was worth a try.

I was unable to purchase mastic gum capsules in Australia, but managed to buy some inexpensively from a US online site.

How did I go? Between April 2012 and March 2014 I had some minor flare ups of colitis, which I found settled within days of taking mastic gum. In March 2014 the real test arrived. I developed a full-blown colitis attack on a Sunday. By Monday morning I was clearly unable to maintain my intake of fluids relative to what I was losing from my back passage. In other words I was dehydrating fast. Hospital admission was arranged so that I could receive some intravenous fluids and the inevitable corticosteroids. I had commenced taking mastic gum capsules on the Sunday evening. By Monday afternoon I began to feel somewhat improved, so much so that whilst driving into hospital my wife and I decided to turn back and try our luck at home. We cancelled the hospital bed. That night proved to be a difficult one and we doubted our decision, but by Wednesday I was much better. By Friday my CRP level (reflecting the inflammation in my bowel) had fallen, from its peak of 116 on Monday, (normal is less than 3) to 16.

The problem I faced was this: neither I nor any of my treating doctors, including my gastroenterologist, Ross, had any experience with using this treatment. So after a week of taking mastic gum when I developed severe constipation, the only guidance I had to manage this was from the original research paper which referred to one of the 10 patients developing a similar problem. They managed the patient successfully by halving her dose of mastic gum for two days and then returning her to the full dosage. So I reduced my two 500 mg capsules twice daily to just one morning and evening. Unfortunately, by the second day on the reduced dosage my symptoms of colitis (fever, bowel cramps, diarrhea) returned. When I increased the dose again it subsided. Over the next week constipation recurred, so I retried the strategy with the same result, colitis re-flaring. I discussed this with Ross and we decided the best approach was to simply maintain the full dose for one month and treat the constipation using laxatives as needed. I used psyllium husks, lactulose, Noni juice and an occasional dose of domperidone for a couple of weeks to restore order. We both agreed that constipation was a far preferable side-effect than suicidal depression when taking prednisolone, and I was grateful for his willingness to monitor me on this alternative treatment.

Retesting my CRP after one month of treatment revealed it to be normal (<2.9) and I was down to just one solid bowel motion per day without the need for laxatives. I was well again, yet I was left with many questions:

- How long do I maintain my dosage of four capsules per day?
- Do I wean down off the capsules and if so at what rate?
- Would there be any preventive benefit in remaining on a small dosage, say one capsule per day?
- If so, would it be safe to stay on this supplement long term?
- Or would it be best to continue to use it episodically as needed?

To answer these questions all I could rely upon was my individual response and trial and error, and hope that further research would be forthcoming. Not a perfect situation, but given my medical options, one I was happy to live with. I was somewhat encouraged about the safety of taking mastic gum because of its long history of use. Fortunately, I succeeded in slowly weaning off the gum over a three-month period without further relapse. In the meantime I have discovered dietary means of keeping my colitis under control. I will share these in a later chapter.

This story illustrates some of the challenges that CM research is faced with. A promising pilot study showing the benefits of mastic gum was funded by a grant from the Chios Gum Mastic Growers Association. The researchers concluded: "Further double-blind placebo-controlled studies in a larger number of patients are required to clarify the role of this natural product in the treatment of patients with Crohn's disease."[37] Unfortunately, the Chios Gum Mastic Growers Association is unlikely to ever be able to afford to support such an expensive trial and no such trial has occurred. The most recent research on mastic gum and colitis was aimed at breaking down the gum into its components, to isolate an active anti-colitis ingredient, which they failed to find, concluding that the whole was more potent than the parts.[38]

It is interesting to note that thus far close to 70 chemical constituents have been identified as components of mastic gum. These constituents demonstrate a wide range of effects, including lowering cholesterol and glucose, antifungal, antibacterial and anti-cancer activity. One of the anti-cancer components, oleanolic acid, also exerts an anti-inflammatory effect and is thought to be one of the main components that helps heal colitis.[39] Let's hope more clinical research is forthcoming.

For now, like so many other CMs, we are left with promising early research (effective in 10 out of 10 active Crohn's patients) without the follow-up needed to consolidate proof of effectiveness and our understanding of how to use it clinically. Yet my experience of mastic gum is that it worked for me, and no matter how much more scientifically solid the trials confirming the effectiveness of prednisolone might be in comparison, my response to both treatments led me to choose the gum (with its Level III evidence) over the steroid (with its Level I evidence). As this story demonstrates, our individual responses and complexities have to be taken into account along with research evidence in making management decisions. Evidence alone may not be the deciding factor.

My heart goes out to the thousands of colitis sufferers, many of whom have needed parts of their bowel surgically removed to save their lives, whose colitis could have been helped with this simple treatment. The conundrum is this: because of the lack of research data I cannot make a global recommendation for mastic gum. All I can say is that mastic gum would be one product I would green-flag for priority research funding.

Colitis is a serious condition, and if a person affected by IBD wishes to try mastic gum treatment for themselves, then I would recommend they do so as I did, under the supervision and careful monitoring of a supportive medical practitioner.

PART II

Chapter 13

DESCENT

*Midway this way of life we're bound upon,
I woke to find myself in a dark wood, where the
right road was wholly lost and gone.*

DANTE THE DIVINE COMEDY – HELL

The hum of the aircraft comforted me as I sat back contemplating the weekend ahead. The five-hour flight from Melbourne to Darwin gave me plenty of time to reflect on my strategy. It was a big moment for me. In my fourth year at Monash University's Department of Community Medicine (General Practice), I had recently been made a senior lecturer. This trip to Darwin was the most responsibility I had been given yet. A dozen foreign medical graduates were waiting for me to conduct a weekend of training to prepare them for the tough examinations they would need to pass in order to practice medicine in Australia. The Federal government was paying for me to do this.

Carousels of slides and multiple handouts filled my suitcase, years before PowerPoint and USB sticks. I would be conducting tutorials and ward rounds in Darwin hospital, teaching not only clinical skills but exam technique, critical to their chances of success in a foreign country. It was a daunting prospect, but a challenge I relished.

Disembarking from the plane onto the tarmac, I breathed in the warmth of the tropics. Ahhh, there's something especially relaxing about that first breath of warm air when you've been living and breathing in a cold winter. It'd been 8°C (46°F) when the plane left Melbourne and arriving to a 24°C (75°F) balmy evening was a definite perk on this trip.

After checking in at the hotel, there was little time to rest; a dinner with local doctors was followed by my first lecture. I loved teaching; it was the reason I went for the job at the University. The weekend was long and demanding, but I was energized and gratified from teaching such an eager to learn group of doctors.

Most exciting of all, my girlfriend, Tori, joined me in Darwin on the Sunday evening. My work done, we lolled around in the hotel pool before a dinner of barramundi, chips and salad. The next day we hired a campervan and began our travels through Kakadu National Park, a holiday that would last for seven days. Perfect weather, camping by and swimming in water holes (picture Crocodile Dundee); it proved to be a holiday of a lifetime. The time was July 1992 and I have selected this part of my story as it was the last time I recall feeling fit and strong.

By December 1992 my energy was beginning to falter. I'd developed pneumonia and asthma for the first time and I'd already decided to halve my workload at the University. It's worth pointing out my workload consisted of a full-time university position that incorporated general practice work, four sessions a week. I had also begun to run stress management groups and presentations and was a board member of the non-profit educational organization, the Whole Health Institute of Australasia (WHI). Focusing on the common ground of caring and a holistic approach to healing, WHI broke down the barriers between people and particularly between various mainstream and complementary health professionals.

My reduced workload didn't last long. By early 1993 WHI had lost its president and I had been asked to step in to fill the breach, which I did. My stress management consultancy work was also expanding and I began to give presentations throughout Australia. I was driven to make a difference to help people and I loved doing so. Tori moved into my apartment and by year's end we were engaged. I attempted to balance my output by practicing an hour and a half of yoga and meditation each morning. I also swam one km three times per week as well as taking a walk with Tori to the beach from our apartment most evenings. Despite these measures, my health continued to gradually decline as I seemed to collect more illnesses each year.

At the end of 1993 I presented a paper at the second Dead Sea Scrolls conference in Tiberius, by the Sea of Gallilee in Israel. On behalf of Dr Craig Hassed and myself, the paper outlined the work we were doing with medical students, introducing them to a mindfulness meditation-based stress management program. Tori had pleaded with me not to attend the conference as she could see I was exhausted and needed my holiday-time to rest. Keen to present at the conference and to catch up with my Israeli relatives, I ignored her sage advice. Within hours of arrival in Israel I experienced back spasms followed by a nasty upper respiratory infection and asthma. I struggled on, managed to present my paper and after the conference took a bus from Tiberius to Jerusalem to visit family and friends. When the bus arrived in Jerusalem I was hungry and purchased a falafel from a street-side vendor. That night I experienced a bout of severe food poisoning, which would turn out to be the beginning trigger for an unrequited relationship with Irritable Bowel Syndrome (IBS). Still, upon my return I carried on my various roles with gusto and a few more visits to the loo!

Tori and I were married on a hot summer's day, December 1994. It was a super mixed marriage; differing cultural and religious backgrounds along with the joining of a medical doctor and a chiropractor. The garden wedding ceremony and luncheon took place at her grandparent's bluestone home in Batesford, just outside of Geelong. It was a beautiful, memorable day, but I was unwell at the wedding. The five-week honeymoon driving tour of New Zealand that immediately followed, was notable for how much time I needed to rest.

I barreled into 1995 'saving the world,' all the while continuing to lose stamina. By year's end I could only swim half of the one km distance I'd previously swum continuously, and even this only by stopping to rest after each lap. My GP had ordered a number of blood tests, but nothing obvious was found to explain my decline. A gluten-free diet did improve my IBS, but by the time 1996 came around, I needed to rest all weekend just to make it back to work each Monday morning.

A mediation role

I'd like to share the following experience in detail as it represented the zenith of a process I'd implemented in WHI for humanizing meetings. In the middle of 1996 I was asked to chair a mediation between two groups competing with each other: The Australian Complementary Medicine Association (ACMA), headed up by Dr Mark Donohue, and the Australian Integrative Medicine Association (AIMA), led by Dr Vicki Kotsirilos. The Federal Government wanted to deal with a single body to represent doctors practicing integrative medicine. Both of these groups were vying for that position and despite several meetings earlier in the year, could not come to an agreement.

My experience with WHI gatherings had shown me the possibility for understanding to develop between competing professionals, like a naturopath and a doctor. This could be amplified many times if each person in the room initially met on common ground. To this end, any meeting I conducted within WHI would commence with everyone having the chance to say something briefly, for example, about their day's highlight or why they'd come along. Even if it was just, "Hello, my name's Bruce. I got my washing done today." Bruce would no longer be invisible, as so many people can be at meetings. Importantly, with everyone's attention, albeit briefly, Bruce would also feel welcomed and encouraged to contribute to the group. Depending on the nature of the meeting this opportunity to speak would be limited to a stated time of say, no more than 30 seconds. Each person could choose to pass on this opportunity if they so wished. Meetings were so much more productive following this formula.

I was curious as to whether this principle would work in such a high-powered setting, and I took considerable time reflecting upon and finding a question that would hopefully bring each participant onto common ground.

The meeting was to take place on a Saturday. Once again Tori pointed out my need to rest each weekend and encouraged me to relinquish my role as chairman of this meeting. In hindsight, I was naive as to the amount of energy I would expend in such a daunting role. Unable or unwilling to see how vulnerable my health had become and convinced of the importance of the meeting, I went ahead.

Forty doctors flew into Melbourne from most states in Australia, each aligned to one group or the other. We sat in a large circle in the ballroom of an old Toorak mansion, named Armagh. Winter sunshine illuminated the garden outside the window as I began with a brief welcome and my customary habit of running a brief meditation. I then explained the approach we were going to take in order to discover common ground, so that the group as a whole would be more likely to achieve a wise decision.

While most of the practitioners in the room had spent many years in clinical practice, I wanted to take us all back to first principles, so I unleashed what I hoped would be the unifying question. I began by asking each person in turn to introduce themselves and briefly share *why they became involved in complementary medicine as part of their medical practice*, a choice that would potentially bring them into conflict with accepted medical practice. Their story would need to be contained within five minutes or less, with Mark the designated timer. One by one, they were heard in turn, many utilizing their full allotted time. Most of their stories related to personal or family health crises, many were heartrending and uplifting. It turned out, as I'd hoped, to be a moving process, connecting all of us in the room on a human level, regardless of affiliations.

At the morning tea break several doctors cornered me. Questioning my strategy they asked me when we were going to get on with the 'real business.' When we re-gathered I told everyone I'd been asked this question. Hoping like blazes I knew what I was doing, I paused, then said with some gravity, "This Is the Business!" The sharing of individual stories continued until it came to a natural end by lunchtime. The rest of the day involved respectful discussion, but ended without an agreed resolution. I knew I was in trouble!

Whilst many in the room were appreciative of the way I'd run the meeting, some were critical, especially when I called the meeting to a close as some members had to leave to catch flights. The critics wanted to continue until a resolution was reached but I'd stipulated at the beginning of the day, and all had agreed, that when one person had to leave the meeting circle, the meeting would end. Besides which, I'd done as much as I was able to do, it was 5:00p.m. and I was completely spent.

The critics need not have worried, within two weeks a phone discussion had ensued between Dr Kotsirilos and Dr Donahue in which the latter conceded that AIMA was in the best position to play the role with the government (a role they still play). All was settled with the type of honest discussion modeled in the meeting.

I, on the other hand, had something to worry about. It reminded me of a slogan I saw on a T-shirt once, "Elvis is dead, Sinatra too and me, I don't feel so good."

The plug is pulled

From my perspective the day had been rewarding but very taxing. I struggled even more to get through the next two weeks at work, culminating in an event that turned my life 180 degrees. It took place on July 17, 1996. Sitting at my desk at the University finishing some paperwork, I was feeling tired but quite content. As coordinator of our department's fourth year teaching program, I was pleased that it was now completed for another year. My workload for the rest of the year would be a little easier for it. It was after 5:00 p.m. and most of my colleagues had gone home and I was about to follow them.

Without warning, I felt as if someone had pulled an energy socket out of the left side of my upper abdomen. (This sudden onset is not uncommon with Chronic Fatigue Syndrome (CFS)) I was overwhelmed with extreme exhaustion and knew instinctively that something was seriously awry. I'm not sure how I managed to drive myself home that evening but when I arrived there, I told Tori I was unwell, collapsed into bed and slept for the next 18 hours only to wake up unrefreshed, my mind racing.

The fatigue reminded me of the experience I'd had in my 20's when I'd suffered from glandular fever (mononucleosis). I'd had anxiety and panic attacks sporadically in the past too, but hadn't experienced these since I'd taken up regular meditation nine years previously. When I tried to return to any work, I quickly became exhausted, anxious and in need of rest. Though I didn't know it at the time, I was suffering from post-exertional malaise, so that any extra effort, physical or mental, that previously I'd have done easily, left me feeling exhausted and unwell. This is the most common feature of Chronic Fatigue Syndrome (CFS). All I knew was something invisible had snapped inside me, a story I would hear many times when later I ran a clinic for CFS patients. While I'd previously had the capacity to juggle many roles at once, it now took all my concentrated effort to hold a single role, even just briefly. I was also finding after periods of standing for any length of time that I would become dizzy and need to lie down. Much later, I would discover the reason for this, a commonly associated problem with CFS, neutrally mediated hypotension (NMH) or Postural Orthostatic Tachycardia Syndrome (POTS), in which heart rate rises and blood pressure falls when sitting or standing upright, so that one frequently needs to lie down or risks fainting (the Yellow Wiggle, Greg Page, was unable to work because of this problem.) Regardless of my own understanding at the time, it became apparent I needed a significant break away from work.

It's a strange and frightening thing: one moment you're traveling along managing all the things you do in your life, next moment you've crossed an invisible line and your previous capacities are gone. Of course, I'd had years of deteriorating health leading up to this moment and yet there was a clear breaking point. It was as if an unseen protective bubble had burst, leaving me vulnerable to the emotional elements. I'd always had the capacity to empathize and had an idea of what others were feeling, but now this was magnified to such an extent that it was like a tsunami. Counseling someone with panic disorder I could no longer separate their panic from my own. Noisy, busy places, like shopping centers, became unbearable. My natural instinct was to seek retreat.

Professor John Murtagh, my university boss, was understanding and once I'd organized coverage for my work roles, allowed me to take my accrued sick leave. It took seven weeks to either cancel or cover my various responsibilities. To give you an idea of what I was juggling at the time, here is a list:

- University - teaching 1st, 2nd, 4th and 6th year students and administrative responsibilities.
- Clinical work - two four-hour sessions of predominantly counseling general practice work per week. Many of my patients had chronic illnesses with poor prognoses and they

would come to see me for one or two consultations to have some hope restored. I was also a regular facilitator for 90 minutes one night per week, of six week-long meditation courses, for groups of up to 10.

- Public Speaking - Grand Rounds, conferences and WHI events.

- Stress Management Consultancy - my regular clients included: air traffic controllers, high school students and teachers, careers counselors and health practitioners of various persuasions.

- Whole Health Institute – at its peak, WHI had a membership of over 640 people Australia-wide. We put on annual events including a conference for the general public, a doctors conference, a student conference for health students of all persuasions (I first met Tori at the 1991 conference), and various one-off speaker events. We published a directory of members and the Healing Currents journal. All conferences included speakers, workshops, entertainment (Tori and I were part of a fun troupe of WHI comedy skit actors) and healthy catering. We also had a regular one-hour community radio slot each week. Meetings included a monthly Melbourne core group gathering and a quarterly board meeting. There was only one paid member of the organization, our administrator, whom I met with at least weekly. We received no advertising income and relied entirely on membership and participant payments.

Whilst we had a board of directors and various subcommittees, the overseeing and direction of all these activities was done by me. I was a passionate enthusiast but dreadful at delegation and did not protect my time with boundaries, so late-night phone calls were the norm. I loved the organization, the people in it and what it stood for, but the truth was I was working virtually a full-time voluntary job, on top of the rest of my work, and had fallen into the trap of believing I was indispensable.

As I relinquished my various jobs, the most taxing and yet the hardest to let go of was my role as WHI president. Paradoxically, when I did, it was a huge relief.

Heading rural

When you can no longer trust your body to cope with situations you previously found easy to deal with, everyday life becomes a challenge. Post-exertional malaise meant crashes into flu-like fatigue for days after minimal overexertion. It could strike quite quickly or be delayed by a day or two. Some days I wouldn't be fatigued, giving hope that I was turning the corner, but whatever energy I had would dissipate very quickly, leaving me with my unwanted friend, overwhelming fatigue, once again.

Convinced I needed a long break to allow my body and mind to recover, I sold my Melbourne apartment, traded in my city car for a second-hand Subaru and went on a three-month camping/driving sojourn around Australia with Tori. She was having struggles of her own at the time and didn't need much encouragement.

Vice president of WHI, Shirley Winter, and her husband Doug, lived in Perth, Western Australia (WA). They kindly offered for us to housesit and for Tori to do a locum job in their chiropractic clinic while they traveled overseas for six weeks. So we had a destination. With three months to get there we took a slow 4000km road tour through Oz. The trip with its simple lifestyle in connection with nature's beauty, along with the friendly people we met along the way, restored some of my physical stamina. A strange symptom that occurred around this time was a significant loss of my sense of smell, something that became somewhat of a joke between us. It would be 10 more years before I would realize that this was an early sign of Parkinson's disease.

At this time I labeled what had happened to me as a 'burnout.' I was more than a little embarrassed that such a fate had befallen me, a meditation and stress management teacher. Over time it became clear that what was happening was a lot more complex than this. Along with my treating doctors, I was bewildered and unable to pinpoint or explain exactly what was going on with me. This contributed to a growing misunderstanding between us and our families. Finding out I fulfilled the criteria for Chronic Fatigue Syndrome (CFS) only magnified this.[1] In those days it was known as 'Yuppie Flu,' implying it was an illness of the middle class and implicating the person with the problem as the cause of their 'fake' disease and of staying ill. Nothing could be further from the reality of this terrible condition, which occurs equally across the population. We'll look more closely at CFS in the next chapter.

After Perth, we moved to the South West of WA where we also had friends from WHI. We rented a rural house overlooking a 20 acre wetland in a town called Vasse, between Busselton and Dunsburough. Wetland birds and kangaroos were welcome visitors, while tiger snakes were less so.

Tori rented a room in a physiotherapy practice in Busselton, where she worked as a chiropractor. For our sanity we turned to creative pursuits: Tori drawing and painting, me writing and photography. All the while I tried many different modalities to improve my health. At one time I had acupuncture twice weekly for six months. Improvement was minimal, if anything. I fell into a deep depression during this 14 month period, as I began to uncover some of the patterns from my childhood family dynamics that had contributed to my driven personality. I went into this dark pit willingly, as I believed that I had to go through it rather than around it and that it held the key to my recovery.

Both my parents were survivors of the Holocaust who gave their all for their three children. Yet I would discover in the ensuing years, that their childhood traumas were unwittingly, epigenetically or otherwise, passed on. The impact on children of survivors, the so-called 'second-generation,' is deep and significant and I was no exception.[2] I received invaluable assistance with this from a psychiatrist who had written a chapter in a book about his own experience as a second-generation child of survivors.[3]

After two years of living in WA, we moved back to our home state of Victoria. I hadn't recovered as quickly as I had expected to, so I was keen to continue living in a less stressful environment. We chose Apollo Bay, a favorite destination from my childhood, and rented a farmhouse overlooking the town. Tori saw clients from home, before moving her business into a natural therapies clinic in town. It was a beautiful place to live and being part of a small community (permanent population of 900) was a unique experience. Highlights included the people we met, being part of the community choir and participating in an amateur theatre production. This said, our seven years there were some of our most challenging. The weather was too often cold and misty for our liking and getting out of town meant at least 45 minutes of driving through winding mountainous roads. As my need for health services beyond the town increased, this became more problematic.

My efforts at creating alternative work and income were also thwarted. A junior novel I wrote, inspired by my nephew Andrew, failed to find a publisher, despite some promising leads. A poster series I created from my photographs taken of wildlife in Vasse, attracted great interest but no distributor. Frustratingly, I lacked the strength and energy to promote these ventures myself.

As my illness and inability to work dragged on for years on end, like so many people suffering from CFS, I was being seen as variously 'not really sick,' 'a malingerer,' 'a retiree,' 'just all in his head,' and no doubt some other choice descriptions!

I saw a documentary once, about a type of seabird, the male of the species with red stripes on its beak. The female birds and the bird community generally were most impressed with the male with the most 'red stripes.' I don't believe we humans differ too greatly from this. As a financially secure, successful doctor, I had lots of 'red stripes.' Unable to work, on a disability pension and renting, with the unsexy label of CFS, my 'red stripes' had faded to grey. My salvation was; not in Tori's eyes.

In 2005 the death of Tori's beloved mother, Carol, and my beloved father, Lee, compounded our sadness and misery. With no improvement in our situation in sight and no assets, our finances reached breaking point. Things looked grim, but help was to arrive from unexpected quarters.

Visitors

The Great Victorian Bike Ride is an annual event in the state of Victoria. In 2005, bike riders passed through Apollo Bay along the Great Ocean Road. Amongst them were Dr Daniel Lewis and his son, Justin. Daniel, a rheumatologist and a friend, had phoned to organize a catch up on his way through. During his visit I discovered that remarkably, he had a special interest in rehabilitating people with Chronic Fatigue Syndrome and fibromyalgia. It turned out his physiotherapist and yoga teacher off-sider, Laurie Lacey, was soon to holiday in our region and so Daniel organized for him to help me out.

I can still recall Laurie striding up our driveway, his 6ft 8 inches (2 meter) tall frame demonstrating perfect posture. He generously visited daily for a week, walking the 10 km from his campsite to our house to arrive punctually at 10:00 a.m. and guide me through a program. Before we look at this, let me paint a brief picture of where I was at during that time:

- I barely had the strength to walk down our 10 meter driveway and back.
- I showered second daily because of my lack of energy for it. If I washed my hair, the extra effort involved meant I needed a plastic shower chair to sit on and rest. Then I'd need Tori's help to dry my hair and get dressed before flaking out on the couch for hours recovering. Most of my day involved resting on the couch.
- I didn't have the energy to brush my teeth properly so I bought an electric toothbrush.
- In order to attend any social events, I would rest for days before and then for days after. At the event I would need to sit down frequently and often lie down on a couch or a bed.
- On one occasion I went to the post office and there was an unusually long queue. I was unable to continue standing and embarrassingly had to get someone to get me a chair to sit on, otherwise I risked fainting.

Within six months of Laurie's carefully prescribed rehabilitation exercise and yoga breathing practices, I was able to walk to the township and back without stopping to rest, a round trip of one km. To give you an idea of what this rehabilitation exercise meant, let me describe how I began. Every second day I would cycle on a stationary bike at its lowest resistance for 60 seconds, my heart rate rising from 40 (an autonomic nervous system dysfunction causing a strangely low pulse rate and low blood pressure being part of my CFS - or was it Parkinson's? - picture) to 60, at which time I became breathless. I then lay down flat on my back allowing my breathing to gradually slow and consciously relaxed for 10 minutes.

I came to call this my rest/activity dance, commonly known as pacing. Initially, for each exertion I would rest for at least twice as long, or until I felt the exercise was integrated and I was no longer breathless. If I overstepped the mark, I experienced post-exertional malaise for three or four days, after which time I got back on the bike and restarted the program, halving the level I had reached for the next week, before increasing again. I discovered I had to keep my heart rate below 110 to avoid a crash. At one point, I think it was after about three months, I felt my energy suddenly lift and I was able to achieve so much more each day. My energy levels were still well below that of a normal person, but were ten times higher than they had been prior to commencing the program. I felt like I'd been released from a low-energy prison.

After my father's death, my mother, Michelle, began to see the truth of our struggles, and her generosity allowed us to move to the city of Geelong and purchase a house in which we could both live and work. Her support, the serendipitous intervention of Daniel and Laurie, along with the invaluable psychotherapy, helped me regain enough physical and emotional strength to attempt a return to some part-time work for the first time in 11 years.

We had good friends in Geelong and they put us onto a reliable builder, Graham, who refitted our newly acquired house, allowing us to shut off our clinic from our living area. A new coat of paint and brass plaques at the front entrance set the scene for a new beginning. A small office near the front entrance connected to a waiting room, which in turn opened to a corridor leading to the obligatory toilet and two consulting rooms. This would allow Tori and me to work simultaneously, both playing the role of receptionist as needed. Working from home would also allow me to rest in between seeing patients. I was nervous and excited about returning to work. Not working, regardless of the reason, had been demoralizing and this was a set up I felt I could handle.

I was passionate about helping fellow CFS patients and so established a special interest clinic, predominantly seeing people with CFS. The Geelong Division of General Practice (later called Medicare local) was very supportive and advertised my availability for this role to the other GPs in the region. I also met with the local CFS support group. By March 2007 I was ready to go. It felt like a monumental step and I was so grateful for the opportunity to work once again, especially to be able to help people who had suffered with CFS as I had done.

My return to work took other forms as well. Between 2007 and 2012, in addition to my clinical work, I produced a stress management CD teaching meditation and relaxation skills and was given the opportunity to return to medical teaching. This took the form of a lecture and tutorial series for first year medical students on self-care and stress management at Deakin University Medical School. Astrazeneca, a pharmaceutical company, also employed me to present sessions on self-care for general practitioners. Life was looking up again.

Chapter 14

A CFS CLINIC

*To have ME (CFS) is to experience hell twice over, firstly
through the devastation of the disease itself, and secondly
through the lack of diagnosis, information and support
that most sufferers are still having to endure.*

CLARE FRANCIS, CFS PATIENT

I would like to begin this chapter with an essay written by one of
my patients, Sue, a bright 24-year-old student and musician. Upon
completion of her VCE, Sue had been accepted into studying music
at Melbourne University, but decided to take a Gap Year before
commencing. It was during this Gap Year, at the age of 18, following
a series of viral illnesses coupled with a stressful employment situation
that she developed CFS with severe Postural Orthostatic Tachycardia
Syndrome (POTS). When I first consulted with Sue, POTS had left
her unable to sit upright for more than 10 minutes before needing
to lie down. Her essay, *An Unexpected Friendship*, was published in
Emerge, quarterly Journal of CFS Australia (VicTasNT).[1]

An Unexpected Friendship

Five years ago, I contracted Chronic Fatigue Syndrome. I would like
to share with you all a rather unusual friendship, which has evolved
over this period of time. I would never in my wildest dreams have

expected something so joyful to come out of being socially isolated and housebound. I hope you can appreciate the humor of it-and may it bring a smile to your face.

For me, it represents the small, simple pleasures in life that I have learnt to appreciate, value and cherish since becoming so ill.

So, with no further ado, I shall begin.

I have a little dog called Jaco. He's a black and white foxy cross with a Jack Russell, and he is absolutely gorgeous (although I do admit I am rather biased!). I don't know how I would have survived without him these past five years. I know that for many of you reading this who have pets, you will understand my attachment.

When I was initially diagnosed, I was constantly dizzy and unable to walk very far without aid. That first winter Jaco spent many days curled up with me at the foot of the couch, snuggled against my feet and cushioned in my warm, green blanket. He was such a comfort to me.

And there he would stay...except for the same time each day, when he would suddenly go crazy, barking like mad. He'd rush to the door in a frenzy to get out. I'd hear him howling fit to burst for two minutes or so. And then, as suddenly as it began, he would come back inside, snuggle right back down against my feet, and go to sleep again.

Now, it didn't take long for my curiosity to become aroused. What on earth was happening each day? Who, or what, was so important for Jaco to see?

Well, the next day I waited for the scheduled time. I was prepared, and had saved up enough energy that morning to make it to the front door off the couch at said time. To my utter astonishment, coming down the street was a big, big man with a fat, waddling black and white Dalmatian by his side. Jaco sprung out to greet them, barking fit to burst. However, what eventuated next perplexed me further...as the man seemed to know *Jaco's name!* He called out to him jovially, started talking to him, laughing with him, and then proceeded to tell him off for his rude, barking behavior. *His* dog, might I add, was impeccably well behaved during this entire episode-he didn't even blink an eyelid at the annoying little dog trying to terrorize him through the fence.

Well, from that day on, this interaction was something that I gleefully looked forward to every morning. Come rain or shine, it was a constant that I could rely on, and that I could *enjoy*, no matter how terrible I felt. I'd wait for the time, and sure enough a chuckle would escape from my lips and a big grin would spread over my face as I peeped through the window, watching for *Mr. Man*-a name I quickly coined for this strange gentleman (to who's real name I had utterly no idea). Every now and then I'd go outside too, if I was feeling strong enough. Over time, we slowly got to the point where we both felt the bonds of familiarity emerge, and we managed a small wave to each other-never a word though, mind you. No, this man, *Mr. Man,* was one of those rare species of men that we like to call *'dog people'*. But that didn't trouble me. After all, the way I saw it, the less talking I had to do, the better.

That year, for the first time in the history of Jaco's life, he received a Christmas card. It was entitled 'Jaco and Family.' I froze. 'It couldn't be,' I thought, and then proceeded to open the envelope with trembling fingers.

'Yes it could!'

Written on a beautiful RSPCA doggie card was a heartfelt message of thanks and gratitude to Jaco and his owners. That is possibly the most exciting Christmas card I have ever received. And best of all...*I finally found out Mr. Man's real name!*

It still amazes me to this day that something so... normal could become a source of such great amusement.

I will return to Sue's story later in this chapter. But now, let me give you a little background briefing about CFS.

Chronic Fatigue Syndrome (CFS) also goes by the names Myalgic Encephalomyelitis (ME), Chronic Fatigue Immune Deficiency Syndrome (CFIDS) and the Systemic Exertion Intolerance Disease (SEID). It is classified by the World Health Organization as a disease of the central nervous system (CNS). It's characterized by debilitating fatigue that is not relieved with rest and is associated with physical symptoms. Like Parkinson's Disease, there is no simple diagnostic test for CFS, so the diagnosis is based on the following clinical criteria: severe (pathological) fatigue, post-exertional fatigue and malaise, unrefreshing sleep, pain (muscle, joint, or headache) cognitive dysfunction (memory and/or concentration impairment), and two symptoms from the following categories: autonomic, neuroendocrine or immune (See Appendix 3 or http://www.iacfsme.org/Portals/0/PDF/PrimerFinal3.pdf p12). The patient needs to have had the illness for a minimum of six months if an adult and three months if a child. The diagnosis is confirmed when other disease processes are excluded (blood test screening for other causes of severe fatigue being negative).[2,3,4]

Fibromyalgia, an illness with similarities to CFS, tends to cause a predominance of muscle pain over fatigue, although the two can overlap. I've included a copy of the Canadian Clinical Criteria for CFS (see Appendix 3 or http://www.iacfsme.org/Portals/0/PDF/PrimerFinal3.pdf) to give you a sense of the breadth of problems a person with CFS can face. This illness is often physically, mentally and emotionally debilitating, and persons with this diagnosis are twice as likely to be unemployed as persons with fatigue who do not meet the formal criteria for CFS.[5]

The cause of CFS is unclear and is likely complex. Research has shown dysfunction of mitochondria (the 'energy batteries' within each cell) along with the immune, neurological and adrenal systems. There is an association with certain genetic markers and a more common history of childhood trauma amongst people affected by the illness. It may be triggered by an infection (the vast majority), chemical exposure or trauma (psychological or physical). In some people, like myself, a series of illnesses precedes the final collapse into exhaustion. It is becoming clear there are many different subtypes of disease contained within the banner of CFS.[6,7]

One way of conceiving how this all fits together is that predisposing factors, like genetics or childhood trauma, set the body up to respond inappropriately to triggers such as an infection or surgery. A healthy person would have an acute appropriate overdrive response to such triggers, before their body systems reset back to normal drive. In a person predisposed to CFS their body systems go into and remain in overdrive, as well as becoming more sensitive to further triggers, which further perpetuates the problem. This eventually leads to a common pattern of exhaustion and the myriad of problems associated with CFS. So while there may be different apparent triggers in different people with CFS, these roads converge into a common recognizable pattern of symptoms.

As part of this pattern, CFS is considered one of the Central Sensitivity Syndromes, where the brain is inappropriately signaling in response to various inputs.[8] Functional brain imaging has recently confirmed over-responsive areas in people with these syndromes,[9] effectively indicating a neurological malfunction.

Prognosis

The prognosis of CFS is variable, with children having a better recovery rate than adults. Most adult patients show some improvement over the first five years of the illness, but usually plateau at a level below their pre-illness level of health. In fact, most people affected by CFS never regain their previous level of health or functioning.[10,11] The statistics for adults with CFS are sobering. A Review of 14 studies found on average that just 5% of patients recovered (range 0%–31%); 40% of patients improved during follow-up (range 8%–63%); only 8%–30% returned to work; and 5%–20% of patients reported ongoing worsening of symptoms.[12,13]

In practical terms at any one time, about a quarter of CFS patients, like Sue, will largely remain housebound due to the disease's severity. About 25% will have a milder condition allowing them to at least participate in part-time work or school, whilst around 50% will be somewhere between these two ranges of functioning.[14,15] Many remain unwell and have frequent relapses for the rest of their lives. During the course of the illness patients commonly have good (remission) and bad (relapse) days with bad days being called 'crash' days.[16] People with CFS who do recover often still need more rest than their contemporaries.

The following factors increase the risk of ending up with a more severe level of illness:[17-20]

- The severity of the illness at the time of onset. Orthostatic intolerance (low blood pressure and feeling unwell upon standing) is an indicator of this.
- The standard of early management of the illness (e.g. late diagnosis or overexertion in the early stages of the illness is likely to lead to deterioration).
- Having a mother with the illness.
- A diagnosis of fibromyalgia together with CFS.

Economic Impact

As a severely debilitating chronic disease, CFS places a tremendous burden on patients and their caregivers, as well as the health care system. Unemployment rates among those with the disorder range from 35% to 69%. One study found that as a result of CFS, individual income losses of approximately $20,000 annually occurred in households.[21,22]

The Canadian Community Health Survey of 2005 and 2010 documented that patients with CFS were significantly impaired compared to Canadians with other chronic conditions, such as cancer and heart disease. People with CFS reported high levels of permanent inability to work, needing help with activities of daily living and high numbers of consultations with doctors (10+ per year). They reported high rates (29%) of unmet health care and home care needs and high levels (20%) of moderate or severe food insecurity, indicating they were unable to access sufficient healthy food. Reasons for this included not being able to afford healthier food and not having the energy to prepare it.

A sizeable proportion report income and productivity loss of $20,000 per patient, and many report an annual household income <$15,000.[23,24,25] In the US between 836,000 to 2.5 million people have CFS, with the direct and indirect economic costs to society estimated to be in the billions, somewhere between $18 and $24 billion annually.[26]

Potential perpetuating factors (modified from McIntyre)[27]

- Repeated overactivity, inappropriate lifestyle, lack of rest.
- Fear of the repercussions of activity, which can lead to physical deconditioning, isolation, introversion and depression.
- Persistent infection- viral, chronic bacterial (eg sinusitis), chlamydia pneumoniae, mycoplasma or rickettsial (such as Lyme disease or Ross River Fever) and/or an autoimmune response triggered by an infection.

- Lack of social support and emotional stress.
- Gastrointestinal - dysbiosis (CFS patients have been shown to have more unhealthy bacteria in their gut compared to healthy people, which can affect mood and immune function);[28,29] food intolerances and a poor diet.
- Exposure to chemicals, environmental pollution.
- Low vitamin D levels (may be particularly significant in fibromyalgia),[30] low vitamin B12 (a number of my patients with low B12 levels, had marked improvements in their ability to concentrate following intramuscular B12 injections)

The Hysteria Myth

CFS is more common in people aged over 40 and twice as likely to occur in women than men, although there is no gender difference in incidence when it occurs in children. It is estimated to affect 0.2% of the population and tends to occur sporadically, favoring neither social class, race nor culture.[31,32,33] It can also occur in epidemics. An example of this occurred in 1955, when nearly 300 members of the hospital staff at London's Royal Free Hospital developed what was obviously an infectious illness over a period of four and half months. Of the ill hospital staff, 255 had to be admitted to hospital. Typical of CFS, many of these staff remained unwell for years.[34]

In 1970, two psychiatrists, McEvedy and Beard, produced two papers in the British Medical Journal: 'Royal Free Epidemic of 1955: a reconsideration,' and 'Concept of Benign Myalgic Encephalomyelitis.'[35]

In these articles, with inadequate research, they proposed that the Royal Free Epidemic of 1955 had been an outbreak of mass hysteria, and that other outbreaks in the world also had features of hysteria. When they wrote these articles, neither of them had bothered to interview or examine any of the Royal Free staff who had been involved, some of whom were still very unwell. In spite of the fact that there were obvious flaws in their reasoning, such as the signs of infection and neurological involvement, which do not occur in hysteria, this psychiatric hypothesis was taken up by the media. Unfortunately it was also accepted without question by many of the medical profession as well. The trivialization and inappropriate management of CFS that has resulted from this has done incalculable damage.

Debunking the myth

Given it's been 46 years since the hysteria hypothesis was proposed, do we now have evidence that debunks this myth?

As I alluded to earlier, laboratory research of CFS patients has uncovered abnormalities in mitochondrial function, inflammatory markers and immune function.[36] Under-functioning adrenal glands have also been demonstrated.[37,38] A recent review looked at whether post-exertional malaise had a corresponding biological basis. Do CFS patients truly respond differently to exercise? This review analyzed 23 studies that had compared the bodily responses to exercise of healthy sedentary people and CFS patients. They found significant differences in the way the immune system responded in the CFS patients.[39] CFS patients who experienced significant symptom flare post-exercise showed increased cytokines (pro or anti-inflammatory chemicals released by immune cells known to cause flu-like symptoms) eight hours post-exercise.[40] These differences could explain the flu-like symptoms that occur in response to overexertion. The problems identified with immune function have been shown to be reflected in specific patterns of genetic expression.[41] The importance of genetic factors is confirmed by the fact that CFS is significantly more common in identical (55% concordance) than non-identical (19% concordance) twins.[42-5]

In 2015 the independent and respected non-profit Institute of Medicine in the United States (now known as the National Academy of Medicine), reviewed the CFS research literature and published a report that concluded there was "sufficient evidence to support the finding of immune dysfunction in CFS."[46,47]

Many aspects of immune function have been found to be abnormal. Cytokine networks essential in balancing immune function for instance, form a different geometric arrangement in CFS patients than in healthy people, a pattern consistent with latent (hidden) viral infection.[48] There is also a clear correlation with disease severity linked to the important Natural Killer (NK) immune cell, which functions poorly in CFS patients. The lower the level of NK functioning, the more severe the illness and more disturbed cognitive function is in people with CFS.[49-53] Daily fatigue severity was also significantly correlated with inflammation in a study of adipokine leptin (a cytokine) in women with CFS and not in the controls. A machine learning algorithm differentiated high from low fatigue days in the CFS group with 78.3% accuracy.[54] These correlations confirm the fact that there are physical reasons why people with CFS are feeling unwell.

Another review has pointed out some of the similarities between CFS and Multiple Sclerosis (MS).[55] Fatigue and post-exertional malaise are shared by both illnesses, along with pathological changes indicated by neuro-inflammatory markers and mitochondrial dysfunction. Poorly functioning mitochondria is now a recognized feature of many neurological conditions. So just as metabolic syndrome is now recognized as a significant but subtler metabolic disease that may or may not progress to becoming type II diabetes, it could be that CFS is similarly a significant but subtler neurological condition than MS. This is supported by the brain scans of people with the Central Sensitivity

Syndromes I mentioned earlier, indicating neurological malfunction.[56] In addition, a positron emission tomography (PET) research study has demonstrated neuro-inflammation in widespread brain areas in CFS patients compared with no such changes in healthy controls.[57]

It's poignant to remember that less than 50 years ago, patients with Multiple Sclerosis were also labelled as neurotic or hysterical.[58] It seems, in English-speaking countries at least, illnesses that are complex and difficult to define are too easily lumped into the classification of hypochondriacal. What we can say is with the research evidence we have today regarding CFS, the lingering hysteria hypothesis proposed in 1970 should be well and truly cremated.

Management

The management of CFS needs to be individualized, but let me broadly outline the approach I took in treating CFS patients referred to my clinic. My initial role was to confirm the diagnosis, explain what the diagnosis meant and how it tied together their experience of so many wretched symptoms. This explanation of their experience would often bring great relief. The next step was to establish, as best as possible, strong social supports, via sympathetic family or friends, or if isolated, via a CFS support group. I'll share more thoughts on this in the next chapter.

I would explain that there was no specific magic bullet, pharmaceutical or natural therapy, to treat CFS, but there were a number of things that could help the body and mind to significantly improve. I would then introduce a comprehensive lifestyle strategy including pacing[59] and gentle rechallenging with new activities, relaxation, sleep management, diet, and deep breathing. Coexisting anxiety, depression and sleep disorders are common with CFS and if present, additional treatment was provided.

Many of my patients also experienced multiple chemical sensitivities in which strong odors, for instance, would aggravate symptoms. Others would find electromagnetic frequencies from devices like mobile phones, iPads or computers would be aggravators. Strategies for avoiding or minimizing exposure would be explored.

Social supports, a lifestyle foundation and pacing strategies in place, we would then look at mind-body therapies and paced rehabilitation, a modified version of the best researched treatment options, cognitive behavior therapy (CBT) and graded exercise therapy (GET). Cochrane reviews confirm that while neither GET nor CBT cure CFS, they are both equally effective in providing moderate improvements in fatigue levels, work and social adjustment, anxiety, and post-exertional malaise.[60,61] However, these positive results are contradicted somewhat by surveys conducted by CFS support groups of their members, indicating a worsening of their condition following these therapies in 25 to 60% of people.[62-4] This problem can be overcome, as I'll explain in my upcoming book *Chronic Fatigue Syndrome – A doctors journey and solutions*, when Energy Envelope Theory and pacing are incorporated (too detailed a discussion for our overview here), so that a different approach is used and disease aggravation can be avoided.

Let's finish with an update of Sue's story with which we started this chapter.

> Having overcome her housebound debility, the last 12 months have been Sue's best since she developed CFS. This said, several attempts at attending university have led to her having to defer, being overwhelmed by fatigue. She is, however, pursuing some online education in Health and Well-Being, doing volunteer work at several art galleries and expressing herself creatively. She has moved from the violin to the guitar, enjoys writing and has had some of her work published. She has also taken up drawing and painting,

but found the fumes from acrylic or oil paints wiped her out physically, so has had to remove these media from her repertoire.

Sue puts her improvement down to many factors: the loving support of her family; counseling with Mickel therapy, that helped her to learn how to acknowledge feelings and ways of being proactive in managing them; creative expression; learning to trust her body, appreciating and accepting its sensitivity; exercise, including Pilates classes; the self-healing that happens with the passing of time; antidepressants for managing her anxiety (she is weaning off these); and a medication prescribed by a cardiologist for raising blood pressure (fludrocortisone), which together with exercise has markedly reduced the impact of POTS. She can now sit upright or stand for prolonged periods without needing to lie down and no longer requires the fludrocortisone.

Sue is now feeling well enough to attempt going for her driver's license, something she was about to do when she fell ill six years ago. (PS. She succeeded.)

Further Resources

https://www.betterhealth.vic.gov.au/health/conditionsandtreatments/ chronic-fatigue-syndrome-cfs (accessed March 2016)

CFS Australia http://www.mecfs.org.au (accessed March 2016)

For doctors - Canadian Clinical Criteria Summary - http://sacfs.asn. au/download/consensus_overview_me_cfs.pdf(accessed March 2016)

http://www.me-de-patienten.nl/CCC Checklist.pdf(accessed March 2016)

FINDING HOPE BY DR. STEVEN J. SOMMER

There are online websites teaching pacing – eg.

Campbell B. The Patient's Guide to Chronic Fatigue Syndrome and Fibromyalgia. 2011 Available at: http://www.cfidsselfhelp.org/library/the-patients-guide-chronic-fatigue-syndromefibromyalgia

http://www.cfidsselfhelp.org/library/managing-your-energy-envelope

Keep an eye out for my book: *Chronic Fatigue Syndrome – A doctor's journey and solutions.*

Chapter 15

VALIDITY AND SOCIAL SUPPORT

*.. to not have your suffering recognized is an almost
unbearable form of violence.*

**ANDREI LANKOV, NORTH KOREAN EXPERT
KOOKMIN UNIVERSITY SOUTH KOREA.**

In 1988 the prestigious journal, *Science*, concluded that having a lack of emotional support in your life was a greater risk factor for disease and death than smoking.[1] This came on the back of research that demonstrated the most lonely and isolated people had three to four times the risk of dying prematurely when compared with those with close social ties.[2,3] To appreciate the magnitude of this, consider the fact that those with close social ties and unhealthy lifestyles (such as smoking, obesity and lack of exercise) actually live longer than those with poor social ties but more healthy living habits.[4] It is therefore of great significance if a chronic illness leads to more social isolation.

Research has uncovered that people with Chronic Fatigue Syndrome (CFS) are less likely to have good social supports than healthy people.[5] This is not surprising given debility leads to social isolation. It is a double edged blade, however, because treatment of CFS is less likely to succeed if there is poor social support.[6,7] In my clinic I observed that adolescents still living at home, like Sue, had a better chance of recovery. They had no bills to pay or work obligations and their parents, seeing the reality of the illness and how it had affected their child, could not deny its seriousness. The months or years needed to bring about recovery could usually be incorporated into the family dynamic. In contrast, older patients were often met with disbelief and struggled to achieve the support they needed to tackle the illness.

> I first consulted with Trudy in 2008. She was 43 years old and married with two young sons. Three years prior to this she had been diagnosed with CFS and Fibromyalgia. This had developed on a background of working in a high-pressure administrative officer's position, postnatal depression and a nasty attack of meningitis that required hospitalization. Following this meningitis attack, she suffered persistent severe headaches, generalized muscle pain and fatigue. Other symptoms included post-exertional malaise, anxiety, unrefreshing sleep, brain fog with impaired concentration, irritable bowel syndrome, an irritable bladder, dizziness, and the loss of adaptability and tolerance for stress. All of these symptoms worsened in the second half of her menstrual cycle, culminating in dreadful period pain.
>
> Post-exertional malaise and fatigue were particularly difficult problems for Trudy. Any excessive physical or emotional exertion would commonly leave her unwell for the next four or five days or longer. For example, a visit from her sister from interstate would be both enjoyable and exhausting. Trudy also struggled to keep up with her two growing sons, becoming overwhelmed by their needs and leaving her, at times, bedridden with pain. This extreme pain and limitation could take the form of migraine, back pain, chronic neck pain, with difficulties lifting, bending and sometimes even showering.

Her situation was seriously compounded by the fact that her husband and extended family did not believe in the severity of her illness and the limitations it imposed upon her. Her attempts to explain the situation were met with sideways looks, changing the subject or an uninformed remark such as, "Get your act together, I get tired too." She expressed feeling 'damaged' by their incongruent responses and wished she had cancer because that would bring more empathy.

Trudy had tried numerous things to get well before consulting with me, including weekly counseling sessions with a therapist trained in 'Reverse therapy.' If anything, her condition had only worsened. Despite these backward steps, throughout the three years in which I consulted with Trudy, I found her to be highly motivated and an active participant in her own management. I introduced her to pacing, stress management and cognitive strategies. After consulting with her and her husband, he developed a greater understanding and compassion for her suffering. During this time, Trudy also attended an exercise physiologist, a chiropractor and a psychiatrist who placed her on antidepressant medication (an SSRI). Trudy also undertook a series of Botox injections into muscles around her head and neck, in an attempt to manage migraine, jaw and neck pain. This gave her some temporary relief. In addition, she underwent a hysterectomy that cured her of painful menstruation, but did not impact upon her CFS or fibromyalgia symptoms.

She had times of improvement, sometimes lasting for several months, but would then relapse in response to a physical or emotional stress. Now nine years since her original diagnosis, she has been unable to return to work and her husband has lost his job. Bravely, they've decided to sell their home and move their young family interstate so as to be closer to a more supportive sibling and further away from destructive family inputs.

For some people, like Trudy, CFS brings with it social dysfunction plus the significant loss of career and independence. For others it can mean the complete breakdown of their marriage or family ties. While the level of suffering and the severity of the illness will vary between individuals, all people with CFS have lost the ability to function in areas of life that healthy people take for granted. Just getting through a day showered and fed can be a major challenge that many with CFS cannot manage alone. As referred to in the previous chapter, at the severe end of the spectrum, people can be bedbound. The measure of disability experienced can be equal to the disability experienced by people undergoing chemotherapy, or with other chronic conditions, such as AIDS, multiple sclerosis, end-stage renal disease and chronic obstructive pulmonary disease.[8] And yet it can attract little or no sympathy or support from family or friends and even members of the medical profession. Like mental illness, the lack of obvious physical abnormalities, they can look well enough, contributes to this attitude. The lack of validity, understanding and support, in people desperately in need of these things, can remove all opportunity for recovery. This, in spite of the fact that most CFS patients are highly motivated (in clear distinction from severe depression that is characterized by loss of motivation), willing to do just about anything to get well, and frustrated by not being physically able to function any more. This is a far cry from the 'lazy' archetype they may have been painted with. The illness simply has them trapped.

Both from personal experience and from observing my patients with CFS, I've come to understand Eva Hoffman's insights into suffering, when she says, "And it may be that suffering shared, suffering respected, is suffering endurable. Suffering that is misunderstood or dishonored can turn on the self in unendurable pain."[9] Feeling guilty or ashamed for having this illness and not being able to 'will' yourself out of it, can lead to depression or worse.

Compounding this effect can be the response of the CFS patient to the lack of recognition they receive. Commonly they will feel a need to tell everyone who will listen about their many symptoms. A problem shared is a problem halved is true enough, but be careful who you share it with! The effect of this on people who do not believe there is a real illness anyway, is to further reinforce their belief that this person is in fact a hypochondriac. Ultimately this leads to the character of the person being seen as in some way deficient or weak, bringing it all on themselves, in effect a character assassination. I recall my own experience of this led me to suicidal despair.

I've experienced no deeper pain than that of having the people I thought loved and cared for me, turn their backs on me. In my limited Western understanding of what the Australian Aboriginal practice of 'pointing the bone' may mean, I can imagine if an entire community turns its back on the person selected so that they effectively become invisible, it can lead to their death. We simply don't appreciate the unseen social glue that holds us every minute of the day until it is diminished or gone.

I found myself looking in the mirror one day saying to myself, "but it's me, why am I being treated so differently? I'm still here! I just have this terrible illness." My mental health was severely challenged as it was, with the loss of my career, sense of purpose and financial security. I was a high achieving, motivated person who loved his job, I would never have chosen to put myself in this situation. I found myself reeling for days after difficult conversations; Tori was on suicide watch for years. In the end, reluctantly in a way, for I longed to be part of the social glue that had supported me when I was well – but to preserve my life, I had to stay away from negative inputs as much as possible.

I have since observed that some healthy people with a lack of personal experience of chronic illness, just 'don't do illness.' That is to say they find it difficult to empathize or to be with a person with a chronic disability. Whether that is because they are deeply fearful of it themselves and don't want any reminder that they too are vulnerable, I can merely speculate. Whatever their reasons, they are emotionally unsafe people to be around if you're feeling at all fragile and not people you want with you in the trenches of life.

Of course any chronic illness can bring out the worst in a person's personality and I was certainly guilty of this at times. Anyone living with a loved one experiencing chronic pain will testify to this. In this situation the illness or injury causing the pain is quite correctly attributed to be the factor that changes the person's personality. This is very different from concluding, as many do with CFS patients, that their changed personality is the problem.

Support groups

Given the many misconceptions about CFS, it's no surprise that a key role that CFS support groups play is in validating the reality of the illness. They also play an invaluable role in directing people towards local doctors and other practitioners with an understanding of the condition. In addition they can provide educational materials that can help to explain what is going on to family and friends. Some groups also provide management education, pacing in particular. Whether or not you are inclined to attend such a group, or participate online, depends very much on your circumstance and personality. When I attended a local CFS support group, I witnessed the overwhelming need of each person to have the reality of their horrendous situation affirmed. This was clearly critical, but I found the experience, paradoxically, to be very tiring and decided not to re-attend.

This contrasted with my experience of attending other support groups for illnesses I developed later, that were recognized as valid and were not being questioned by the medical profession. Here, even though the illnesses were disabling, the focus in these groups was more relaxed and fun. We didn't have to waste energy on restoring validity, that was a given. The fact that my ensuing illnesses had a range of established pharmaceuticals and/or surgical treatment options created an easy point of focus too. CFS had none of this.

These fundamental differences go some way to explaining the research finding that CFS patients often do worse if they attend a CFS support group.[10,11] It's likely that the group attracts those people with the least amount of social support who would have been even worse off without them. I certainly found this in my clinic. In fact I only recommended a support group for those in dire need of it. Those who had good supports, after having their illness validated, were able to take the next step and focus their limited energy on ways to recover their health.

To finish this discussion about support groups, let me just say that each individual group will have a different dynamic, so the only way to fully know if it will be helpful for you or not, is to do what I did and check it out. Like me, you may decide to only attend once, or you might become an occasional or regular attendee; you be the judge of what works best for you.

A Twist in the Tale

Running a CFS clinic was both challenging and rewarding. Hearing the difficulties my patients were facing was at times heartbreaking, whilst on the other hand, seeing them benefit from the strategies I was teaching was gratifying. While many of them were on the journey of recovery my own journey was becoming more complicated. I'd developed some worrying new symptoms: uncontrollable shuddering in my right leg at night, a tendency to trip on my right foot, the lack of arm swing in my right arm whilst walking and the occasional tremor in my left hand. My handwriting was also decreasing in size. My medical eye had a fair idea of what this meant, but I did not want to believe it!

In February 2009 Tori and I were referred to the office of neurologist Dr Peter Bachelor. It did not take him long to pronounce, "you have Parkinson's disease." Tori broke into tears. I felt the blow of it, but was not the least surprised. What did surprise me was that the 13 preceding years of ill health labeled as CFS, was at least in part, early Parkinson's disease (PD). It is now recognized that an illness similar to CFS can precede the classic Parkinson's symptoms by up to 20 years.[12] It is now labelled as early-stage Parkinson's disease. I've since met several fellow PD patients who were diagnosed as having CFS for many years prior to the obvious unfoldment of their PD.

My response to this revelation was curious. I knew, medically speaking, PD was considered to be a chronic progressive disease and that this was not good news, yet all I could think of following the years of ridicule and disbelief about the legitimacy of my CFS struggles, were the words comedian Spike Milligan had engraved on his tombstone; "I told you I was sick!" With Parkinson's, finally I had a label that people would believe, a terrible admission from a doctor who has championed and continues to champion the legitimacy of CFS patients. The need for appropriate validation is so, so important.

When a dear 88 year old friend, Caspar, developed a multitude of vague symptoms, along with a mild but unusual headache and more trouble reading than usual, he saw several doctors over a period of weeks before they took him seriously enough to look beyond the obvious and order a brain scan. A brain tumor was detected. His response was relief. "Not being believed," he said, "was one of the worst experiences of my life."

With no definitive test to make the diagnosis, it is little wonder then that people with CFS express feeling damaged by the response of treating doctors and their closest family and friends when for months and often years their struggles are not taken seriously.[13,14]

Given fatigue and other autonomic nervous system symptoms are a feature of neurological disorders, like PD and MS, it suggests to me that the World Health Organization recognition of CFS as a type of neurological disorder is correct.

While my PD was a blow, it was not the knockout punch that took me out of the workforce once again. That came out of left field in the form of two new illnesses, Ulcerative Colitis and Graves' disease. We'll pick up that tale in the next chapter.

Further Resources

Prof Sir Michael Marmot, President of the World Medical Association, speaks on Social Justice and the Health Gap: https://itunes.apple.com/au/podcast/boyer-lectures-fair-australia/id206589427?mt=2

Chapter 16

A NEARLY DEAD EXPERIENCE

We can use our pain - emotional or physical -
as a catalyst to begin healing not curing. To me curing
means only getting back to the way we were before we
became diseased. Healing is when we use our pain or
illness as a catalyst to begin transforming our lives -
healing our inner pain and our relationships, our hearts
and our souls.

DR DEAN ORNISH

I realize now that those tiny molecules of hope became
the foundation for my survival.

JOEL ROTHSCHILD - LONG-TERM AIDS SURVIVOR

Near death experiences: I'd read about them and had some of my patients tell me about theirs, but when I was lying in a hospital bed in April 2012, facing my own, I was in uncharted territory. The previous two years had been a nightmare of continuous recurrences of colitis (Ulcerative Colitis), each acute attack slashing four to five kg (10lbs) of my already low body weight. Having to rush to the toilet six to 14 times a day for weeks on end, especially when struggling to do so with Parkinson's disease, was no fun.

By April 2012 my weight had dropped to 40 kg (88lbs) giving me a Body Mass Index of 12, I looked like a survivor from a concentration camp. Barely able to stand, I required assistance with the most basic activities. This admission, unlike my previous three, was different in that the high-dose intravenous cortisone treatment did not slow the colitis down. After my second week in hospital, my gastroenterologist, Ross, sat down and said, "we could operate, removing your colon, but I doubt you would survive surgery; we could give you immunosuppressants, but these could very well lead you into kidney failure or we could keep you on intravenous hydrocortisone, but that should have worked by now." The feeling of being close to the edge was brought into fearful focus. The nurses on my ward were giving Tori hugs in preparation for what they thought was my inevitable demise.

My fear surprised me. In my late twenties, deeply spiritual moments in meditation had left me fearless of death, certain of the timelessness of life in some or no form. I recalled the story of an Indian guru who when approaching his imminent death shocked his disciples by pleading, "I don't want to die!" I was screaming these very words on the inside. I was freaked out by the prospect of dying, my life felt unfinished and ending it now felt wrong. This said, part of me had had enough of the endless cycle of suffering that had been my life of ill health for the previous 15 years and slipping off into endless sleep was on one level attractive.

At this time I was light in more ways than just my body weight. Dreams and visions, some of them profound, occurred in my daytime experience. In one of these moments I asked for spiritual release; the response was a clear message that this was not my time. It was also apparent to me that in the end you suffer and die alone. Both are internal experiences. While others can comfort and distract you from your suffering, they cannot experience it for you. It is for you to face. In the situation I was in I could either fight for or give up and surrender my life; there was a level of choice.

Did I reflect back on my lifetime? Not really, not then. Did I think of all the people I'd helped during my medical career; lectures given as a teacher; workshops I'd run; the money I'd made? No. I was consumed by the ever-present struggle and what became apparent to me was that the most important thing, for whatever life I had left, was my connection to people who loved me. My wife, Tori, was foremost here, always by my side (sleeping on a foldout bed beside me throughout each admission).

My best friend, Pete, was a welcome visitor, full of love and strength, he willed me to keep fighting. Cousins, Natalie and Tania, also arrived at a critical time and in their response to me I felt how much I meant to them. Through this experience I was reminded I meant something to others unseen: family and friends, such as my good friend Judy interstate. Di and Ron, Robert and Ingrid, along with Therese were also invaluable, supportive friends who sat by my bedside. Nonetheless, my prospects were not looking good and this was reflected in the eyes of my friends and hospital staff. Then something extraordinary happened.

Let me paint the scene. Desperate, with hope fading, Tori flew to Sydney for a consultation, on my behalf, with Professor Thomas Barody, a gastroenterologist and a pioneer in the use of fecal transplantation for treating colitis. Meanwhile back at my hospital bed in Geelong, I was having a difficult day. With the assistance of nursing staff I was back and forth to the toilet and the pain in my abdomen was nasty. Then there was a moment, with Tori away and free from attendant nurses or visitors, I did what I had been avoiding, I allowed myself to feel and enter completely into the pain in the left side of my abdomen.

I had experienced some form of physical or emotional pain in this area ever since my health collapsed in the middle of 1996. I'd used mindfulness techniques in the past to connect with this pain and received significant insights. However, on this occasion, something unique happened: I experienced a daytime vision complete with wise commentary.

The vision was of a massive brown tangled mess, like an early Universe, within which was a tiny bright dot. It was made clear to me that I was this dot and that I had been born into this tangle. The tangle represented my family traumas from the Holocaust, a scene of Nazis marching confirming its meaning. In a flash the utter nonsense of taking on a role of somehow healing this tangled mass was made known to me. I was simply an innocent dot born into the middle of it all. As we all were.

I had done years of psychotherapy to understand this and thought I'd dealt with the issue, but when this vision occurred and ended in a matter of seconds, a huge release in my psyche took place, a release from a burden of responsibility I'd unconsciously taken on all those years ago. It was truly not mine to fix after all, and every cell of my being knew it fully for the first time. An invisible tie, that somehow had ensnared me for as long as I had memory, was broken.

One month after this, reflecting on this experience, I wrote this poem.

Tangle upon tangle
Into it I am born
Generational Trauma

Nazis
Dislocation
Migration
And what came before?
Terror unexpressed
My being needs to feel
A conduit I've become.

Tortured and wracked

My body succumbs
Till the light of revelation
Sweeps self-blame away
This is not mine to fix after all

It just had to be felt
So that I could be free

I cannot overstate the experience of relief and release I felt. As I said to Tori on her return from Sydney, if I die now at least I feel at peace and it was worth going through all of the hellish ill-health to reach this point.

But I wasn't done yet; now the fight to recover my health really began.

Checking out, checking in

The longer I was going to stay in hospital the more likely I was going to die there. After two weeks, against the advice of my physician Ross, but with Tori's agreement, I signed myself out. While on the one hand Ross was reluctant to commence further treatment, on the other, he thought I was too frail to cope at home. My thinking was that if I stayed, he would eventually have to treat me further and that this would not end well. My best chance I felt was to recuperate at home. Besides this, if I was going to die, I preferred to do this in a quiet, familiar space. "You're one of the 10 toughest people I've met," were Ross's parting words. This meant a lot to me as I'd thought of myself after my breakdown as somehow weak.

In the days leading up to leaving hospital, Tori and I did our best to organize as much practical assistance as possible. With the help of an Occupational Therapist we arranged for the hire of a hospital bed with an alternating air pressure mattress, bought a portable commode and hired a bed-pole. In the months prior to my admission we had also received four hours a week of Council respite care for Tori, so we contacted them to arrange extra hours of help. Good friends, Robert and Therese provided invaluable further backup respite for Tori, so that she could continue her Fine Arts degree. We also called on another friend at the time who was a competent cook and a very willing helper in the kitchen. He produced large batches of colitis-friendly food during his weekly visits. Our neighbor, Phil, offered to shop for our groceries and other friends, Monica and Liz, were willing shoppers too.

Despite all of these measures, we were like army novices entering a major battleground, thankfully unaware of the toll life was about to exact upon us. While I was acutely unwell in hospital it was easy to overlook my serious mobility issues. Frail and unable to tolerate the medication to relieve my Parkinson's disease, now that I was home, this became frightening. My world had contracted to the most basic of concerns: wanting, but unable to adjust my pillow; trying to reach for a sip of water; needing help to toilet. My frustration levels were extremely high as I had to ask for assistance each time I needed any little thing. I became more insular in my thinking and a demanding pain in the bum, at times uncharacteristically aggressively so. Invariably the person I kept asking was Tori and this wore her down.

While it took me some time to realize this, the high dose of prednisolone prescribed to treat my colitis was affecting my personality. I'd witnessed this effect on other people, most notably on a close friend of my mother's, whose sweet, gentle nature became aggressive and inappropriate whilst on this drug. As the weeks went by, prednisolone also began to cause me to experience panic attacks and suicidal depression, but I'm getting ahead of myself.

Let me return briefly to some significant experiences during my final days in hospital.

When a person is under overwhelming duress, they can experience 'Third Man Syndrome.' First noted in explorers when at the brink of exhaustion, as when Ernest Shackleton approached the South Pole, the experience is of sensing the presence of a benevolent being.[1] In my final week in hospital I believe this happened to me. It took the form of images that appeared in my mind during quiet meditations. The most ever present of these was the appearance of a golden, smiling, Buddha-like face, which in my mind's eye surrounded my abdomen. I felt very still with this experience, and the intuitive message I received from this being was that no illness could continue whilst I was connected to this state of mind. I found this very comforting and reassuring; it eased my fear.

Another significant event from this time relates to Una, a 95 year old lady in a room two doors up from mine, who had suffered a cardiac arrest two nights before my departure. To the surprise of both hospital staff (who'd resuscitated her) and her family, she did not die. The evening following this, Tori was drawn to speak with her and knocked on her open door. Happy to have company, Una related a near death experience she'd had the previous night. In it she described being in a peaceful garden where she had met with deceased relatives. Despite its attraction, she told these relatives that she was not ready to go yet, as she wanted more time with her grandchildren.

During the previous 10 days, Una had seen me shuffling up the corridor with Tori, using my walker. Whilst Tori sat by her bed, Una held her hand and told her that she was too young to lose her husband and that she wanted to speak with me. So on the day I left hospital Tori pushed me in my wheelchair into Una's room. Una took my hand, squeezed it tightly with considerable strength, looked me in the eye and said, "If you want to live, you've got to want to be here and you've got to pray. Now say it five times – 'I Want to Be Here!'" I did.

I arrived home on a cloudy autumn Thursday, April 19, 2012. The plan was to continue on oral prednisolone, gradually reducing the dose over many weeks. If I ran into trouble, I was to contact the hospital immediately and return. In the meantime I was to maintain phone contact with Ross. The colitis continued unabated for the next three days with fever, abdominal pain and diarrhea. All this occurred during the chaos of trying to cope in a less controlled environment. By Sunday lunchtime we doubted the wisdom of our choice to come home. At this point I was lying in my bed, practicing Una's instruction, whispering, "I want to be here, I want to be here…" Then, awkwardly, I began to pray.

Prayer is not something I'd ever done much of. Like my father, I was never a religious person. *So who did I pray to?* I thought about this for a moment, and then decided to pray to the *loving energies*. Sincerely, with all my heart, I prayed for their help. Almost instantaneously I experienced one of the most remarkable events of my life. Flowing down from above my head with the volume of a surging stream, came a blissful energy. It washed through my entire body and was so intoxicating that I just lay there smiling, soaking in bliss, never wanting it to end. I think this lasted for about 10 minutes, until Tori called out that lunch was ready and the spell dissipated. I knew from that moment on, I was going to be okay. That night my fever broke and the colitis began to subside.

While the acute crisis had lessened, the battle to rebuild my body was well and truly on. Using digestive enzymes liberally I ate a wholefood diet with high calorie foods, including bone broth chicken soup, salmon, sardines, overcooked pureed vegetables and whey protein smoothies, all in frequent small doses. I gained 2kg in 10 days and Ross was happy to hold back on inserting a feeding tube, something he believed would ultimately be necessary. With a little more energy my immobility became even more frustrating, I wanted to scream with anguish until I remembered a device I'd seen my aunt Rosina, who'd also had Parkinson's disease (PD), use. It was a foot cycle. I also remembered seeing one in the showroom of a local medical supplier, so I rang and purchased it. To my delight I discovered that Parkinson's disease does not inhibit the ability to cycle one's legs. When my legs moved freely it seemed to liberate my mind as well, releasing some of the tension, both emotional and physical. These brief interludes were a daily highlight and sanity saver; they inspired this poem:

The Foot Cycle

Frail, frozen, immobile
every movement stifled
trapped inside fuming frustration
I'm helped into the cycle
feet strapped in
they move, legs move, slowly at first then faster ...
faster exhilaration, release, relief
I tire, two minutes of daily freedom cherished.

An Unpopular Disease

Colitis is not an illness many people know about for good reason. Imagine having a bout of gastroenteritis (gastro) that just doesn't stop. This is not a topic for dinnertime conversation. Thought to be an autoimmune condition, my first attack of Inflammatory Bowel Disease (IBD) occurred in November 2010. Following 10 days of unremitting fever, abdominal pain and diarrhea, I'd become dehydrated and was admitted to Geelong Private Hospital. Severe patchy inflammation of my entire colon was eventually discovered on colonoscopy. A diagnosis of IBD, either Crohn's Disease or Ulcerative Colitis (UC), was made, biopsy results inconclusive as to which of these two diseases I had. In the ensuing two years recurring attacks every three to four months required four hospital admissions and led to a progressive debilitating weight loss of 20 kg. Complicating matters, and contributing to my debility and weight loss, was an undiagnosed overactive thyroid gland condition known as Graves' Disease. An appropriate name for the way I was feeling!

There was a serious question as to whether my Parkinson's medication had triggered the initial colitis. The day I increased the dose (of levodopa) being the day my bowel started having conniptions. So I chose to remain unmedicated for PD over this period. A rare side-effect, but my neurologist has since had two other patients with colitis triggered by levodopa.

As I've alluded to, the combination of PD, where quick movement was impossible, and colitis, where being able to rush to a toilet (urgency) was essential, was interesting! The portable commode chair saved me here. I would jangle a little bell and Tori would arrive, 'throne' in hand, to the rescue. Still urgency, too often became an 'emergent -cy'and I had to wear nappies at night. It took months before I was able to venture away from home.

Unfortunately, mesalazine, a medication used to treat colitis, had the opposite effect on me, aggravating the illness further. Rechallenging my body with this medication during one of my hospital admissions in December 2011, confirmed this. The only medication that had worked was high-dose corticosteroids. Immunosuppressants, such as Imuran, were the next line of therapy open to me. In Ross's words, "these medications are pretty awful." Given my propensity to look outside the medical square, naturally I attempted to find other ways of managing my colitis.

The first ray of hope in this regard occurred when I met a fellow called Adrian, an organic farmer who delivered a box of vegetables to our door each week. We got chatting one day and I discovered he'd suffered from Crohn's Disease. Adrian was solidly built and looked remarkably healthy, so I was surprised to discover that part of his bowel had been removed and his weight had fallen to 48kg (106lbs) during his only hospital admission with Crohn's colitis eight years ago. Since that time he'd taken to an organic vegetarian diet, avoided fried foods, sugar, dairy and gluten and taken probiotics. This approach had kept him well with only minor flare ups not necessitating medication or surgery. His weight had returned to a healthy 85kg (187lbs).

I emulated Adrian's approach but continued to have serious attacks. When my colitis flared up in March 2012, I even attempted a high calorie liquid diet, that trials had shown could successfully treat attacks of Crohn's Disease but not UC.[2,3] While I did not lose any more weight during this four week period, the colitis continued unabated, providing some evidence that my underlying disease was Ulcerative Colitis, a diagnosis Ross concurred with.

Despite four gastroenterologists who had managed me at different times advising me that diet had no effect on colitis, along with my own unsuccessful attempts to manage it this way, intuitively I still felt it must be important. Colitis is inflammation of the lining of a very large tube, the large intestine. It made sense that what you placed into that tube would influence the state of that lining. In the week prior to my April admission I looked for clues on PubMed and the Book Depository website. Searching for titles that might provide inspiration and insight, I came across two books that I promptly ordered. The first book, by Tracie Dalessandro, was entitled, *What to Eat with IBD*.[4] Tracie was a dietitian who had suffered from Crohn's Disease. A second book, by Virginia Harper, was entitled, *Controlling Crohn's Disease the Natural Way*.[5] Virginia had also suffered from Crohn's Disease and remarkably, after three years of countless attacks, had found a way of managing her illness for the next 20 years without medication or surgery. This got my attention. Both books were waiting in a stack of mail collected by our neighbor when we arrived home from hospital. They provided hope and direction while we were floundering in uncertainty.

Tracie's approach was to avoid any abrasive or irritant foods. It made sense to treat a raw, inflamed lining in this way. Obvious foods to be avoided were nuts, seeds and anything high in fiber. All of her recommended list of vegetables needed to be overcooked. We did this as well as then puréeing them for the first three months after I arrived home. Virginia's approach was different again. She embraced a macrobiotic diet with a Japanese influence. I had previously discovered that Japanese people on their traditional diet had the lowest incidence of colitis in the world.[6-8] If they took up a Western diet with an emphasis on a high intake of saturated fat, sugar and protein, their incidence of colitis increased accordingly,[9-12] evidence one would think of the importance of diet in colitis management.

Apart from diet, Virginia also emphasized the importance of resolving emotional difficulties, something my recent daytime vision had gone a long way to accomplishing, but stress management was needed to help me cope with the ongoing ordeal. Contributing significantly here was a small dose at night (7.5 mg) of the medication mirtazapine which helped me to sleep, quelled my anxiety and acted as an appetite stimulant.

Another important recommendation from Virginia was to use digestive enzymes liberally with food to make digestion easier and to enhance weight gain. I found these to be very helpful, especially the gentler non-acid containing ones. A key feature of her diet was the use of cultured foods, such as miso soup and pickled vegetables. As I've mentioned, IBD is considered to be an autoimmune condition, and the influential role of the bacteria in the gut on the immune system is now more evident, as we will explore in a later chapter. For now let me point out that IBD sufferers are known to have 25% less biodiversity amongst their gut bacteria than non-sufferers.[13]

In her book, Virginia gives an example of entering an acute colitis episode which settled with hourly miso and seaweed soup. It seems likely to me that just as a healthy garden can be achieved through composting, cultured foods promote the health of good bacteria in the gut, thus influencing the immune system and reducing inflammation. I added a daily miso vegetable soup to my diet along with pickled vegetables, such as umeboshi plum. I also continued a daily probiotic supplement. Research supports the use of particular probiotics in the treatment and prevention of acute Ulcerative Colitis.[14,15]

The medical consensus in 2014 was that the incidence of Inflammatory Bowel Disease was rising and that this may be due, at least in part, to dietary influence, especially westernization. However, to date there was not enough research evidence to support particular dietary triggers or diet as a therapy.[16,17] This said, the issue seemed to be that there simply had not been enough research, rather than the likelihood of a negative correlation. What is known is that genetic predisposition plays a significant role along with environmental triggers such as smoking, antibiotic usage and almost certainly diet. In my case, I found eliminating sugar and refined grains, such as bread, cakes and biscuits to be helpful. Apart from hearing of Adrian's success in modifying his diet, I also heard of another local doctor who had had many admissions for Crohn's disease. His Japanese partner had placed him on a more traditional Japanese diet that drastically decreased his exacerbations. I'm aware of one research study which supports the benefits of the semi-vegetarian Japanese-style diet (meat once a fortnight) in helping to manage IBD.[18]

In time, perhaps we may discover that diet needs to be individualized depending on genetic profiles. While I have heard gastroenterologists express their dismay at the restrictive nature of many of the diets being recommended to treat IBD, from the patient's perspective this can be such a dreadful and life-threatening condition with potentially harmful treatments and no known cure, that if modifying one's diet can bring relief, it's worth trying.

Challenging the Consensus: the Specific Carbohydrate Diet

A recent case series (published in 2015) thoroughly studied 50 IBD patients who had followed a restrictive diet known as the Specific Carbohydrate Diet (SCD), and flagged its potential.[19] This diet, whose main features include the exclusion of sugar, all grains, many dairy products and some starchy vegetables, such as potato and sweet potato, was developed in the 1940s by gastroenterologist, Dr Sidney Haas.[20] It long predates the similar, but different, modern Paleo diet.

Haas developed the diet as a treatment for celiac disease, before it was understood to be caused by the grain protein, gluten. At this time, it was postulated that poor digestion of carbohydrates led to an overgrowth of inappropriate gut bacteria that perpetuated an inflamed, diseased gastrointestinal tract. Placing people on the SCD, which included easily digested (predominantly monosaccharide) carbohydrates only, would give the gut time to heal. He recommended that following the diet for a minimum of one year was required for this to occur, after which a person could go back onto a normal diet. Anecdotally it was a highly successful treatment and Haas was lauded for his work.[21] Only when it was discovered that a simpler gluten-free diet would restore the health of most celiacs, did Haas's more restrictive diet (which was also gluten-free) fall out of favor. The diet, however, did not go away because it appeared to have a broader application, with numerous anecdotal accounts of its success in treating IBD.[22] Backing these up, the researchers have found that in the 50 IBD patients they studied, the SCD did indeed maintain remission, with 92% rating it effective in doing so and 91% rating it effective for managing acute flare ups.[23]

The main reason patients gave for taking up the SCD was fear of the consequences of using medication long-term (the immunosuppressants used to treat IBD increase the risk of lymphoma and skin cancer), with the ineffectiveness of medication and adverse side-effects being other common reasons. Sixty-four percent also found the SCD more effective than medication, and 22/50 people studied were able to cease all medications and have the disease controlled completely by the SCD alone. They also found, contrary to what might be expected, that despite the restrictive nature of the diet, quality of life in those in remission was high. The difficulty in maintaining the diet rated a very modest 4/10; not having to worry about where the nearest toilet is, medication side-effects, or whether you may need bowel surgery, in my experience, motivates one and more than offsets the downsides of dietary restrictions. Mind you, those suffering with less severe disease, or a disease profile that responds well to medication, would naturally be less inclined to change their diet to this extent.

Other interesting findings from this research study were that the average time to see some improvement when following the SCD was 29.2 days (range=1 to 180 days) and that in the 33 patients (66%) who noted complete symptom resolution, this occurred after an average time of 9.9 months (range=1 to 60 months) after starting the SCD.[24] Earlier research studies on the SCD had found that the diet had led to a change in the pattern of bowel flora (gut bacteria) and that this may have been a mechanism to explain the diet's effectiveness.[25,26]

Weighing all this up, the researchers conclude: "If following the SCD changes the microbiome significantly and/or reverses some of the dysbiosis (abnormal gut bacteria patterns) reported in patients with IBD, this may be a low-cost intervention to induce and maintain remission with little or no known adverse reactions. As such, further interventional studies of SCD and diet therapies in general for IBD are urgently needed."

If I put on my doctor/scientist hat, I see the potential limitations of this research study. In particular patients were recruited by advertisement, so that perhaps only those enthusiastic about the benefits of the SCD would have volunteered for the research. This could bias the results in favor of the diet's effectiveness. A true indication of its potential would only be obtained through a randomized double-blind intervention trial and I could only recommend this diet with confidence if such trials were done.

If I put on my informed patient hat, I recognize that this 50 patient case study research is the best available evidence to date, and demonstrates a real possibility that this diet could help my disease management, give me more of a sense of control over my IBD, and avoid the possible long-term complications of taking immunosuppressant medication. Coupled with the fact that there is minimal or no risk involved in trying the SCD, I'm excited by the possibility. As my disease is current, I need to make decisions now rather than wait for intervention trials that may never eventuate, given the dearth of research funding for this type of dietary intervention. I believe I have more to gain than to lose by trying it.

Hopefully you can see from this example that it's easier to make decisions based upon mathematical algorithms when one isn't involved. But life is rarely like that in clinical medicine, so that a number of things need to be weighed up in making choices, a recurring theme of this book.

For those of you interested in exploring the SCD further a good place to start is Elaine Gottschall's book, *Breaking the Vicious Cycle: Intestinal Health Through Diet*.[27] Elaine championed the benefits of the SCD for IBD, celiac disease (especially if poorly responding to a simple gluten-free diet) and for other conditions, including autism. Elaine's interest in this area was sparked from near personal tragedy. Her daughter had been diagnosed with Ulcerative Colitis at the age of five and following three years of worsening ill-health treated with corticosteroids and sulfonamides, was facing imminent surgery. It was 1959, and anxious for another answer she took her daughter to see Dr Haas. Dr Haas placed her on the SCD and two years later her condition had completely resolved. After several more years on the diet, her daughter was able to return to normal eating patterns and more than 20 years later continued to be well.[28] This stimulated Elaine to become a university-based research scientist with an interest in nutrition and IBD.

Therapeutic versus maintenance diets

Let me finish this chapter by clarifying something about diets. Therapeutic diets, such as those recommended for managing diabetes or high cholesterol, are designed for specific purposes. The SCD is another example of a therapeutic diet, this time for Inflammatory Bowel Disease, the general teaching here being that after one year without symptoms one could change to a less restricted diet. The SCD, if done well, may be balanced enough to be continued as a maintenance diet (a diet balanced and healthy enough to use lifelong e.g. the Mediterranean diet),[29,30,31] but it is worth keeping in mind that other diets, especially cleansing or weight loss diets, may be okay for a short period as a therapeutic diet, but may not be healthy for the longer term. If in doubt consult a nutritionist or dietitian.

Chapter 17

SEARCHING FOR THE BOTTOM LINE

All disease begins in the gut.

HIPPOCRATES

In treating active colitis medically, the dosage of prednisolone (an anti-inflammatory) must be reduced slowly, usually over three months. There are potentially dangerous consequences if one just stops. It eventually became clear to me that each morning, 30 minutes after taking my prednisolone tablets, I would begin to experience panic attacks followed by suicidal depression. Like a passing storm, this would all subside in the late evening when the medication wore off. It became a ritual torture session, feeling normal when I awoke in the morning, knowing that I had to place this medication in my mouth, swallow it and wait for hell to arrive. It was awful. I felt like Dumbledore in one of the scenes from Harry Potter and the Half-Blood Prince, where in order to uncover a Horcrux, he had to drink a potion that was increasingly tormenting him.

At this time some help arrived from a surprising quarter. Danita, a delightful friend from our time of living in Apollo Bay, phoned. We hadn't heard from her in years. Ascertaining my situation she offered loving support and involved her step-father, Daryl, a well-known healer in Colac. Refusing any payment, he 'tuned' into my plight and told me to focus upon and slow down my breathing. This was invaluable advice. I'd given this very same instruction many times to anxious patients of mine, but in my own state of panic, I needed someone else to remind me.

From an initial dose of 37.5mg daily, I weaned off the prednisolone over seven weeks. Only when I reached a 10mg dose did my panic begin to diminish. When this awful time was over and my panic dissolved, I vowed to do anything possible to avoid taking prednisolone again. It motivated the search that led me to the discovery of the benefits of mastic gum (see earlier chapter on Complementary Medicine) and dietary management approaches.

As I have alluded to, the combination of fighting for survival, frustration with my disability and the effect of the prednisolone made me, all too often, an unpleasant person to be around. It was as if I was possessed; at times I could see myself speaking aggressively but couldn't stop it. Confined by illness and reliant upon others for my basic survival needs, I'd become incredibly self-focused and I loathed my own behavior. This further exacerbated the depression I was experiencing as a side effect of the prednisolone. I'd always seen myself as a kind and compassionate person and it was hard to reconcile this self-image with my grumpy demeanor. Tori was being distressed and our marriage stretched by this.

From the moment Tori and I met in 1991 she had been my soul-mate. Even though my ill health had dominated the time in which we'd been married, we'd always loved being together. These two years of severe colitis attacks, however, on top of the many difficult years preceding it, brought us to breaking point. It wasn't helped by the fact that physical intimacy between us had been prohibited by my weakened condition and that so much of our time was now dominated by day-to-day survival issues. As a result of all this Tori's and my deep wish for children was never to eventuate.

With all these challenges going on, there was a lot of work to be done to reinvigorate our marriage. The truth was I'd taken too much for granted and I needed a wake-up call. The very act of making an appointment with a marriage counselor triggered some necessarily pointed communication. It was clear we both wanted to stay together and were willing to work to make this happen.

Thank goodness there was some light appearing as our strategies for the colitis were succeeding. By September I reached 47kg (104lbs), I'd avoided the insertion of a feeding tube and I felt ready to travel to Melbourne for a much-needed nurturing meal with my family. However, I still suffered from urgency (the sudden need to go to the toilet) and the main anxiety was that there were only two potential toilet stops on the 70 km (44 mile) highway between Geelong and Melbourne. Being anxious of course triggered the very problem I was worried about. It made for a pretty distressing and sometimes messy trip for me and driver Tori. Over the next month, with the combination of continued dietary restriction and probiotics, my urgency began to settle, a blessed relief.

Two minor flares of colitis occurred during this period. These were easily dealt with by drinking umeboshi kuzu tea and taking several days of treatment with mastic gum capsules. Thankfully, each flare settled within 24 hours.

When Christmas arrived, I had regained 10kg (22lbs) - to 50kg (110lbs). Once again we were able to participate socially, go to the movies (albeit in a wheelchair) and generally bring more joy into our lives. As things improved we were able to reflect back upon and acknowledge the extraordinary context that had strained our relationship. We had both felt a level of shame, but this was being replaced by gratitude and understanding.

Reflecting upon the key things that I believe helped me to come out of my self-absorbed state and back into my truer personality, I came up with the following list:

- A decreasing dose of prednisolone allowed more daylight into my mind.
- My improving health and rising body weight (when I reached 47kg (104lbs) my sense of humor returned).
- The challenge to my marriage, a precious jewel that I never thought I could lose, making me more honest about my behavior and my struggles.
- The realization that with intention and effort, I could still remember (I relived past hugs in my mind) and therefore connect to the kinder, more considerate side of my personality.

Realizing I could consciously choose to find (remember and feel) the compassionate side of myself and act from there was a turning point. This had always come easily to me in the past and now I had to actively reclaim it. Later I would discover the work of Kristin Neff and her book, *Self Compassion*,[1] which helped me to anchor this strategy. The four steps that she suggests you use when facing any struggle are:

1. Acknowledge to yourself that this is a moment of suffering.
2. Know that other people in the world are experiencing similar suffering.
3. Say to yourself, "may I hold my suffering with tenderness and kindness."
4. Say to yourself, "may I give myself the compassion that I need."

I find this approach helps me in tough moments to nurture myself and paradoxically stay open to others. Kristin's research has shown that people who practice self-compassion can more sustainably be compassionate towards others, that is, they are less likely to experience compassion fatigue. If you are struggling with this, then you might like to try it.

A word about Graves' disease

Like IBD, Graves' disease, a disease of the thyroid gland (located at the front of the neck), is considered an autoimmune condition, several of which can occur, as in my case, in the one person. My Graves' disease proved tricky to diagnose as it began its life presenting as a low thyroid activity problem (hypothyroidism), for which I was treated with thyroid hormone tablets, before it changed its mind and went to its inevitable overactive (thyrotoxicosis) form. During my first hospital admission for colitis, iodine within a contrast injection I was given for a CT scan of my abdomen, probably kick-started the thyrotoxicosis, iodine being the favorite mineral of the thyroid gland, excess intake of which can overexcite it.

It's a very unpleasant illness giving one a range of symptoms including palpitations, breathlessness, muscle wasting and weight loss, restlessness and anxiety. Untreated it can lead to a 'thyroid storm,' a massive outpouring of thyroid hormone causing heart failure and death.

When it was finally accurately diagnosed, the condition was brought under control with the medication, carbimazole (or methimazole), but continuing my seemingly endless ability to develop adverse drug reactions, three quarters of my body became covered in a weepy, raised, red, extremely itchy rash. I could not stop the medication because of the potential for a thyroid kickback, so I saw a skin specialist who treated me with an approach known as soak and smear. For five consecutive nights I was instructed to soak in a warm bath for 20 minutes, exit and whilst still wet, have my entire body smeared with a large tube of cortisone cream. Not quite as thrilling as it sounds.

Tori, of course, did most of the work, with my PD making the exercise of getting me into and out of the bath almost a Paralympic sport! Covered in cream, Tori would then help to dress me into my sexy (not) pajamas. Surprisingly this whole rigmarole only gave me a small amount of relief from the itchy torment that greeted my nightly sleep. This went on for months only improving a little when I was changed onto a different medication, propylthiouracil (PTU).

In a small percentage of people the thyroid resumes normal function after one or two years of treatment with medication. This did not happen in my case. So In October 2013 I underwent radioactive iodine treatment, which involved me swallowing a capsule containing radioactive iodine that was then taken up by my thyroid gland. This effectively destroyed the gland, meaning I now need to take thyroid hormone tablets for the rest of my life.

After several days delay, the radiation therapy left me feeling very ill, aggravating my Parkinson's so that my ability to move around was drastically curtailed for a couple of weeks. In addition, my singing voice, singing being one of my great pleasures, already weakened by my PD, seemed to leave town completely, my 2 ½ octave range reduced to a sad, single note. (This has partly recovered). At least I could take some solace in the fact that Graves' was one disease I now had under control.

By March 2014 my weight had risen to 60 kg (132 lbs). However, a course of antibiotics and/or the slackening of my dietary restriction (was it the bowl of white rice?), triggered a major colitis relapse. Having previously suffered major relapses three to four monthly, it had been 22 months between relapses of this magnitude and I'd gained 20 kg (44 lbs) in the meantime. How I dealt with this episode using a mastic gum supplement is outlined in the earlier Complementary Catch chapter.

During my travails, increasingly I was coming across bits of information and research that suggested a common origin for my various illnesses: the gut. Let me share some of my discoveries with you.

The Human Microbiome

Hippocrates' idea that illness begins with an unhealthy gut may turn out to be true. Seventy percent of the body's immune system resides in the walls and surrounds of the gastrointestinal system and is known as the Gut Associated Lymphoid Tissue (GALT). The importance of the interaction of this tissue with the microorganisms that live within and upon the gut lining is increasingly recognized by researchers. The bacterial, archeal (a newer category of microbe), fungal and viral intestinal communities are referred to as the gut microbiota. Their collective genomes (genetic codes) are referred to as the gut microbiome.[2] Eons of co-evolution have selected those species that bring no harm (commensals) and those that confer benefit to us (mutualists).[3]

This new understanding about the gut flies in the face of the popular belief that all bugs are bad and are to be feared, an attitude that has spawned the overzealous use of antiseptic products. As opposed to the benefits given by sanitation, there is a new and accepted counterbalancing theory, called the Hygiene Hypothesis. It essentially states the under exposure of children to bugs makes them both in childhood and in adulthood more prone to allergic, autoimmune and possibly many other diseases. This hypothesis has broadened our perspective from simply decreasing exposures to 'external' infectious microorganisms, like those on our skin,[4,5] to a more specific look at a lack of gut microbial exposure. The importance of this for normal immune development and regulation has become increasingly apparent.[6]

Until the 21st century it had been difficult to quantify the number and variety of bugs that live in our gut and throughout our bodies, as culturing them in the laboratory proved difficult (most of the gut bacteria are anerobes – they thrive in an oxygen free environment). It is estimated that only 20 to 30% of the bacteria present in the gut were able to be identified by culturing.[7] New techniques and technologies, such as DNA sequencing of the microbiome, give a much more accurate picture (much like the Hubble telescope did for astronomy), and have brought into clear focus the vast array of co-inhabitants we share this body with. Now, by reading the various DNA sequences present in our poo, we can identify precisely the variety of bugs we live with. The numbers are striking:

- For every human cell in our body there are 10 microorganisms. They reside on our skin and throughout our body, with the greatest collection in our large bowel (colon), which harbors the most densely populated ecosystem known, with approximately 10^{13}(that's 10 followed by 13 zeros!) bacteria.[8] This includes about 500 species and 30,000 subspecies and weighs 1 kg (60% of the dry mass of feces being bugs).[9]
- Collectively the gut microbiota contains approximately 3.3 million genes, almost 150 times more genes than the 23,000 contained within our human DNA.[10] So from a DNA perspective we are more than 99% microbe!

It's early days and there is so much more to learn, but we already know that these bugs play an important role in assisting with food absorption and positively or negatively modifying immune function and metabolism. When there is an imbalance of this system (dysbiosis), disease can follow. Dysbiosis is already implicated in diseases such as obesity, type 1 and type 2 diabetes, inflammatory bowel disease, and colorectal cancer. In addition to these diseases, abnormal patterns of microbial presence are being matched with many other diseases, implicating them as either a cause, a contributing factor, or an effect of the disease. I'll present more specific examples shortly, but for now let's start at first contact.

A relationship begins

Contrary to earlier beliefs, the womb is not a sterile environment. As a fetus we meet our first bacteria there.[11,12] But our most critical inoculation occurs at birth where, traversing through the birth canal and out into the world, we receive exposure to trillions of bugs from the vagina and perianal (around the anus) regions. Shortly after delivery the gut microbiota of a vaginally delivered infant resembles that of his or her mother's vagina.[13] In contrast, infants delivered by means of cesarean section (CS), initially acquire microbial communities typically found on maternal skin, followed by the gradual acquisition of a more complex microbiota, although usually more slowly than vaginally delivered infants.

Infants born by means of CS have a higher incidence of respiratory distress[14] and appear to be at higher risk for asthma and atopy,[15] obesity[16] and type 1 diabetes.[17] While cesarean section can be a life-saving procedure, these potential unhealthy effects on the child are a concern as the rates of CS deliveries are increasing globally.[18,19] It is postulated that a lack of early exposure to bugs that appropriately prime the immune system is the main cause of the deleterious impact of CS on a child's future health. For this reason, some mothers and some hospital birthing centers choose at the moment of delivery by CS, to place a swab into the mother's vagina then into the newborn's mouth, inoculating them with helpful bugs. A sensible idea, one would think, that is currently being trialed in some hospitals.

By the age of three or four years a fully established gut microbiome settles. Environmental influences such as diet and antibiotics are particularly important in this early period of life, breastfeeding initially and minimizing or avoiding antibiotics if possible, being ideal. While we know there are only a handful of bacterial groupings (phyla) that survive and colonize the human gut, the presence and variety of various species and subspecies differs greatly between individuals. So, each of us has our own unique colony of microbial 'friends.' Whereas we share more than 99% of the same 23,000 or so gene codes in our human cells with most humans on the planet, our gut microbiome may vary from our neighbors by more than 90%, showing us just how extensive the variety of microorganisms is. Identical twins don't have identical microbiomes, in fact they have as much similarity as non-identical twins in this regard. This suggests genetics plays less of a role than environmental contact when it comes to deciding which bugs we end up carrying around with us.

In healthy people the gut microbiota remains relatively stable throughout life, until they become elderly at which time diversity decreases. The reduction in diversity corresponds with and may account for the commonly seen increased susceptibility to infection, decrease in immune function (immunosenescence) and increase in chronic inflammatory diseases (inflammaging) as people age.[20]

Tending our bugs

While for most of us our gut microbiota is established by age four, the relative proportions of bugs are widely variable. Which of the bugs are in predominance at any given time is still dependent on many factors. Diet is the most obvious factor and a change of diet can dramatically alter the balance of power amongst those vying for a little bit of gut wall (mucosal) real estate. Antibiotics, stress and infections can also significantly impact this balance. Our understanding of how all this works is very new, but I believe it's worth thinking about attending to our microbiota as we might tend to our garden or our pets; feed and treat them well and they'll flourish.

One thing most researchers agree upon is that the best food for our gut microbiota is plant-based fiber. So we need to eat plenty of veggies, salad and fruits. It's useful to try and include the most fibrous bits like the stalk of the broccoli, the green leaves of leeks, the base of the asparagus and the skin of potatoes and pumpkin. Fiber promotes a healthy fermentation process in the colon producing short-chain fatty acids, like butyrate, propionate and acetate, considered good for health. Vinegar contains acetate and there is some evidence it could positively impact our gut microbiota as well.[21]

The good news is, changing our diet can change the balance of power within days or weeks so that health benefits may not take long to appear.[22]

Who's in charge?

There are many reasons why it can be difficult to change our eating habits. A novel one, recently recognized, is the influence of our gut bugs themselves. It seems they can manipulate our dietary choices through chemical messengers. It is thought that they do this by directly influencing our mood via the production of neurotransmitters (brain influencing chemicals), generating cravings for us to eat the sorts of foods which promote their survival and/or suppress their competitors.[23]

For instance, my wife and I can attest to the difficulty of removing sugar from our diet; we went cold turkey and found it took two weeks before the sugar cravings began to subside. How did we overcome the will of those tetchy, sugar-loving bacteria? All I can say is it wasn't easy and it involved having a small amount of protein, such as nuts or seeds, with every snack and sourcing alternative sweeteners, such as stevia, rice syrup and evaporated coconut nectar. We both found that if we ate just one sugary biscuit, the cravings for sugary sweets restarted and would last for at least a day or two. Fortunately, the longer we stuck with it, the more we craved healthier options, suggesting a successful leadership challenge had occurred in the gut microbiome, with the fruit and veggie loving bacteria now predominating.

Just how important the behavior changing influence of these bacteria can be, is evidenced by research involving obese and healthy rats. When the feces of the obese rats were transplanted into the gut of the healthy rats, the healthy rat's behavior changed; they began gorging on their food in the same way as their obese colleagues. This, along with metabolism changes, also triggered by the newly acquired bacteria, led them to becoming obese as well.[24]

When things go wrong

The following examples illustrate some of the associations that have been discovered between disease and our gut bacteria profiles:

- Healthy children in developing and tribal cultures have a greater diversity of microbes in their microbiome than healthy children in developed countries.[25,26] Our Western lifestyle with its high fat, high sugar, high-protein diet and widespread use of antibiotics, seems to be the culprit here. Research is implicating this diminished diversity as a contributing factor in the increasing prevalence of obesity, chronic disease and our decreasing resilience to infections.[27]

- In the human gut approximately 80% of the bacteria belong to either the major phyla of Firmicutes or Bacteroidetes. People with a higher proportion of Firmicutes are more likely to be obese. Interestingly, upon losing weight over 12 months, this relative misproportion of bacteria reverses.[28,29]

- Antibiotics have been given to farm animals to fatten them up for decades now. It seems they are capable of doing the same to us. Broad-spectrum antibiotics, which can alter the microbiota of the gut dramatically, when given to infants up to 23 months of age, significantly increases their risk of developing obesity as they grow older.[30]

- On the subject of obesity, of particular interest, and backing up the rat experiment presented earlier, is the fact that obese mice, who have the same microbiota pattern linked to obesity as we do, lose their tendency to obesity when the feces of thin mice are consumed by them (mice being coprophagic, i.e. they eat each other's poo).[31] This occurred independently of the amount of calories they consumed, suggesting a metabolic effect was at play here. So one important angle for tackling obesity will almost certainly be to help change the microbial balance in the gut.

- While it is unlikely to replace chocolate mousse on the menu any time soon, capsules containing healthy, frozen human feces are currently being used to successfully treat a serious gut infection caused by the bacteria, Clostridium Difficile.[32] Their use is likely to widen in future. It seems healthy poo may be powerful medicine. We'll tackle this subject in the next chapter.

- Children with lower than usual numbers of Firmicutes and a decreased microbial diversity are more likely to develop type 1 diabetes.[33] Rats who present a similar gut bacterial pattern that also makes them prone to diabetes, had their incidence of diabetes reduced by giving them antibiotics that altered this balance. This raises the wonderful possibility: could we prevent diabetes in children by improving their gut microbiota pattern?[34]

- High levels of the gut bacteria Prevotella have been strongly correlated with new onset untreated rheumatoid arthritis patients.[35] On the flipside, low levels of Prevotella have been correlated with autism.[36,37]

- Seventy-five percent of kidney stones contain oxalate. A bacteria found in the gut known as Oxalobacter Formigenes, helps to metabolize oxalate and those people with this bacteria are less likely to develop kidney stones.[38]

- As I mentioned in the previous chapter, inflammatory bowel disease (IBD) patients have 25% less diversity, based upon the number of microbial genes present, than healthy subjects. Patients with IBD have reduced numbers of the phyla Firmicutes and Bacteroidetes and increased numbers of Actinobacteria and Proteobacteria. However, it is not clear whether these differences are a cause or consequence of the development of IBD.[39-41]

- Bowel cancer and many other diseases including Parkinson's disease, have complex, specific patterns of dysbiosis associated with them.[42-47] Watch this research space for developing understanding of how these patterns emerge, understanding that will hopefully bring with it innovative treatments.

In the next chapter we'll look at one of these innovative treatments, Fecal Microbial Transplant (FMT).

Chapter 18

FECAL MICROBIAL TRANSPLANT (FMT) - REVITALIZING OUR GUT MICROBIOME

It was believed that the only good bacterium was a dead bacterium and their importance in maintaining health was unimaginable. We now appreciate that a well-balanced and diverse community of bacteria is crucial to the health of the host and we are learning that to restore such a balance once it has been interrupted can result in a miraculous cure.

DR LAWRENCE J BRANDT

Picture this; a nurse places fresh human poo into a blender with a bit of salty water (saline), blends it, then strains out larger impurities, sucks it up into a syringe and presto, trillions of bugs are ready for insertion. After healthy fecal donors are carefully screened, this is the nuts and bolts preparation behind FMT. It can then be inserted into the upper gut via a naso-duodenal tube, as is commonly done in Europe, or via the backside through a colonoscope or a simple rectal enema kit. More recently, as mentioned previously, it has also been given in the form of double encapsulated frozen capsules (*crapsules*) to be swallowed (you'd want to make sure it was 'double' encapsulated!). Regardless of which route it is taken by, it seems to be the ultimate probiotic.

Growing an enormous number of different vegetables in your vegetable patch so that there is little room for weeds, is the principal behind FMT. But, I hear you say, "someone else's poo, inserted into where? Disgusting!" It may have a high 'Yuk factor,' but inserting the healthy feces of one person into the unhealthy bowel of another person, so that the healthy bugs overwhelm the unhealthy ones, can be life-saving.

History

In 400 B.C. Hippocrates stated that, "...death sits in the bowels..." and "...bad digestion is the root of all evil...." Fecal transfer from healthy donors to the sick in order to treat disease has been described in the ancient medical literature.[1,2] In the 4th century in China, Ge Hong described the use of human fecal suspension by mouth for patients with food poisoning or severe diarrhea. The first literary record of the application of fecal transplantation was reported in the Chinese handbook of emergency medicine *Handy Therapy for Emergencies*, and at that time it was considered a medical miracle that brought patients back from the edge of death. Later in the 16th century, Li Shizhen described using fermented fecal solutions, fresh fecal suspensions, dry feces, or infant feces for treatment of severe diarrhea, fever, pain, vomiting and constipation. Alternative medicine doctors labelled these products with unique names such as 'yellow soup' to avoid patients' repugnance. In the 17th century, fecal transplant was used in veterinary medicine orally and rectally, and was termed 'transfaunation.'[3] Much later, Ralph Lewin reported that "...consumption of fresh, warm camel feces has been recommended by Bedouins as a remedy for bacterial dysentery; its efficacy was confirmed by German soldiers in Africa during World War II."[4]

A decade or so later the rise of a killer infection led to human donor feces being placed back on the medical menu. Clostridium difficile (CDiff) is a bacteria that can cause a serious bowel infection, most commonly as a result of a side-effect of antibiotic treatment. The incidence of this infection is rising globally.[5] In 2011 almost half a million people in the United States were documented to have CDiff infection, 29,000 of whom died from it.[6]

In terms of modern medicine, it wasn't until the late 1950s in the US that FMT was tried. It involved a man with CDiff who was not responding to other treatments and whose next stop would have been the morgue. Remarkably, he rapidly recovered, so much so, he was able to go home within 48 hours.[7] FMT continues to be used to treat CDiff, its efficacy confirmed by trials and now widely accepted.[8] Currently CDiff is the only condition for which FMT is approved by medical authorities, although this may change as it has recently been tested affirmatively as a treatment for Ulcerative Colitis.[9] In addition, pioneers in the field have made some serendipitous observations, yet to be confirmed by trials, in which FMT seems to benefit other conditions as well.

Beyond Clostridium Difficile

My interest in FMT was awakened in 2011 when I read an article in *New Scientist* magazine referring to the work of Prof Thomas Borody.[10] Borody, a pioneer in the broader use of FMT, had been using this treatment for severe cases of irritable bowel syndrome and inflammatory bowel disease (IBD), as well as CDiff, since the mid-1990s. The article in question referred to a gentleman who was receiving treatment for chronic constipation and was incidentally also suffering from Parkinson's disease. Incredibly, not only was his constipation resolved, but his Parkinson's symptoms disappeared too! Borody had also documented cases with other serious illnesses, including MS,[11] which had inexplicably resolved following FMT treatment.

There are other diseases documented in the medical research literature that have been observed to resolve or significantly improve following FMT: idiopathic constipation,[12] nonalcoholic fatty liver disease,[13] sclerosing cholangitis,[14] idiopathic thrombocytopenic purpura,[15] myoclonus dystonia,[16] insulin resistance and metabolic syndrome,[17] chronic fatigue syndrome,[18] autism,[19] and stress-related behavior and anxiety.[20]

The intestinal microbiota in these diseases requires further investigation before conclusions can be drawn about their role, if any, in pathogenesis (disease causation). The therapeutic role of FMT in particular opens up exciting new angles of research.

Diving in

If FMT is having a therapeutic effect beyond the gut walls, how might this be so? The most obvious proposition is that changes in immune function are triggered by an altered microbiome. Given, as I alluded to earlier, that 70% of the body's immune system is located in and around the gut, along with the fact that gut bacteria have been shown to interact via chemical messengers with immune cells, thereby altering their function,[21] this seems likely.

Another possible mechanism comes from research suggesting that Parkinson's disease originates in the gut, with a toxin being transported via the vagus nerve. This nerve collects into a bundle, nerve fibers from the entire gut wall and carries their messages all the way up to the brain.[22] Could altering the microbiome and thereby preventing toxins from feeding up into the brain from an unhealthy gut, allow the nervous system an opportunity to heal? Even from the incurable Parkinson's disease? This was too important a possibility for me to ignore, so along with the huge potential for resolution of my debilitating Ulcerative Colitis, this was my hope as I embarked upon an FMT.

When I discovered that gastroenterologist Dr Paul Froomes was performing FMT in Melbourne, my heart leapt. I'd considered it for a number of years, but the impracticality and the expense of doing it through Dr Borody in Sydney had been insurmountable. The very real chance of getting on top of my Ulcerative Colitis (UC) and the outside chance of improving my Parkinson's disease had been tantalizing, and now it suddenly seemed within reach.

A friend also put us in touch with a physiotherapist, I'll call Sally, who'd benefited greatly from the procedure with Dr Froomes. Sally's 20+ year history of Irritable Bowel Syndrome and chronic fatigue had left her only able to work part-time. Three months after the FMT her energy began to build, so much so that six months later she had taken on a Master's degree whilst continuing part-time work. Sally assured me this was the best thing she had done to improve her health in 20 years. I wanted some of what Sally had! (Note: Her story appears at the end of this chapter).

The plan drawn up for me was to have the initial dosage inserted via colonoscopy, followed by nine fecal retention enemas (with useful instructions from Paul's nurse Danielle). The regimen involved an enema daily for four consecutive days following the colonoscopy, then one fortnightly for 10 weeks. (Note: A patient with less chronic health problems than myself may require less FMTs to establish their new gut microbiome. There is not enough research to confirm the ideal regimen as yet.)

My preparation involved two weeks of antibiotics to, in theory, clear out as many of the old unhelpful bugs as possible to make way for the new ones. This left me feeling ill but at least I knew it was for a good cause. The usual bowel prep formula was recommended prior to the colonoscopy to complete the job.

We booked a self-contained apartment in Melbourne near Essendon Private Hospital, where the procedure was to take place. Inexplicably, the bowel prep, which all my friends with prior knowledge assured me would involve at least 20 explosive visits to the toilet, failed to fire. Dejected, we had to cancel the procedure. It took a further 10 days, in which I was particularly wobbly on my feet, for the prep to leave my system and then several months to get my strength and confidence back to face up to it all again.

Some months later, on Paul's advice, we tried an alternative preparatory approach: 48 hours of nothing but clear fluids along with colonic irrigations on those two consecutive days. Taxing, but it worked. We arrived at the hospital on a hot North wind day at 8.30 a.m., some 30 minutes after the healthy donors had delivered their precious poo, that soon would be inserted into my colon. In order to maintain a healthy bacterial content, these samples would need to be used within six hours or frozen for later use. Paul used the fresh stuff. I was fifth on his list that morning and the whole procedure took less than half an hour, so that I found myself awakened from the anesthetic by 12.30 p.m.

The first thing I noticed was my colon felt settled, more settled than it had felt in years. Sally had used the same expression to describe her initial experience to me. In the five years since I'd developed UC a background irritability threatening and/or developing into a bowel motion was with me most of the time. Now it was gone.

The follow-up fecal retention enemas were more challenging than I'd expected, being both exhausting and at times difficult to retain. The idea was to hold onto the enema for at least 35 minutes, but ideally up to four hours, to allow the new bugs to attach to the bowel wall from where they could spread to the rest of the colon.

After we'd spent the initial week in Melbourne for the first four enema FMTs, Tori had to drive a three hour round-trip to pick up a fortnightly fresh sample and deliver it to my rear. The enema was contained within two full 60 ml syringes and ejected via a long, thin rubber tubing. A practical tip: I found the further the tubing was inserted, the easier it was to retain the enema. We also discovered administering it on two separate occasions, by freezing one syringe for later, also increased my chances of retention. Due to the Parkinson's limiting my flexibility, Tori had to do the honors (so to speak), but most people manage to self-administer the enemas.

In the initial weeks following FMT my bowel felt foreign to me. What do I mean by this? It's just that I was unfamiliar with the signals it was giving, leaving me at times unsure whether I needed to go to the toilet or not. Rather than colitis, with its characteristic loose stools, the first two months were characterized by constipation. The key to managing this, along with maximizing the chances that the new microbiome would develop healthily and settle in, was to increase my fiber and water intake. I welcomed my trillions of new friends with a predominantly plant-based, wholefood diet, including a raw food smoothie with fruit, green leaf vegetables, nuts and seeds each morning.

Blissfully, I had none of the mouth ulcers that had plagued me whenever colitis threatened. To our delight my general stamina was also increasing, allowing Tori and me to get out and about more without the anxiety of having to rush to the nearest loo. Two weeks before my recommended three monthly top up enema, I did notice an increased bowel irritability which settled following the additional FMT. These three monthly top ups apparently can be lengthened to 6 monthly and eventually will not be required. Paul indicated it would take nine months for the improved immune system benefits to be fully apparent, so that I could yet see benefits for my Parkinson's symptoms. At the seven-month point, as I'm writing this, there may be some signs of minor improvements. I remain hopeful.

Research confirms potential

Seven and a half months after I received my first FMT, the largest research study yet to look at the potential of FMT in treating Ulcerative Colitis was presented. This took place in San Diego at the Digestive Diseases Week 2016 conference. Lead researcher, Dr Paramsothy, a gastroenterologist from the University of New South Wales, and his team, had enrolled 81 patients across three Australian study sites. Forty-one of the patients received FMT treatment and 40 received placebo, or non-active treatment. All had active Ulcerative Colitis and were resistant (as I was) to standard treatments, such as corticosteroids. Patients received their first FMT or placebo treatment through a colonoscope. Subsequently, participants were given enemas that were self-administered five days per week for eight weeks. "By using fecal microbiota transplantation, we aim to treat the underlying cause of Ulcerative Colitis instead of just its symptoms, as opposed to the majority of therapies currently available," Dr Paramsothy said.

After eight weeks, more than three times as many FMT patients had responded to treatment than those in the control group. Specifically, 11 of the 41 FMT patients (27 percent) achieved the study's primary goal — patients reporting no UC symptoms and doctors determining the lining of the digestive tract had healed or substantially improved, by viewing it on colonoscopy. Only three of the 40 patients (8 percent) in the control group reached this goal. When researchers looked at just the number of patients who reported being symptom-free (and discounted clinician observation of the colon), they found that 44 percent of FMT patients reported improvement versus 20 percent in the control group.

Dr Paramsothy concluded: "Our study has been able to show definitively that fecal microbiota transplantation is an effective treatment for Ulcerative Colitis. This is important because there are millions of people worldwide seeking alternative treatments for their condition." I would add this is especially so when patients are no longer responding to Western medication, as was the case with all the patients in this trial.[23]

Hopeful as this research may be, particularly for those people affected by inflammatory bowel disease (IBD), one still has to acknowledge that in this study less than half of the patients responded with improvement. It is unclear why some patients with IBD respond so impressively after FMT while others fail to respond. It is clear however that FMT is not a 'one size fits all' and there appears to be many factors that play a role in the success of this modality in the treatment of IBD. More investigation is required to increase our understanding of how to use it most effectively.[24]

Further research linking the gut to Parkinson's disease is also continuing. The key pathological finding in PD is the abnormal build-up of a protein known as alpha-synuclein in the cells of the nervous system. This abnormality is found in nerve cells surrounding the gut prior to it being evident in the brain. It is thought to lead to gastrointestinal dysfunction in the form of constipation, which characteristically precedes the cardinal symptoms of PD by many years. This has led to the hypothesis that PD begins in the gut and may relate to the microorganisms that reside there. A study which looked at the microbiome of 72 PD patients and compared them to 72 healthy people, found evidence of specific patterns of bacterial presence that were predictive of PD. For example, a relative abundance of the bacterial family Enterobacteriaceae was positively associated with the severity of balance and gait difficulties in people with PD.[25] This research might provide some reasoning as to why FMT could positively influence PD and I eagerly await trials to test this hypothesis.

A Microbiotic Revolution?

We could be on the brink of a paradigm shift in the way we treat disease.[26] Just as the antibiotic revolution changed the practice of Medicine in the middle of last century, finding friendly bugs with which to both prevent and treat disease may soon do the same. Perhaps it will even help us to fight the so-called antibiotic resistant superbugs by using the FMT model of overwhelming them with helpful competitor microorganisms. In future, we may very well be spraying our hospitals and our homes with helpful microorganisms rather than with antiseptics.

This should not be too strange an idea, given most of us have ingested helpful microorganisms as a part of our diet in the form of probiotics. Probiotics are foods (eg yoghurt, kefir, sauerkraut) or products that contain live microorganisms that can benefit us. Complementing these are prebiotics like fructooligosaccharides (FOS), galactooligosaccharides (GOS), xylooligosaccharides (XOS), inulin and pectin. These are indigestible fibers that are not absorbed by the gut, but which act as a healthy food source for the good bacteria in the colon. Both prebiotics and probiotics (termed Synbiotics when combined) are considered to be food supplements, known as functional foods. Prebiotics have a potentially positive effect on health beyond basic nutrition. Functional foods have been demonstrated to alter, modify and reinstate the pre-existing intestinal flora.[27] If one stops ingesting them, their presence in the gut is undetectable within weeks.[28] This is unlike FMT which is thought to permanently implant a changed pattern in the gut microbiome.

While there are many probiotics on the market, there is a lack of large research trials to back up their effectiveness. This said, meta-analysis of several randomized controlled trials has confirmed benefit for the administration of the bacteria, Lactobacillus rhamnosus GG, and the yeast, Saccharomyces boulardii, to prevent antibiotic-associated diarrhea and to treat acute infectious diarrhea.[29,30] Individual studies have also suggested the benefits of probiotics to prevent acute gastroenteritis (eg. when travelling overseas) and to serve as a useful adjunctive treatment in Ulcerative Colitis, pouchitis, antibiotic-associated diarrhea, CDiff, functional abdominal pain, Irritable Bowel Syndrome, and colic in breastfed babies. Although promising, larger well-designed studies need to confirm these findings.[31] If you have to have a course of antibiotics, however, it seems reasonable to follow this up with an increase in your intake of cultured foods and /or a course of probiotics.

Beyond the broad brush strokes of probiotics, prebiotics and FMT, scientists are trying to harvest specific key bacteria from healthy human feces, to be grown up to a standardized dose and used as a targeted therapy for particular conditions. For example, traditional native peoples, still on their traditional diet, have healthy bugs in their bowels that we lost long ago. While this research may reveal invaluable treatments in future, I suspect that the broad treatment of FMT, with its complete diverse ecosystem replacement, will remain an important option. Beyond this, the ultimate long-term treatment and the key for maintaining our good health is our diet.

Sally's story (in her words)

"My name is Sally, and I am 47 years old. I have had 'bad tummy problems,' eczema and other allergy symptoms since age 9 which gradually worsened over the years and I became quite sick in 2007/8, when all my symptoms multiplied and became very severe. This is despite numerous conventional (strong cortisone and other creams, U/V therapy) and natural treatments (diets, herbal medicine, homeopathy, etc). I drew the line at internal cortisone and immuno-suppressive drugs, considering them not addressing the cause of the problem.

From 2009 I started seeing an integrative medicine GP and we found out eventually that I have multiple food sensitivities, multiple chemical sensitivities (notably all scents including perfumes, essential oils, etc); candida overgrowth and leaky gut/intestinal dysbiosis. This explained why diets excluding single or just a few food items never worked for me as I was still reacting to other items, and why herbal medicines, juicing, concentrated food supplements and fermented foods never helped me, in fact, they only made me worse and this has puzzled many a naturopath. However, finding the cause(s) did not really lead to a permanent solution. I still had a lot of symptoms on a daily basis despite major changes to my life. Things were still up and down. Fatigue was such a big issue; I stopped working as a naturopath (also because of disillusionment) and had to reduce my work hours as a physiotherapist drastically.

At the end of 2014 I decided to have an FMT – fecal microbial transplant. It's been the single item that has made the most consistent and most global results to date. I have been told I will improve over several years with regular top-ups. (Following my initial five FMTs in December 2014, I have had a total of seven top ups in the past 12 months.) It is still experimental at this stage for IBS and there are a lot of unknowns. I have noticed improvements in many of my symptoms including – sleep, memory/cognition, moods (calmer/able to handle stress better), energy and motivation, skin, gut and digestion, hair, joint and muscle pains, weakness, immune system, sinuses, etc. I have also been able to stop or reduce some medications/supplements that I couldn't do without before. The list is not exhaustive and the improvements are not always immediate. I started studying Masters part-time this year – I would not have been able to cope if it were not for the FMT. However, I am not there yet, 'it's a long, long road...' (as my favorite lyrics go!). Recently I had severe exacerbation of all my symptoms in Spring – traditionally a bad time for me.

Thankfully an FMT enema top up, whilst not returning my health to pre-Spring levels, again significantly improved my symptoms. It was amazing to see the rash on my body fade away within a few days, retreating back to its 'normal' areas. The FMT is the only thing I've found that makes that big a difference.

Throughout the years, I have never doubted I would ever 'get there.' Of course I had and still have bad days/periods where I feel defeated but I never lost sight of my goal. I have always considered myself lucky despite being plagued with ill-health all these years: I can walk, I can work (even though part-time), I have a very stable family life with supportive husband and others, I can find the money to access expensive treatments like FMT, there are good medical services in the area I live. I have always found gratitude a very good recipe for happiness. Oh, and having fun/laughter and daily meditation help tremendously."

Chapter 19

PARKINSON'S DISEASE - MY EXPERIENCE

This is a very important lesson. You must never confuse faith that you will prevail in the end - which you can never afford to lose - with the discipline to confront the most brutal facts of your current reality whatever they might be.

VICE ADMIRAL JAMES STOCKDALE, POW SURVIVOR
AFTER 7 YEARS OF BRUTAL CAPTIVITY IN
HAO LO PRISON, NORTH VIETNAM.

Don't deny the disease. Just defy the verdict that is supposed to go with it.

NORMAN COUSINS

The disabling experience of chronic disease can be unrelenting. My own experiences with Chronic Fatigue Syndrome, Irritable Bowel Syndrome, Inflammatory Bowel Disease, Graves' disease, frozen shoulders, severe physical deconditioning (muscle and weight loss), adverse drug reactions, depression, severe eczema and Parkinson's disease (PD) have tested my capacity for enduring suffering and sheer frustration. At times it has sucked the will to live out of me. As a doctor I'm aware that people, who have multiple medical assaults either from disease, medical treatments, or both, can come to a point where enough is enough. Many times I've been close to giving up the fight and I've needed to dig deep into the basket of hope to find reasons to carry on.

Perhaps if I had been born with a disabling condition it would be different, but for a good part of my first 35 years I took for granted that my body basically did what I asked it to do; most of us live this way. A bout of acute illness, such as gastro, may for a short time remind us of our vulnerability, but this is quickly forgotten when everything returns to health. Chronic disease does not provide one with this delicious gift.

Two of my chronic diseases were now well-managed. Graves' disease conventionally with radioactive iodine and thyroid hormone replacement, Ulcerative Colitis more outside the medical square with mastic gum, diet and FMT. This allowed me the opportunity to see what could be done to improve my experience of PD. It had been deteriorating significantly in the background as I spent years dealing with survival issues.

In order to give you some insight into what it's like to have PD, let me start by sharing the following essay, originally written for family and closest friends. Writing this helped me to be honest about the reality I was facing with Parkinson's disease, especially whilst I was unable to tolerate appropriate medication (an ongoing issue). A caveat here - for at least the first seven years after diagnosis most PD patients who tolerate medication do not experience this level of PD severity.

Sweet Movement – A Reflection on Parkinson's disease
July 6, 2013

Have you ever thought how wonderful it is to be able to walk or grab a mouthful of food? Do you ever reflect upon the many amazing movements your body can make without a conscious thought; from swiftly hopping onto a train, to picking your nose? I never did, but I do now. Parkinson's disease (PD) has made this so.

Just initiating a movement can make me appear like a frozen computer screen. Waiting for a signal to pass through. I stand bent forwards, statuesque, willing my legs to move, but they do not. When I do move, it is in slow motion or in an overbalancing quick-step, unsteady as if intoxicated. The effort required to walk any distance, at times, can feel like walking through wet cement carrying a 50kg pack. Functional Magnetic Resonance Imaging (fMRI) confirms this. A healthy person uses only a fraction of their brain's activity to walk, while a PD sufferer needs just about every brain cell firing.[1] The automatic pilot has left the control room, so movements, like walking, that barely required a thought, now need my maximal concentrated effort.

Dexterous, speedy, fluid and graceful do not describe my movement. Frozen, hesitant, shuffling, shaky, clumsy and slow are closer to the Bulls Eye. The medical facts indicate the cardinal features of PD to be slowness of movement, rigid stiff muscles,tremor at rest, and posture, balance and gait problems, creating a high risk of falling. This does not tell you about other 'motor' (movement) features, like a loss of manual dexterity. I find typing these words and using mobile phones extremely difficult, while brushing my teeth is now impossible without an electric brush.

As is typical, to start with, one side of my body was affected more than the other. A right-sided drooping foot, eye-lid and smile told my story. I rarely shake, however, as not all people with PD do. This is a blessing as it allows me to sit in a public space unnoticed, apart from my Botox-like expressionless face. "Free plastic surgery," I hear some of you say, yet this anti-ageing face mask of PD feels like a cage to me. Other so called 'non-motor' features include loss of one's sense of smell, frozen shoulder, constipation and severe fatigue, all of which I experience. These features can precede the full development of PD, with its cardinal features, by many years, as it did with me. In these early years, it is difficult for a doctor to make a diagnosis. Not surprisingly, fifty percent of Parkinson's sufferers also have depression, both a response to the disease and as a result of the disease, which affects mood centers in the brain.

To try and bring across more of the impact that Parkinson's has had on my life, I thought I'd share some of the things that I miss being able to do. Like getting out of a chair without great effort; rolling over in bed without assistance; drying myself after a shower; dressing without assistance; walking more than 100 meters (or yards) unaided; driving a car; using a fork and knife without making a complete mess of myself; and swimming, one of my great loves. Oh, and don't ask me to turn around quickly, as I can't and if I try, I am liable to fall over. Because I once did all of these things thousands of times with ease, each time I attempt them now, I am still surprised and then frustrated by my body's inability to respond to my request. Only in my dreams, or in deep meditation or when engrossed in a TV show can I forget I have PD. As soon as I need to move, it's back.

PD occurs in about 2% of the population aged above 50, although 5% of PD patients are aged between 20 and 40. It's classified as a Neurodegenerative Movement Disorder. While symptoms can be improved with treatment, it is a slowly progressive disease with no known cure to date. Communication issues between brain cells (neurons) are the problem. The neurons most affected are those producing the neurotransmitter, dopamine. Most of the dopamine producing brain cells are located in an area of the brain known as the basal ganglia, within a region called the substantia nigra. It is only when 70-80% of the dopamine producing cells of the substantia nigra lose their ability to function, that the cardinal PD symptoms appear and it can be diagnosed.[2]

The ongoing brain damage of this condition leads to my lack of physical flexibility, difficulty walking and poor coordination. Walking whilst carrying something is like walking on a tightrope. Hence, if I wish to bring a glass of water from one spot to another or a plate of food for that matter, I risk significant fallout. I've learnt to either ask someone else to do so or to use my walker as a carrying surface, not always a successful option.

Some days are better than others, but regardless of how I'm going, I tend to try and walk without any aids whilst inside my home. This sometimes means that I career, in a semi-controlled fashion, from armchair into kitchen bench then into the nearest wall, using my arms to keep me upright. My wife has learnt to find this amusing, but new guests can be alarmed and sometimes lurch towards me to break my apparent fall.

I have had a few spectacular falls over the years resulting in some seriously bruised ribs and lacerations. Often these have happened on my good days, when I become a little too overconfident with my walking ability. In my most recent fall I started gaining pace walking towards the back step to our deck; building forward momentum is one of the potential problems with Parkinson's. My drooping right foot clipped the final step and like Superman, I hurtled forwards releasing my walking stick and rotating in midair. Unfortunately, I landed like Clark Kent, hitting my right shoulder, ribs and head. Bringing up the rear with the shopping, Tori had a 'terrorific' view and she was certain I'd broken my hip. Being winded, I was unable to reassure her for some time. I knew it was either my shoulder or my ribs and soon realized neither were broken. Still, for the next three weeks rolling over in bed was accompanied by some choice vocalizations.

One of the biggest adjustments I've had to come to terms with is a loss of independence. Even when I fall over, I am unable to return to an upright position without assistance. In order to give Tori a break from having to constantly be my carer, I've needed to allow other carers into my home. This has been both a challenging and enriching experience; I've met some fine human beings. I'm now much less proud about asking for help and have been delighted to learn how willing so many people are to offer assistance in any given moment.

Losing independence and physical abilities has confronted my self-image. In the past I had not reflected much upon this. Now, if I stumble or drop food from my mouth in a public space, I'm acutely self-aware. Having to 'rush' to the nearest loo with Inflammatory Bowel Disease doesn't help. Combined with the excessive effort it takes to get out and about, the temptation has been to avoid public spaces and even friends altogether. Isolation and depression result. As much as I enjoy my own company, I have discovered how much I also need people contact and times out in the community. When I was well, these events happened effortlessly, now I have to overcome my aversions and make the effort to interact. To buffer against feelings of embarrassment, I carry my sense of humor with me and try to relate from my bright unchanging self, the part of me behind the PD mask that never ages.

The battle for my sanity does not end here. Appreciating and focusing on what I can do rather than what I can't do has been invaluable advice. Unable to work, I must find meaning and purpose in other activities. Sharing my insights through writing, like this, is definitely one of these. To this end I have joined a writing group. Working towards a healthier life, a future foreseen where my body will once again allow me to be more participatory in the world, is another. Currently, there is no proven cure for PD. Medication can ameliorate symptoms effectively for some years, but can also be problematic as it has been for me. Hence, Deep Brain Stimulation surgery is under consideration. Apart from medication, the things I've found most beneficial include a good night's sleep, stretching, exercise, such as on a Pilates Reformer, treadmill or stationary bike, meditation, cranial osteopathy, and a regular Bowen massage.

Being proactive and making sure I do activities that bring me joy has also been vital. Regular dates with Tori and cuppas with friends who like to laugh tops the list. Singing helps to lift my spirits too and keeps my voice strong, while dancing any old way to music, even for just a couple of minutes, feels liberating and loosens rigid muscles. Balancing all this activity with meditative short rests in my armchair helps maintain my energy. This said, making sure I don't sit in one position for too long prevents me from stiffening up. Getting trapped in front of the TV is a challenge, so I try to stand up in the Ad breaks.

Innovative therapies for PD are being developed and I am exploring the ones that make sense to me. Wishful thinking or not, they give me reason to get out of bed, stretch and exercise my body, for as I have learnt, hope is the blood of the soul.

Tracking down a cause?

While the exact cause of Parkinson's disease is unknown, it's thought that genetic predispositions 'load the gun,' while exposure to environmental factor(s) 'pull the trigger.' In my case, both my father and my aunt (my father's sister) developed PD. Due to the Second World War I'm unaware of any records of PD amongst past family members who lived in Romania. All I know is my grandfather was killed in a concentration camp, while my father's older brother, Carl, died in a forced labor camp aged 14. There is no known history of PD on my mother's side of the family tree (also from Romania).

My father, Lee Sommer, prior to his diagnosis in his mid-60s, a little like myself, had a 10 year history of diminished energy and drive, which led to him retiring early and selling his floor-covering retail business. My aunt, Rosina, was diagnosed in her 70s following a five-year illness that had been diagnosed as Fibromyalgia. Both Lee and Rosina spent more than 30 years working in a floor covering retail environment. This has significant implications that I will get to in a moment.

Having a family history of PD and/or specific identified genetic patterns increases one's risk of developing it. Environmental factors have also been identified, including pesticide exposure, rural living, well-water drinking, and having a farming occupation. Conversely coffee consumption, cigarette smoking, and some genetic patterns have been found to decrease one's risk.[3,4] I have no regrets about being a non-smoker, but do wish I'd developed a taste for coffee! As presented in the previous chapter, amongst all these factors we need to consider dysbiosis of the gut microbiome as playing some kind of role as well.

Of all the chemical exposures that have been linked to Parkinson's, the most consistently reported have been pesticides. One of these, permethrin, used to deter dust mite, has been identified as a part of the chemical cocktail sprayed onto new carpets.[5] Another chemical linked to PD development that has been used in many industries, including the floorcovering business (in carpet cleaners and glues), is Trichloroethylene (TCE), a solvent and known neurotoxin that's also the most common organic contaminant in groundwater.[6,7] Novel ways of assisting people with Parkinson's to clear out the buildup of toxic proteins in their brain cells is a promising area of research, but it's early days.[8]

As a kid I spent hours playing in my father's carpet shop, climbing and rolling over new carpet and vinyl rolls, breathing in the chemical fumes, smells I can recall to this day. The lag period between such chemical exposure and the development of PD can be up to 40 years.[9] Whilst other people with this level of exposure would probably not develop PD, my familial susceptibility may have ensured that I did. There was a further specific genetic reason for this.

In recent years the importance of the B vitamin folate has become apparent in disease prevention. It is a vital substance in a process known as methylation. Methylation plays a role in many important functions including DNA repair, detoxification, and energy metabolism (you may recall its critical part in epigenetics – see Epigenetics chapter). Defects in epigenetic methylation are considered a possible trigger mechanism in the development of neurodegenerative diseases, such as PD and Alzheimer's disease.[10] The effectiveness of folate utilization in promoting healthy methylation is largely determined by how efficient an enzyme in the body known as Methylenetetrahydrofolate Reductase (MTHFR) is operating.[11] If it is sluggish, then any folate absorbed by the body will be less effective in preventing the build-up in the bloodstream of a chemical known as homocysteine. High levels of homocysteine produce inflammation via oxidative stress, a chemical process which is damaging to various body cells, including those of the cardiovascular system and the brain.

In 2014 a research paper reported that PD patients with a particularly sluggish version of MTHFR (the C677T variety, found in 5 to 15% of the population)[12] were much more likely to develop PD at an earlier age (mean age of onset 49 years, compared with the average age of onset of 61 years).[13] Other research supports this finding, discovering that early-onset PD patients have decreased methylating abilities.[14] When I had a blood test to determine my MTHFR status, I discovered that bingo, I had the C677T homozygous variety (i.e. the sluggish version that operates at 30% of the efficiency of the healthiest version). Another piece in my causation puzzle found. To improve my body's methylation performance, I now take an MTHF supplement, although this has not been tested by PD researchers as yet.

Putting a timeline together

Born 1961	Genetic predisposition to PD from my father's side, along with the sluggish version of MTHFR (C677T) making me prone to developing PD at an early age. Second-generation Holocaust traumas underlying.
Childhood	Exposure to floorcovering industrial chemicals linked to PD development.
	• Bullied (childhood bullying increases the risk of developing CFS) • Head injury (knocked unconscious playing Australian Rules Football aged 14) can be relevant to developing PD.
1992	Multiple health problems begin: due to overstretching my work capacities and excessive internal drive? Or just bad luck?
1993	Food poisoning triggers Irritable Bowel Syndrome (IBS).
1996	Comprehensive health breakdown: Chronic Fatigue Syndrome (CFS) and/or early PD?
1997	Depression, severe constipation and loss of sense of smell; first symptoms of PD?
2002	Loss of the ability to rapidly rotate my wrist whilst brushing my teeth (another sign of PD).
2004	Left frozen shoulder.
2007	Right frozen shoulder.
2009	PD diagnosis aged 47.
2010	Inflammatory Bowel Disease (IBD) - Ulcerative Colitis initial attack.
2011	Graves' disease diagnosed.
2012	Life-threatening acute Ulcerative Colitis episode.
2015	Fecal Microbial Transplant (October).

Parkinson's – the back story

Let me present to you how the management of my PD evolved.

Following 15 months of trying, with minimal success, to manage PD without medication, I commenced the most effective treatment for this condition, levodopa/carbidopa, under the supervision of neurologist, Associate Prof David Williams. It must be emphasized that levodopa treats the symptoms but does not stop the underlying disease from progressing. Hence it becomes less and less effective over time, and side-effects, including sudden abnormal movements (dyskinesias), become more likely as the dose is increased.

After slowly increasing my dose of levodopa over two months, I reached a dosage of one tablet twice a day. To my delight, my energy levels returned to a point I had not experienced in 15 years. My other PD symptoms also improved markedly and I was able to walk far more easily. Unfortunately, a skin rash developed and as I've outlined earlier, my bowels went into conniptions. I was soon in hospital, seriously ill with colitis. Levodopa was the suspected trigger and I discontinued it. Since then Prof Williams has had two other PD patients with this rare colitis side-effect.

Further medication trials (apomine infusion, rasagiline) followed, but my body failed to tolerate them. So my next step was to consult with neurologist Dr Sanjay Raghav. I'd heard he practiced integrative medicine. He emphasized the importance of yoga exercises and taught me some useful breathing and sounding techniques. Under his guidance I was referred to an Ayuvedic natural therapist who prescribed Macuna Pruriens, a legume (velvet bean) containing levodopa, used in India to treat Parkinson's for thousands of years. Although large trials have never been conducted on Macuna, its potential is acknowledged by medical researchers. It is considered a viable low-cost alternative to levodopa medication for treating people affected by PD in poorer countries.[15,16] After three weeks taking the recommended dose I developed a serious allergic skin reaction that required five days of high-dose prednisolone to settle.

An old medication revisited

By this stage my balance was worsening and I could barely walk without assistance; all outings required a wheelchair. I was beginning to despair that I would ever find a PD medication that I could tolerate, when Dr Raghav suggested amantadine. Amantadine was originally approved in 1966 as a treatment to prevent influenza A, a form of the flu. In 1969 it was accidentally discovered to improve symptoms of Parkinson's disease as well. Its benefits for PD are variable and often short lived, so it is not often the first medication of choice. In fact, a Cochrane review in 2003 concluded there was insufficient evidence in support/or against its efficacy and safety as a treatment for PD.[17] Nonetheless, it works for some people and I had a history with this little pill. Let me explain.

Back in 1988 I did a stint as a Resident Medical Officer at Fairfield Infectious Diseases Hospital. During this time there was an outbreak of Influenza A. All staff members were instructed to take amantadine. I experienced no problems taking the medication and never came down with the flu. I also rang Dr Peter Bruckner, who was the club doctor of my favorite Australian Football League (AFL) team, Melbourne, and tipped him off. (Note: amantadine is not on the World Anti-Doping Agency (WADA) list of banned drugs in sport).[18] You see, football is a winter sport. So, Dr Bruckner subsequently placed all the players on amantadine for the winter. That season, many of the other teams were ravaged by the flu, detracting from their performance, whilst all Melbourne players remained flu-free.

I was amused when I read a newspaper article that talked about a mystery caller who'd advised the Melbourne Football Club to use a secret flu-preventing medication. Melbourne went on to make the Grand Final (Australia's version of the Super Bowl) that year and I was invited to and attended their training sessions leading up to it. I was also one of a hundred thousand screaming football fans that packed the MCG stadium for the big game. Unfortunately, they stumbled at the final hurdle and received the biggest shellacking in history (to that time) from the Hawthorn Football Club!

So when Dr Raghav suggested amantadine, I wasn't sure I was going to win the Grand Final with it, but I was at least confident that I would tolerate it. The good news was that not only did I tolerate it, it improved my symptoms significantly; balance, gait and dexterity all improved. It also allowed me to increase my exercise routine as I was taking longer to tire. What a relief; it was like finally being released from the constraints of a maximum security 'body-prison' into a more spacious correctional facility. Sadly, three weeks later, I developed severe generalized muscle pain, a side-effect. It worsened with any physical activity and I had to cease the medication on Dr Raghav's advice. Perhaps the Grand Final shellacking was an omen after all. What can I say? The search continues.

Chapter 20

PARKINSON'S - LOOKING BEYOND MEDICATION

... it may be one step forward and two steps back, but after a time with Parkinson's, I've learned that what is important is making that one step count; always looking up.

MICHAEL J FOX

Electrical treatments

Beyond medication, the main medical option available for me to consider is Deep Brain Stimulation (DBS) surgery. DBS can be as or more effective than levodopa. It involves about six hours of open brain surgery whilst you are awake. Wires are carefully inserted that can electrically stimulate specific areas of the brain damaged in PD. These wires connect to a single wire which runs underneath the skin to attach to a container housing a battery and an Implantable Pulse Generator, much like a heart pacemaker. This is usually located under the skin of the upper chest.[1]

The intensity of the stimulation can be adjusted wirelessly and it can take some months to find the settings most suited to an individual. I have come across people affected by PD who have benefited greatly from this procedure, but have also come across others whose condition improved very little or had worsened following it. Research suggests it is very good with helping improve movement ability, can markedly reduce tremor and benefit overall quality of life.[2] Most people with Parkinson's undergoing the procedure will need to continue taking some medication, although this is usually far less than prior to the procedure.

On the flipside, it is expensive and does have potential risks. Like any brain surgery it carries the risk of stroke, infection and seizures. Other potential side-effects include headaches, lightheadedness and difficulty with balance. In people with PD it also has a tendency to accelerate problems with speech, swallowing and cognition.[3,4] The electrical stimulation can cause psychiatric side-effects too. These include mania, depression and personality changes.[5,6] Many of these side-effects improve when the settings on the device are adjusted to suit the individual better.

Like levodopa, DBS does not cure the underlying condition and therefore invariably loses its effectiveness. A consensus as to its overall benefit versus risks and side effects has not currently been agreed upon.[7] Importantly, the wires can be removed and the procedure reversed if anything goes wrong.

Staying open to the possibility of DBS but with a belief that PD was not completely irreversible, I looked for other options. In my search I discovered Dr Norman Doidge's book, *The Brain's Way of Healing*.[8] I found it inspiring and was particularly spellbound reading both the second and seventh chapters. I'll come back to chapter two in a moment, but let's first focus on chapter seven.[9] In it we are introduced to a new technology known as a PoNS device. It is a non-invasive electronic stimulating machine that is simply placed on the tongue like a lollipop for 20 minutes three times a day. Preliminary research shows that this device, if used whilst participating in an activity, like walking on a treadmill, doing a relaxation exercise or a cognitive challenge, stimulates the development of new pathways in the brain.[10]

This neuroplastic effect can bypass the damaged areas of the brain and recruit new areas to take up the slack. To my way of thinking this provided hope for a more permanent and non-invasive solution than DBS. Early testing has demonstrated its effectiveness in MS, PD and Traumatic Brain Injury (TBI).[11] I contacted the researchers at Wisconsin-Madison University directly by email and they informed me it was in its final trialing (Phase 3 research trials for TBI). I volunteered to be a research subject but alas have yet to be contacted. They hope that it will be available on the market within a year or two.

Neurogenesis brings hope

The discovery that the adult brain produces new brain cells (neurogenesis), especially in two distinct areas, the hippocampus and the supra-olfactory regions, has raised new possibilities for managing Parkinson's.[12,13] Despite the discovery of adult stem cells in the brain as early as the 1960s, indicating neurogenesis could be occurring, this didn't become an accepted medical fact until the 1990s.[14] We now know that via the activation of these adult stem cells, we produce hundreds of new brain cells every day, cells that are capable of replacing old or damaged cells or simply creating new connections.[15]

This understanding has led to an experimental treatment approach for PD whereby medication has been injected into the brain to stimulate particular areas to grow more new cells. While these new cells do not directly produce more dopamine, they apparently can encourage existing cells to produce more in the damaged areas present in PD.[16] This is different to the approach of injecting pre-grown laboratory cultured stem cells as a treatment for Parkinson's, a treatment that seemed promising a decade ago, but had serious safety issues, including the development of brain tumors, which researchers are still hoping to overcome.

While it may be some years until therapies like these become available, we do know that there are things we can do ourselves which stimulate neurogenesis. In her TED talk, Dr Sandrine Thuret lists the following: learning, exercise, good sleep, good sex, calorie restriction, intermittent fasting, essential fatty acids and flavonoids from foods such as, blueberries and dark chocolate.[17] I've indulged in all of these (not at the same time!) and found definite transient improvements in my movement, sometimes lasting for hours, sometimes for days, especially with exercise, good sleep, and a 15 hour fast (7 p.m. to 10 a.m.). The concept of Hormesis seems to be relevant here. Challenging oneself appropriately, such as finishing a shower with a brief burst of cold water is another example I've found useful. Activities that bring sustained joy, such as singing in a choir or a meal with friends, can also impact positively.

This concurs with research involving Parkinsonian mice. Mice in a socially enriched environment that included a running wheel delayed the onset of their Parkinson's, compared to those mice in a less advantageous environment. The preservation of their brain's function was assisted by the production of two chemical growth factors that act like fertilizer for brain cells: glial-derived neurotrophic factor (GDNF) and brain-derived neurotrophic factor (BDNF). These growth factors triggered the mice brains to form new connections between neurones and greatly reduced the loss of dopamine producing nerve cells. In particular, the concentration of GDNF and BDNF increased with exercise.[18-21]

Could this apply to humans with PD? Clinical trials into exercise (stretching, aerobic, resistance,[22-26] dancing,[27,28] yoga,[29,30] tai chi,[31] speech therapy,[32,33] cognitive training[34]) and PD are showing significant improvements can be achieved. The benefit produced, whether it be better balance, gait, strength, louder clearer speech or general well-being, depends on the exercise undertaken. Hence a good mix of exercise strategies tailored to each individual's needs and preferences is recommended.[35] Furthermore, there is growing evidence from brain scans and blood testing of PD patients, that exercise (physical and mental) leads to new brain formation (neuroplasticity) and increases in the concentration of BDNF.[36] Importantly, the benefits obtained can be lost within weeks or months of ceasing exercising, so an ongoing, preferably challenging program is recommended.

> The most extraordinary example of how exercise can impact positively on PD is presented in chapter two of Dr Doidge's book.[37] In it he refers to a gentleman by the name of John Pepper, a successful South African business and family man who was diagnosed with PD in 1992, aged 58. In retrospect it was clear that symptoms of his illness began in his mid-30s, which also corresponded with him taking up 90 minute gym exercise sessions following back surgery. His six days per week exercise routine included 20 minutes on treadmill, 20 minutes cycling, 20 minutes step-climber and 30 minutes strength work. This intensive program may not only have strengthened his back, but may have delayed the progression of his PD. Eventually, a gradual reduction in his capacity to exercise and the development of the cardinal features of PD, led to his diagnosis by a neurologist. PD medication brought improvements, but over the next two years his condition worsened and he became increasingly depressed.
>
> At this time his wife, Shirley, was participating in a walking program known as Run/Walk for Life and suggested he join her. The program very gradually increased a participant's walking capacity and John found it frustratingly easy to begin with. Fortuitously, the person supervising the program knew nothing about Parkinson's disease and kept telling John off for walking so awkwardly, urging him to stop stooping and to straighten up. This got John thinking and by slowing his walking down to a meditative pace, he was

able to analyze in minute detail the subtle movements, which put together created fluid walking.[38]

The first thing he noticed was that when walking, weight is temporarily fully supported on one leg and then the other and that he was unable to do this confidently with his left leg. This meant that if the right foot did clear the ground, he could never straighten his rigid right knee fast enough, so that his right foot landed heavily. Following three months of concentrated, effortful, slow motion practice, he was able to get his left foot to support his body weight, so that his right foot could now land normally. Through close observations he began to work on other aspects of his gait, such as stride length, posture and arm swing. It took him over a year of practice to internalize all these changes, but as long as he paid attention and concentrated on each action, his walking normalized. He appeared to have bypassed the damaged brain areas, and created new and/ or reactivated old conscious pathways, to reclaim a normal gait.

Using this conscious walking method he increased his walking training to eight km (five miles) three times per week, having a rest day in between walks; adequate rest he found to be a key component. When he trained, he walked at a brisk pace keeping his heart rate above 100, so that it was challenging enough to break into a sweat. John developed other conscious techniques to bypass some of the other symptoms of PD, such as lifting a glass and gripping it firmly to stop tremor. Pepper realized his new techniques involved "using a different part of my brain to control an action, which was normally controlled by my unconscious." In practice, this meant consciously performing tasks in slightly different ways. This worked for him as long as he didn't become too stressed or distracted.

Remarkably, many of his Parkinson symptoms, especially those related to movement began to reverse. By 1998 under the supervision of his neurologist, he was able to cease all medication. When Norman Doidge visited him, John was 77, had been off medication for nine years and yet showed no obvious signs of Parkinson's disease. Dr Doidge spent time with John, reviewed his medical records and spoke with his neurologist, confirming the veracity of his story. He also witnessed John assist other Parkinson's patients to improve their posture and movement within minutes by teaching them some of his techniques. (Note: The researchers looking into the PoNS device are also very particular about getting the walking technique correct before applying the electrical neurostimulation that creates new pathways.)

In 2008 John tore a ligament in his left foot that took four months to heal. This stopped him from walking. The PD symptoms that had been controlled re-emerged with full force. When he eventually got back to walking seven km in just over an hour, his symptoms were controlled once again. It suggests that unlike in stroke, where neuroplastic interventions like exercise can lead to permanent gains, in PD the brain damage is ongoing. Therefore, neuroplastic interventions need to be consistently applied in order for the gains to keep pace with the losses.[39] John Pepper tells his own story in his book *Reverse Parkinson's Disease*.[40]

Dr Doidge believes that whilst every form of exercise that a PD patient can manage can be beneficial, walking (if able) is the most pivotal, especially if the gait can be kept as consciously normal as possible. Not surprisingly, he suggests that every Parkinson's patient should be sent to boot camp as soon as they are diagnosed. I echo this sentiment as I have observed, whilst dealing with Graves' disease and UC, my declining capacity to exercise contributed to my PD progressing. Now that my general health has improved, I am slowly rebuilding my exercise regime and I am noticing benefits even from small amounts of conscious walking, yoga stretching, treadmill (holding on), stationary bike and lightweights. But I have a lot of catching up to do. If we put PD patients onto an appropriately individualized exercise training program (supervised by practitioners experienced with PD) as soon as they are diagnosed, it may be possible for all of them to benefit. Some may even exercise to a level that maintains their health without the need for, or with minimal, PD medication. It may also be neuroprotective, as mice studies[41-4] and John Pepper's story suggest, preventing disease progression; a fascinating area of future research.

The Power of Dropping

With all the excitement about exercise's potential, it is easy to forget the importance of balancing this with deep rest. More is not necessarily better as John Pepper found; he discovered he needed rest days between his exercise days. Apart from building one's exercise routine gradually and integrating rest days, I found specific approaches to relaxation very helpful, whether it be a treatment such as a Bowen massage or craniosacral balancing, or a deep muscle relaxation or meditation. The common experience one hopes to have here, is the feeling of dropping deeply, both physically and mentally.

If you have a partner willing to learn Bowen techniques this could be very helpful. Of late, Tori has offered me a brief Bowen massage along my back whilst I lie on my side in bed before falling asleep. Remarkably, this seems to be decreasing the level of tension throughout my body generally (the rigid muscles associated with PD) as well as stabilizing my balance and gait.

Completing an exercise session with yoga stretching/breathing and a deep relaxation or meditation, something I used to teach my CFS patients (the rest activity dance), can have the same effect. Don't underestimate the restoring powers of deep rest.

(For those of you looking for a comprehensive mainstream text on PD I can recommend: *Parkinson's Disease - A Complete Guide for Patients and Their Families 3rd Edition*, by Weiner WJ, Shulman LM & Lang AE.)

Chapter 21

JUDGEMENT AND ENLIGHTENMENT

We are all vulnerable and naked before the mysteries of life.

JOHN ROBBINS

One of the dangers of discovering you can contribute to or alter your illness through your own efforts, is that you can become frustrated and judgmental of yourself if you do not achieve perfect health. For years, I accused myself of causing my health breakdown, focusing on the fact that I overworked. In time I've come to see this was a narcissistic point of view. While taking responsibility for what we can change is healthy, we can also delude ourselves into thinking we are invulnerable and more in control than we are. For instance, I did not choose the genetic predispositions I was born with nor the second-generation Holocaust tensions. Exposure to environmental toxins, such as those I received whilst playing in my father's carpet and vinyl shop, and the food poisoning that triggered IBS, were also incidental. Life can throw us curly ones that we are oblivious to at the time.

Judgement is not an easy thing to write about, but I've experienced it so intensely as an unwell person in judging myself that it would be remiss of me not to address it.

Some of my judgement of myself came from embracing philosophies, summarized by some as the 'law of attraction'[1] (made popular in the book *The Secret*[2]), that teach we are totally responsible for creating our own reality. The philosophy itself is simple enough: the 'vibe' you exude relates directly to the content of your thoughts and this attracts matching 'vibes,' or something like that. (As the old saying goes, 'you make your own luck.') It does have echoes of a deep truth, which if received in a balanced way can engender a healthy sense of personal responsibility, especially for our thoughts and actions. This can profoundly impact our lives in a myriad of positive ways.

During the events outlined in the chapter entitled, Meditation as Medicine, I felt the truth of this philosophy as opportunities opened up for me, seemingly in response to my being true to myself. That said, I've experienced how much trickier it is to apply this theory when things are not going so well, particularly in relation to sickness.

My observation is this: while exploring the psycho-emotional-spiritual connections involved in any illness can be fruitful, and even lifesaving, an imbalanced belief in the 'law of attraction,' one that is simplistic and lacks a holistic view, can make people who are sick feel an unhealthy level of responsibility for their illness. Expressed at its extreme you end up with Pol Pot's callous words: "the sick are victims of their own imagination." Unwell people stuck in this perspective can find themselves tangled in mental fishing line, forever trying to reel in the 'right' healing insight from their subconscious, feeling ashamed for not being able to succeed, all the while missing out on the simultaneous benefit of something they can change, such as diet or lifestyle.

As I have discovered, this sense of shame is massively compounded if one loses one's ability to work, along with friendships and family support. Medical sociologist, Aaron Antonovsky, called these Generalized Resistance Resources (GRRs). Things such as access to healthy food, water and shelter, a loving childhood, family and social support, a job, adequate finances, strength of personality etc. These GRRs are critical to our ability to handle and thrive in the face of stress. But, just as a happily swimming fish may be unaware of the water that supports it until it is gone, these resources are often unappreciated. They cushion us and help to prevent misfortune, until they are overwhelmed, in which case illness often results.[3]

The other problem I have observed is this: believers in the 'law of attraction' philosophy who are relatively well, may take for granted that they have a job, friends and support (i.e. a healthy cushion of GRRs), and run the risk of attributing their good fortune (karma) to the fact that they must be more 'enlightened' than the sick. This is falling into the trap of using what psychologists call false attribution. In this case, attributing health and good fortune entirely to strength of character, an important, but only a single GRR, which is in fact most effective when it stands on the shoulders of other GRRs.

The corollary for either the sick or the well person who has this belief is that sickness is judged as a weakness of character rather than as a result of complex circumstances. I've heard similar judgements made about the poor, believing the fact that they are poor to be entirely their own fault, rather than as a result of social circumstances and lack of opportunity. Many a human hierarchy has been justified upon such judgements.

One of the most bizarre examples of this type of thinking was expressed to me when I was attending an art exhibition with Tori. I was sitting in my wheelchair admiring a piece of art when a young lady, whom I had only met briefly once before, knelt down beside me and said, "You know, you're sick because you're a bad person." I would have liked to have dented her theory by pointing out to her the large number of psychopaths in the world experiencing excellent health, but I was completely taken aback.

Also annoying is the mantra to "just think positive," usually from well-meaning healthy people who don't realize how hard you're trying to do just that.

All of this makes me wonder if we humans, behind our facade of modernity, still believe that certain sick and sensitive people, like those unable to work because of mental or physical illness, are somehow inferior or cursed in some way and are to be shunned. I suspect this is driven by an underlying fear of illness, the need to make sense of it in a way that doesn't feel threatening, and wishing to avoid facing the inevitable conclusion: there is no guarantee it can't happen to me.

I've come to reflect that while our thoughts and choices are very important, our genetics and psyches are complex, as are the contexts and interdependent relationships we find ourselves in at any given time. All this plays out as part of a milieu, determining our GRRs, which is a lot bigger than us as individuals. Bad things can happen to any of us, yet none of us like to dwell on this. For those of us who are well and assume this is so purely because we feel we are in control, psychologist and author Rick Hanson has the perfect antidote: "Don't take your success too personally."[4]

In the lead up to my health collapse in the 1990s I thought I was buffering myself against illness. I was not overweight, was a non-smoker and drank an occasional glass of wine. I ate healthily, swam and walked regularly, enjoyed weekly singing lessons and I practiced an hour and a half of yoga and meditation daily. I was happily married with many good friends and family and was dedicated to helping people in my work. In summary, my GRRs appeared to be pretty healthy.

Yet there were many factors playing out that I was unaware of: a genetic methylation defect and susceptibility to Parkinson's disease; exposure to environmental toxins; and unconscious forces fueling a driven behavior pattern, the source of which proved difficult to unearth and come to peace with. Understanding the source of one's drivenness is a task I believe we can only tackle when we are mature, ready and supported enough. For instance, one of my weaknesses was being unable to say "no" to helping others. This led to me overstretching myself, a character trait that I would spend many years exploring and overcoming.

Could I have done more to prevent my health going downwards? Maybe, but I thought I was doing the best that I could at the time. It is worth noting that even today there is no known preventive treatment to stop PD from developing. Yet for all this when things went badly awry, I judged myself as being inadequate and responsible for my ill health.

In contrast, my experience of being with many sick and dying people, such as Ron and Mrs Smythe, is that they are some of the wisest, most content and together people I've met. Their ability to respond to hardship with dignity and humor in the face of unrelenting suffering, is a mark of human achievement worth emulating. In the presence of such people it's possible to glimpse through the facade of human hierarchies to see that we are all no more and no less than each other. That is an enlightenment I can get with.

Chapter 22

DYING WELL

Dappled light so gentle
shadows dance upon tree trunks
untouchable braille.

Growing up, my only experience of death and dying involved family pets. The death of my beloved Siamese cat, Pandy, my study companion and playmate throughout high school and medical school, was a powerful introduction to grief.

My first experience of a dead human being was in medical school where we had to dissect cadavers as part of our anatomy training. While these bodies were gruesome, they had been pickled in formalin for some time and there was something a little unreal about them. It wasn't until my hospital training days that I would witness someone who was alive one minute and dead the next. It was a shock. Often these deaths involved failed attempts at resuscitation and were traumatic, leaving indelible memories that can still make me shudder. Not surprisingly then, I place myself among the 60 to 70% of Australians that surveys show would prefer to die at home.[1,2]

This wish, however, may not be easy to achieve. Over the past century, the proportion of deaths at home has declined and that of deaths in hospitals and residential aged care has increased. Today, only about 14% of people die at home in Australia. Fifty-four per cent die in hospitals and 32% in residential care. This does not match up very well in comparison to countries like New Zealand, the United States, Ireland and France, where close to 30% of people die at home.[3]

In practical terms, to improve this statistic one needs skillful community palliative care teams working beside family members. Everyone must be willing and supported enough to go the distance. In general practice I experienced this combination. In these circumstances gentleness and periods of silence held the dying person in a way that just felt right. This was in sharp contrast to the many jarring hospital deaths I witnessed. Perhaps a little more congruence could be achieved if hospital resuscitation team leaders, after a failed resuscitation attempt and before tidying up and packing away equipment, were to introduce, say, a five to ten second silent pause to acknowledge the life just lost.

Carol's story

Tori's mother Carol was a delightful, intelligent woman much loved by those who knew her. At the age of 46 she was diagnosed with breast cancer, which heralded the beginning of a 23 year battle with this disease. Bouts of surgery, chemotherapy and radiotherapy were faced with stoicism, as she and her husband Mike continued to run a jazz club and pub, the Limerick Arms, for a further 10 years. Eventually they retired to the coastal town of Anglesea, where Carol tended to her magnificent veggie patch and involved herself in the local community. Finally, the cancer spread to her lungs and bones causing distressing pain and breathlessness despite home oxygen and assistance from a palliative care nurse. Needing more support and expertise Carol decided to move to a palliative care facility in Geelong. Within 48 hours the right balance of pain and anxiety relieving medication, along with oxygen, was found to make Carol comfortable, whilst keeping her conscious and alert. In this way, in between periods of rest, Carol was able to receive many close friends and family, each of whom she seemed to have something wise to contribute. Her clarity, compassion and wisdom at this time was something to behold.

Two days before her death nursing staff organized for her to sit outside in the beautiful gardens that surrounded the building. At this juncture Tori and Carol were able to have a private extraordinary conversation. Carol was able to see deeply into my wife's distress and Tori was able to acknowledge something of Carol's nature and life story, to which Carol expressed with relief and conviction, 'YES!' The unburdening effect of this conversation on Tori, at a time when she was suicidally depressed, was life-saving. As for Carol, something seemed to settle in her and she surrendered with a sense of contentment and peace over her final 48 hours to her death.

Opportunities that dying can bring

My own close call with death and my experiences with Carol and my father Lee, who also had a much better time of it during his final five days in a palliative care hospice, has made me reflect on the opportunities that dying can bring. In an appropriate, gentle environment in which everyone realizes that time is just about up, qualities like honesty, compassion and humility can be squeezed to the surface, in both the dying and those who come to visit them. Communications can be had, both verbal and non-verbal; a smile, a tear, a hug, something deeply meaningful transmitted. This is not a time to hold back and it can remind us what it feels like to be deeply human and humane.

For the person who is dying there is, in this environment, a special opportunity of surrendering to one's frailty and coming closer to one's comforting inner world, one's spirit (or nature of mind – see Mind-body weaving. Also known in western psychology as 'the oceanic feeling').[4] Having a regular practice of meditation, contemplation or prayer can help familiarize you with a similar experience, so that when the time comes, you know and can let go in to this feeling.

For these reasons I believe the inevitability of death and the organic slowness and relative comfort, with which it can unfold in good palliative care situations, is truly one of the unsung advancements in modern medicine.

Making a choice

It is worth clarifying the distinction between active (acute) and palliative care from an experiential point of view. The former involves ongoing treatment and interventions, such as chemotherapy, radiotherapy, antibiotics, blood tests, x-rays and the insertion of invasive tubes of various sizes and descriptions. Constantly being poked and prodded in this way day in day out can build trauma by attrition, especially in the frail. This said, the aim here is a worthy one: keeping people alive hopefully at a level of health in which life is worth living.

By contrast, palliative care, which can be home, hospice or hospital-based, is all about letting nature run its course and supporting the dying person to be as comfortable as possible while this occurs. The environment is unrushed and family and friends can gather easily to share precious moments. In this scenario, things like lung infections, a common result of being bedridden, rather than being seen as the enemy to be actively treated, are seen as a friend; a friend that can help a person to die in a peaceful way (hence pneumonia has been known as the 'old person's friend').

Most people believe they have to choose between active care and palliative care, where in truth the two can work concurrently. This was highlighted in a study that looked at 151 people with newly diagnosed metastatic lung cancer. These people were randomly assigned to one of two groups: oncology care (active cancer treatment chemotherapy/

radiotherapy etc.) plus palliative care or oncology care alone. Those patients who received both oncology care and palliative care experienced less discomfort and depression, and were less likely to receive aggressive therapies within two weeks of their death. But the most remarkable finding from this study was that they also lived an average of three months longer than those who received oncology care alone.[5]

This concurrent treatment approach is desperately needed. I have witnessed too many terminally ill patients who have not been exposed to palliative care options and therefore continue to choose more aggressive treatments alone, treatments which can effectively bludgeon their frail bodies to death in quick time. The addition of palliative care in this situation can allow the question of the suitability of more aggressive treatment to be discussed, reduce suffering and in so doing can also extend life. Perhaps it's time that oncologists and radiotherapists provide a mandatory palliative care referral as part of their treatment approach whenever their treatment is unlikely to be curative. In this way, the palliation team can focus their skills on alleviating suffering, while the cancer specialists focus on reducing the effects of the cancer; the patient suffers less and lives longer; a win-win for all.

Of course there comes a time when people need to stop active treatment altogether and focus entirely on end-of-life care. I admire people like Carol and Lee who were both able to say enough is enough to active medical treatments that were increasingly traumatic for them to cope with and unlikely to succeed. With this decision the pressure of making further choices about ongoing medical heroics came off and a space opened up into which dignity took center stage. There was a palpable release of tension amongst all concerned when they were at last receiving adequate alleviation of their suffering. This quality care took place in an unhurried, nurturing environment that allowed their true personalities to shine forth once more.

The relief on my father's face when after months of chemotherapy, operations, episodes in Intensive Care and generally being pushed, prodded and injected, he settled in a palliative care hospice, is something I will never forget. His physical symptoms were managed beautifully and in between periods of deep rest his cheekiness and warmth returned for all of us to savor, one last time.

We can't always choose how we die but in my experience, in obviously terminal situations, the decision to switch to palliative care from active care is often left too late. It takes a maturity and courage to admit it is time to pull up stumps. In this situation unfortunately, the seemingly endless choices for active management and the medicolegal fears of not doing everything possible to keep life going can get in the way of a good death, a life enriching opportunity that is being forgone.[6] Currently, there is a lack of structure in the medical system to assist doctors to shift gear and bring in the palliative experts, so that it is often left to the patient or their nearest family, who are already vulnerable, to find the strength to say, 'stop!' The option for palliative choices needs to be presented earlier so that people know it is a real and valid (not a copout) possibility. Predetermined (Advanced) Care Plans developed by patients prior to their need are a response to this problem in the health system. They can be a useful starting point, but should be seen as one element in a system that requires change to support patient's needs and decision-making as the actual situations arise.

What's really needed, when dying is inevitable and near, is increasing courage with discussing death and the palliative options available. Pastoral care workers, who are employed in some hospitals to assist people from all religious or nonreligious backgrounds, are trained in this area. They can be called upon to provide emotional support at these times, helping to facilitate these decisions. While such assistance may not be readily available, if you are facing a situation like this, I encourage you to exercise your right to ask your doctor to include a palliative care referral (community-based or hospital-based) as a part of your treatment plan. In the end, you may need a well-qualified and authoritative health professional (e.g. nurse or doctor) to act as an advocate for you to get the care you need.

Re-visioning the bucket list

When someone reaches the bedridden stage of their terminal illness, visiting close family and friends can feel awkward and unsure as to how to behave around them. The idea of the dying person having a bucket list may seem absurd at this time; trips to the Himalayas aside! The truth is that there is still the opportunity for a more subtle bucket list. It may be spoken or unspoken and look something like this: just sit quietly with me; help me sip water; squeeze my hand; help me to eat a piece of chocolate; select my favorite piece of music. It may not be a grand list but it is no less important.

When my sister and I asked Lee three days before he died if there was anything special he wanted to eat, he asked for apple strudel. We promptly hopped in the car, drove to his favorite cake shop and returned with the strudel. He only ever ate two or three mouthfuls, but boy, did he savor them and we in turn his enjoyment.

They may not always be able to tell you what they want (though it's worth asking), but a frown or a smile can help guide you to the right offering. The world of the bedridden contracts into a small range of concerns, so that inadequate as you may feel, remember, you don't need to do much to be of help. In the end, if you let them know they are loved, you'll be making the world of difference.

Can we prepare for the inevitable?

"Everybody has got to die, but I have always believed an exception would be made in my case."

WILLIAM SAROYAN

"Death smiles at us all; all we can do is smile back."

MARCUS AURELIUS

In the introduction to his interesting book, *Final Chapters – How Famous Authors Died*, Jim Bernhard points out that it has been estimated that since the beginning of the world, about 107 billion people have been born. Of that total, only a little more than 7 billion are alive today, so that out of everyone who has ever lived, 93% of them have died. It seems the odds are not in favor of the remaining 7% of us! Death is both inevitable (so far as we know) and unpredictable (in most circumstances),[7] yet despite this, evidence suggests we are good at avoiding the topic; 45% of people die without a will and nine out of ten people never tell anyone their end-of-life wishes.[8]

Given we're all going to face it and we're not sure when, is there anything we can do to prepare ourselves so that we can 'smile back?'

Apart from getting my affairs in order, such as a will, the obvious lesson I have learnt from my 'nearly dead experience,' is to prioritize the important things in my life while I'm still around. In this way I can experience the satisfaction and joy that these things can bring, such as building relationships with those I care for most, more often. The other thing it has helped me with is not putting off the completion of projects I most value, such as writing this book. Hopefully this will mean when the Grim Reaper comes knocking at my 'final chapter,' I will be ready to go with her and die feeling more complete, without, or at least with less, regrets.

I've heard it said by several sources that if you live well, you'll die well. I'm not sure if this is true but it does bring me some comfort. While I don't practice the Buddhist meditation of imagining one's death in order to become more fearless and appreciative of each day, I continue to find my daily meditation into stillness dissolves my fears and gives me a hint of where I may eventually be going.

If you are struggling with this death-stuff, simply talking more about death and dying without ignoring it, can make you more comfortable with it.[9] If you want to explore further the wide range of issues involved in death and dying, including end-of-life planning, or find other suggestions of how you can become easier with the subject, some useful websites I've found are: http://www.thegroundswellproject.com/ and http://www.deathtalker.com/

FINDING HOPE -
SUMMING UP

*... the person who forgets the language of gratitude can
never be on speaking terms with happiness.*

JOHN ROBBINS

I may not be totally perfect, but parts of me are excellent!

ASHLEIGH BRILLIANT

Finding hope is a proactive activity, hardest to do when we turn to face our darkest hour. I wrote this book to inspire hope in you the reader and me the author, as well as to stimulate discussion about health and health care.

For those of you, like me, who have found yourself falling into decline before you believed it was your time, it's my hope that in these pages you have found reasons to believe things can get better. I may not have returned to perfect health, but I'm still here and I've come a long way since 2012. Tori likes to claim my surname has made me a happy summarizer, so let me conclude by pointing out some of the principles of hopefulness that have been clarified and revealed to me in the writing of this book:[1]

- As I learnt from 95-year-old Una, you've got to want to be here. Find reasons to stick around, engage with life and fight on.
- Prioritize your most important needs and find time and ways to have these met.
- Also prioritize your most important feelings, relationships and activities so that they find a rightful place in your life. Mrs Smythe's story (start of Chapter 1) shows us just how powerful a medicine this can be.
- Accept and learn to work within current limitations due to energy levels, pain and disability, knowing that these can change in time.
- Know that you can influence your health and the course of disease by your own efforts. This is underlined by our knowledge of epigenetics. Our genes do not act in isolation but respond to environmental triggers, triggers that we influence not only through treatments but through our thoughts, feelings and behaviors.
- Lifestyle change cannot only prevent disease but can treat even serious disease. Changing to a more plant-based wholefood diet, for instance, can improve angina and alter the gut microbiome within weeks. Moderate exercise and sunlight can elevate your well-being within hours. Like a healthy diet, healthy levels of exercise can also benefit a wide range of medical conditions and even improve the prognosis of people with cancer. Take time to learn and introduce any new lifestyle skills you may need.
- Remember the concept of hormesis; appropriate physical and mental challenge can help to restore health and build resilience.

- Give yourself permission to make mistakes and learn from them.
- New understandings about how the body works such as epigenetics, how we interact with our microbiome, and neurogenesis, will in time open up completely different approaches to the management of disease.
- Discoveries are being made at an ever-increasing rate, bringing new treatments to light, like FMT. As Ron's story illustrated (start of Chapter 9), if you hang in there long enough, not only can you find meaning in your life, but you can also benefit from these new discoveries.
- Remember, you can utilize both 'zooming in' specific treatments (e.g. medication) whilst participating in 'zooming out' holistic strategies (e.g. diet, exercise, meditation, social support, laughter, doing what you love etc). Both approaches can complement each other. As Mrs Smythe's story demonstrated, if specific treatment options have been exhausted, there are always more possibilities that can be introduced holistically to improve a situation.
- Social and moral support is the foundation upon which any attempts at overcoming serious disease are built. Honor and remember to work on building these relationships if you can. Spend time with others who are encouraging and inspiring.
- Remember to ask for help, for we need others, but be mindful not to overload your carers.
- Set yourself short and long-term goals like getting through the morning or making it to a family event.
- Be honest about your deepest feelings and give them time and space to be creatively expressed (written, drawn, painted, shouted, danced etc). You may like to keep a journal or

simply tear up or delete the piece once you've got it out of yourself. If possible, find a confidante with whom you can share your feelings; someone who can listen to, hold and honor them.

- Effective treatments exist outside of modern medicine, as I discovered with mastic gum. While complementary medicine is best practiced with an evidence-based approach, the absence of research evidence does not equate to an absence of effectiveness. Trial and error and some expense may need to be risked. Decide what you are prepared to invest. Balancing the science, the risks and potential clinical benefits are all good considerations when making decisions for your treatment.

- If trying an unproven treatment, this is best done whilst being monitored by a willing medical practitioner (as I did with mastic gum for Ulcerative Colitis). Fortunately, some medical practitioners are open to this. In my ideal world, not a world agreed to by all of my colleagues mind you, general (family medicine) practitioners would be trained to include this type of monitoring as part of their role.

- Don't underestimate the power of the therapeutic encounter. It is worth searching for the right practitioner(s) that you can relate to. Seeking out second or third opinions may be necessary.

- Prioritize meaningful activity, for if you can find meaning in your life it can serve as a buffer to the many challenges that life, and illness in particular, presents. You may find this in helping others or voluntary work.

- Enhance any treatment you take by activating the meaning (placebo) response.

- Counteract stress with problem-solving, helpful discussion and regular meditation/relaxation/prayer; anything that brings you to a state of deep calm.

- In that state of deep calm, each morning and evening imagine a healthier future you.
- Invoke the ultimate stress buster and immune stimulant, laughter, as often as you can, by looking at the funny side of life's everyday situations and exposing yourself to people or comedy that cracks you up.
- Mindful self-compassion can help you through the toughest times. It's okay to be gentle with yourself.
- If you are moved to do so, pray for assistance.
- Hope inevitably needs renewal. Setbacks are inevitable; we have good days and not so good days. It helps to anticipate this and have some plans to deal with the lows. For instance, it can be helpful to keep a 'Reasons to Be Hopeful List' easily visible (on the fridge for example). Include on this list only things that you find give you hope. These can serve as backup plans, so that if Plan A fails, you know you have a Plan B, C or D to trial next.
- Keep adding to your list as you discover new activities/possibilities. Refer to this list, especially on bad days.
- Keep an eye out for more inspiring stories and research and/or remind yourself of those inspirations that you already know of. Record these on your fridge list.
- When times are tough, it can be helpful to set yourself a short-term goal, like getting through the morning as mindfully as possible. It may also help to remind yourself that 'this too will pass.'
- Illness slows us down and contracts our world; there is a gift and an opportunity in this. Taken out of our busyness there is time to cherish a smile, a joke shared with a friend,

the sparkle of early morning dew, a meal sat down with family or friends. These things which we simply missed or may have taken for granted in the past, now have a chance to receive our appreciation. It is a time to take stock, to enjoy what you do have rather than focusing on what you don't have. Appreciate the little improvements. Gratitude is a gift for all.

- Share your insights with others who may need to hear it.
- Become comfortable with the imperfect. Paradoxically, whilst my hope has been buoyed by striving for as close to perfect health as I can imagine, at the same time, coming to terms with the imperfections in this quest, as well as those glitches within myself and others, has given me peace of mind. Perfect expectations are rarely met, and that's okay.
- Illness can be a difficult beast, yet through the brakes it has put on my life, I've come to see that accepting its interwoven complexity along with love of one's self, with all one's failings and problems, has been its gift. Together with exorcising the demons I'd inherited from the Holocaust, this has been the journey my illness has taken me on.
- You can strive for health, success or whatever you like as much as you want, but you'll never feel complete if unaccompanied by deep self-acceptance.

Surfing the Wave of Our Existence

As we age it becomes more and more apparent that our lives dance between entropy and renewal. There is a time to strive and explore and a time to savor and accept; a time to seek out new treatments and a time to say that's enough; a time to live and a time to die. Ultimately we need to trust our intuition will guide us as to which of these states is the best one to serve us at any given period of our lives. Sometimes it is obvious, like the example of a friend's mother in her mid-90s who quite lucidly chose to reject medical treatment knowing it was time for her to go. Other situations are less obvious and can depend very much on the personality making the choice, so that prescriptive advice has limited value.

As we face the challenges in our lives and surf the wave of our existence, with all its highs, lows and occasional wipe outs, hope is the surfboard we return to time and time again, until our time is done.

I wish you well.

Appendix 1

MEDITATION BASED STRESS MANAGEMENT

(This is a transcript from Dr Sommer's MP3 download recording, *Restoring Balance* available at www.drstevensommer.com)

Unwinding, Resetting Your Thermostat

We all have a stress thermostat, a barometer if you like, which determines how easily or not we become stressed. When it is raised high, we can become anxious very easily, when it is set low we are more resistant to stress. Our genetics, our upbringing and life traumas can all affect our thermostat. Fortunately the choices we make in the way we live from day to day can influence it as well.

Do you ever find that your day runs a bit like a paragraph without a punctuation mark?

For instance, take a look at how one of your average day's runs. How much time are you spending getting wound up? How does this compare with the time you allow yourself to wind down? Is there a balance?

The basis of the stress management approach I am teaching here is restoring balance to the way we go about our lives. It is as simple as learning to punctuate our day with commas and full stops. Commas are brief pauses that can take as little as *thirty seconds*, while full stops require a minimum of *five minutes*.

Your Breath Barometer

The way we are breathing at any one time can tell us a lot about our state of mind.

Right now, if your hands are free, I'd like you to place one hand on your chest and your other hand on your belly. Just let your hands rest gently and breathe normally. …Notice how your hands move with your breath. ……….. Are both hands moving as you breathe? Or just one? If both are moving, is one hand moving more than the other? Or are they both moving equally. There is no right or wrong here, we are simply noticing the pattern of our breathing.

Now, leaving your hands where they are look directly in front of you. Keeping your head still, look upwards with your eyes. Maintaining this position for a few breaths, notice if there is a change in your breathing pattern.

Now return your eyes back down and rest your hands.

This is your breath barometer and you can use it to check where you are at, at any time.

Rapid shallow breathing is a sign that we are stressed. In the exercise we just did, this would display itself as more air moving into our upper chest, than lower down. Hence when we are anxious, the hand we place on our chest will move more than the hand on our belly. What this means is that the diaphragm, the sheet of muscle that divides the chest from the abdomen, is not flattening out as we breathe in. Hence, little air moves down into the lower parts of the lung, leaving our belly unmoved or only moving slightly.

If you watch a baby breathe while it is playing happily, you will notice that its belly moves easily with each breath it takes. Most of us inevitably lose this ability. We can however relearn how to breathe more deeply. Why is this important? Well, when the diaphragm flattens out it triggers a relaxation response. Chemicals are released into our nervous system that instantly help us to relax. So taking two slow deep breaths is a bit like self-medicating without the medication.

A Brief Pause (A comma in your day)

Two or three slow deep breaths can be taken at any time in your day, helping you to rebalance. This is what I refer to as a pause or comma. Don't be too fussed about the way you take your deep breaths, doing it is the main thing.

Practice this now. Breathe in as slow and low as you can.. maybe even give a sigh as you breath out. ...and again, slow and low. ...If you are struggling to shift your breathing down towards your belly, try gazing upwards while you take your deep breaths. It will get easier in time. But as I said, just doing it is the most important thing. Try that once more. A slow deep breath....Really focus on the feeling of the air, as it flows in and out. Good. That's it. A simple way to pause.

Of course knowing how to rebalance like this is one thing, remembering to do it is another. My suggestion here is to introduce some common everyday events as reminder triggers. For example, any time you are waiting, such as when being stopped at a red light, standing in a queue, while placed on hold on the telephone, waiting for your computer to connect, sitting in traffic, in a waiting room or on the loo. Another good trigger is before or after food, where two deep breaths can aid digestion. You might want to set a reminder on your mobile phone.

Reflect on your day. Are there any obvious moments that you could use as pause triggers? Jot these down. It might help to review some of the suggestions I just made and then keep adding ideas as they come to you.

Obviously you will need to choose common events that occur in your day. Importantly many triggers can be found in events that might otherwise cause us irritation. So next time you find yourself having to wait, instead of getting annoyed think - 'GREAT! A chance to unwind' and take two slow deep breaths.

How many times should you pause during a day? I would suggest at least three to five times, but experiment and see what works for you. A good way to start is to place reminder stickers or comma signs around your home or work place.

Regular pauses can help to check the wind up that occurs during a day and the longer restoring exercises will enhance your wellbeing and build your stress resistance. Let's look at these now.

Restoring Exercises (Full Stops) – also see Appendix 2.

Restoring exercises are time outs. Times to be, rather than to do. Times to renew, to drop our load, to rest. They are times when we leave our worries behind for a little while, knowing that they will be there to pick up later if we choose. Regularly practiced these time outs can bring us so much.

I'd suggest you begin with a five minute Senses Exercise (see Appendix 2), twice a day. If this seems too daunting then start with once a day and build from there. Consolidate with this for a month then try to extend it to 10 minutes. The other two exercises, Soften and Flow for easing emotional or physical pain, and the Deep Muscle Relaxation, which can also be used to aid falling asleep, could also be used for regular practice (see Appendix 2). Feel free to try each one.

The main instruction with the Senses and Deep Muscle Relaxation exercises is as you become mindful, that is aware, of thoughts or feelings during your practice, one simply learns to observe these, allow them to be, and then to return one's focus to whatever it is you are meditating upon. This process is repeated as often as you become distracted or drift off into daydreams. Importantly, you're not trying to empty your mind of thoughts, but simply stepping back from them for a while. In this 'stepping back' you receive restorative rest. In time, as you cultivate your ability to be mindful of what's going on both inside of you and around you, you'll find it easier to maintain your attention.

The approach with the Soften and Flow exercise is different, in that the point of attention becomes the pain or the feeling that we find. You then breathe into this discomfort, at the same time both acknowledging and soothing it. Once again we keep returning our attention to this focus as often as we are distracted from it until it eases.

Guidelines for Practice

These restoring exercises are best practiced with your body placed in a balanced and symmetrical position.

Sitting upright in a basic kitchen chair is ideal, but if this is too difficult, try lying down on supportive ground with a flat pillow for your head, knees bent if need be. The idea here is to stay awake during the exercise. If this is not possible then by all means try out different positions and see what works best for you.

An extra layer like a shawl or a jumper might be needed. Other general guidelines include practicing before food rather than after, and you might even consider a gentle stretch for your body before you start. Before breakfast and before dinner are good times. It might mean waking up 10 minutes earlier, starting out your day on a clear note, then leaving behind the day's events by full stopping before dinner. If this is not possible then any time is better than missing out. The key here is timetabling it as a priority time just for you. Other members of your household may need to be told that you are off limits during your restoring breaks…and leave the phone off or on mute.

There is no right or wrong or success or failure with this. Just like washing your teeth, regular practice is the main thing.

Further Applications

The key to this program is simply practicing the commas and full stops each day. You may like to just leave it at that. However, once you have established a regular practice for a month or more, then you might wish to read this section. Here I explore the restoring exercises further and look at ways of applying them in everyday life, the simplest way being to link them with the deep breath commas.

The Senses restoring exercises are sometimes referred to as mindfulness practices. In these we are simply giving our attention in turn to one of our senses - touch, smell, taste then listening. Cultivating our ability, if you like, to just observe without comment. In doing this we bring our mind out of its worries and into a simple experience of what is happening now. In time, you may find you can use this skill to connect with your senses during everyday activities. For example, when standing just connect with the weight of your body, when walking try feeling your feet as they take each step. Other ways of applying this mindfulness approach include, really giving your full attention to tasting food as you eat it or just listening to all the sounds around you. Give it a try. You might like to combine it with the deep breathing commas. A simple way would be to take two slow deep breaths and feel your body's weight.

The Soften and Flow exercise is also a mindfulness exercise that helps us to tune into, acknowledge and ease uncomfortable feelings. It is easy to lose touch with our feelings. When we do they tend to build underneath, urging us to pay them some attention. Often all we need to do is to acknowledge them, sit with them and they settle. This can be one of the most important steps in restoring balance. In time as you practice the Soften and Flow exercise you may find that you develop the ability to check in with yourself during the day and ease building tensions in this way. Of course some feelings will be more persistent carrying important messages for us that we may need to address. This exercise can also help you to realize this.

The Deep Muscle Relaxation exercise helps us to become aware of when and where physical tension is building. As your skill with this exercise improves, you may find that when you pause to take two or three deep breaths you can also scan for tension and let it go. For example, relaxing and dropping shoulder tension on your out-breath. This is another way of preventing tension building up in your body during the day. It can be a great way of preventing problems such as headaches.

Variations in Experience & Long Term goals

Importantly, like the weather, your experience will vary from day to day. Some days will feel clear and sunny, others might feel stormy. In other words, you might feel calm one day and agitated the next. This is normal. Other experiences you may have include feeling tired or feeling like you've just stepped off a merry go round. This is also normal. The key here is just doing it each day regardless. If you do, the restoring benefits will flow into the rest of your life, even on days when your time out feels like a waste of time.

As you become more confident with these full stops, try to practice without a recording. In this way you'll become more independent. You might even like to build your practice time. For example, some of my patients enjoy doing 20 minutes once or twice a day. Another future challenge you can try is practicing a full stop in a noisy situation, like seated in a shopping centre. Being able to renew yourself wherever you are is a wonderful skill to cultivate. But the first step is establishing a regular practice at home.

Further Reading

Meditation: An In-Depth Guide, by Ian Gawler and Paul Bedson

The Wise Heart, by Jack Kornfield

The Mindful Path to Self-Compassion, by Christopher Germer

The Art of True Happiness, by Sharon Salzberg

Wherever You Go, There You Are, by Jon Kabat-Zinn

Freedom from Stress and Anxiety, by David McRae

Appendix 2

RESTORING EXERCISES ('FULL STOPS')

(This is a transcript from Dr Sommer's MP3 download recording *Restoring Balance* available from www.drstevensommer.com)

Senses Awareness Meditation (5 or 10 Minutes)

Let's start this exercise sitting upright in a chair, your feet resting flat on the floor and your back straight. Keep your head upright as well so that it's balanced, taking any pressure off your neck muscles.

Now, gently close your eyes and take two slow deep breaths letting the chair take your body's weight completely as you breathe out. [pause]

....Maybe take one more of those deep breaths and if you like, give a sigh as you breathe out.

Good, now become aware of your feet where they touch the floor. Wriggle your toes if this helps, then rest them....

Become aware of the weight of your body in the chair....Feel where the chair is pressing against your buttocks and your back....

Perhaps you can become aware of the clothes where they touch the skin....

See if you can feel the play of air on your face and your hands.

Let any sense of smell come into your awareness as you breathe in through your nose.

Allow any tastes present in your mouth to be detected.

Now shift your attention to listening. Take in all the sounds you can hear both near and far, moving from one sound to the next....

If you become aware your mind is focusing on other things, like thoughts or feelings, not to worry, just let them be and whenever you are able, return your attention to simply listening....

Let the listening stretch right out into the distance.

Good....good.

Now take another slow deep breath returning your attention to the feeling of the weight of your body sitting in the chair.

Wriggle your toes and your fingers and just in your own time when you're ready, gently open your eyes.

Soften & Flow Meditation

Once again find a balanced position either sitting upright in a chair, or you can lie on your back on a firmish surface with a pillow beneath your head; body straight; legs either resting straight or bent at the knees.

Now, gently close your eyes. Let's start by taking 2 slow rich breaths, letting the air flow out fully with each breath. **[pause]**

Maybe take one more of those deep breaths, letting the chair or the floor take your body's weight completely as you breathe out.

Good. Now we are going to scan our body, becoming aware of any areas where we might be holding tension. Just observing these areas noting any physical or emotional tension, without the need to change them, just acknowledging what's there.

So let's start with our legs. Observe your feet....Are your feet holding any tension?...What about your calves?....or your thighs? How do they feel?

Now shift your awareness to your buttocks....Acknowledge if there is any tension there. [pause] Now to your back? [pause] Your shoulders?... [pause] Your neck?... [pause] Your head? .... [pause] Your face? [pause]

Become aware if any tensions are held in your chest....what about your abdomen [pause]. It is common to find emotional tension held in our belly or chest areas; perhaps tune into these areas again....

Now choose one area that you have found where you might be holding some emotional or physical tension. Observe it again.... acknowledge it.

Now gently breathe into it, and as you breathe out say in your mind - "soften and flow....soften and flow"....Continue to gently breathe into it and every now and again as you breathe out say, "soften and flow, soften and flow."

[BIG pause]

Acknowledge it again. Sit with it if you like. There is no need to resist it, just be with it, breathe into it and .... "soften and flow, soften and flow."

[BIG pause]

If you find your mind wandering, not to worry, just as often as you are able, bring it gently back to the area of observation and .... "soften and flow....soften and flow."

[BIG pause]

You might find the tension is easing off a little now.

If you'd like to continue to rest quietly, do so.

[brief pause]

Otherwise just begin to deepen your breath a little. Wriggle your toes and your fingers. And in your own time when you're ready, open your eyes.

Deep Muscle Relaxation

Let's spend some time now tuning into and relaxing our body. Find a balanced position lying on your back with a pillow beneath your head; body straight; or you could sit upright in a chair. If you are using this as an aid for sleeping then lying on your back in your bed ready for sleep is fine.

.... Now, gently close your eyes. Begin by taking two slow, deep breaths. Breathing in as fully as is comfortable and letting the air flow out fully each time.

.... Now allow your breathing to return to its own natural pace. Become aware of your whole body. Feel your body's weight. You might like to adjust your position, so that it feels balanced and comfortable.... Now take another slow deep breath, allowing the surface you are lying on to take your weight completely.

.... Clearly picture your feet in your mind, wriggle your toes if it helps and let your feet relax, soften, loosen, allowing a deep relaxation to flow into your feet.... Turn your attention to your calves, notice how they feel, is one calf tighter than the other, just observe how your calves feel without the need for judgment or comment and allow the calves to relax. Let the relaxation flow deeply through the muscles of the calves - softening, loosening, releasing.

.... Turn your attention now to your thighs. Notice how they feel, feel the back of your thighs, feel the front of your thighs, allow them to release, letting go. Allow your thighs to relax..., soften..., loosen. **[pause]**

.... Bring your attention now to your buttocks. Allow the muscles to relax. Letting go of any tension, let it flow down your legs and out through the tips of your toes....

.... Focus now on your belly. Notice how it feels, allow it to soften. Feel a relaxation spreading around your belly to your lower back.... Feel the relaxation spreading right through, calm and ease....ease and calm.

.... Shift your attention now to your chest, notice how it moves with your breath - as you breathe with your own natural rhythm.... Feel the chest wall soften; loosen, all the way around to your back.

.... Become aware of your arms. Feel the weight of your arms, relaxing your upper arms, your elbows, your forearms, your wrists and your hands.

.... Bring your attention to your shoulders, notice how they feel, allow your shoulders to hang loose..., soften..., release.

.... Become aware of your neck, feel your muscles soften, relax, release....

.... Allow the jaw to hang loose, the lips to part slightly, relaxing the mouth..., your cheeks..., softening and releasing.... Feel your eyes relax..., your forehead smooth over..., feel the top of your head loosening and releasing..., the sides of your head..., the back of your head.

.... Rest with your body's weight....

.... Let's take a further mental inventory of the body, deepening our relaxation as we send a message to let go and relax to the:

Toes of the feet..., soles..., heels..., back of the feet,

Send a message to let go and relax to the:

Ankles..., calves..., shins.... and your knees.

Send a message to let go and relax to the:

Back of the knees..., thighs..., back of the thighs.... and your buttocks.

Send a message to let go and relax to the:

Lower back..., middle back..., upper back.... and your shoulders.

Send a message to let go and relax to the:

Upper arms..., elbows..., forearms.... and wrists.

Send a message to let go and relax to the:

Palm of the hands..., back of the hands..., fingers and your thumbs.

Send a message to let go and relax to:

Your belly..., chest..., neck.... and your jaw.

Send a message to let go and relax to:

Your mouth..., nose..., cheeks.... and your eyes.

Send a message to let go and relax to:

Your eyelids..., eyebrows..., forehead.... and your ears.

Send a message to let go and relax to:

Your temples..., top of your head..., sides of your head and the back of the head.

Feeling waves of relaxation passing through your whole body, as you simply let go and relax.

.... Resting with the ease of it all....the ease of it all.

[BIG Pause]

(Silence for as long as desired.)

(Feeling the weight of your body and the ease of it all....the ease of it all.)

[BIG Pause]

Gently deepen your breath..., wriggle the toes a little..., and your fingers.... and just in your own time when you're ready, gently open your eyes.

Appendix 3

ME/CFS CANADIAN CLINICAL DIAGNOSTIC CRITERIA SUMMARY

To diagnose ME/CFS the patient must have the following:

- Pathological fatigue, post-exertional malaise, sleep problems, pain, two neurocognitive symptoms, and at least one symptom from two of the following categories: autonomic, neuroendocrine and/or immune.
- The fatigue and the other symptoms must persist, or be relapsing for at least six months in adults, or three months in children. A provisional diagnosis may be possible earlier.
- The symptoms cannot be explained by another illness.

Improved diagnostic accuracy can be obtained by measuring the severity and frequency of the listed symptoms.

Symptoms	Description of Symptoms
Pathological fatigue	A significant degree of new onset, unexplained, persistent or recurrent physical and/or mental fatigue that substantially reduces activity levels and which is not the result of ongoing exertion and not relieved by rest.
Post-exertional malaise	Mild exertion or even normal activities followed by malaise: the loss of physical and mental stamina and/or worsening of other symptoms. Recovery is delayed, taking more than 24 hours.

Symptoms	Description of Symptoms
Sleep problems	Sleep is unrefreshing: disturbed quantity - daytime hypersomnia or night-time insomnia and/or disturbed rhythm – day/night reversal. Rarely is there no sleep problem.
Pain	Pain is widespread, migratory or localized: Myalgia; arthralgia (without signs of inflammation); and/or headache - a new type, pattern or severity. Rarely is there no pain.
Neurocognitive symptoms	Impaired concentration, short term memory or word retrieval; hypersensitivity to light, noise or emotional overload; confusion; disorientation; slowness of thought; muscle weakness; ataxia. (Two required)

At least one symptom from two of these categories:

Autonomic	Orthostatic intolerance: neurally mediated hypotension (NMH); postural orthostatic tachycardia (POTS); light headedness; extreme pallor; palpitations; exertional dyspnea; urinary frequency; irritable bowel syndrome (IBS); nausea.
Neuroendocrine	Low body temperature; cold extremities; sweating; intolerance to heat or cold; reduced tolerance for stress; other symptoms worsen with stress; weight change; abnormal appetite.
Immune	Recurrent flu-like symptoms; sore throats; tender lymph nodes; fevers; new sensitivities to food, medicines, odors or chemicals.

ACKNOWLEDGEMENTS

Thank you to all my patients and friends who shared their stories with me so that I could share them with you. I offer particular thanks to Tori Sommer for her role as a sounding board, editor and one-person cheer squad. Vicki Kotsirilos, for being such an inspirational friend, acting as a medical editor and for writing such a beautiful Foreword. Michael Keary for reading the full manuscript and providing invaluable grammatical suggestions. My sister Dianne Sommer for proof reading assistance. David Manks, for reading specific parts of the manuscript and offering suggestions. My good friend Judy Singer for tracking down research articles for me. The 'Powerful Poets' luncheon lines group: Caspar von Diebitsch, Therese van Wegen and Tori; our monthly meetings where I could share my writing were precious and kept me on track. Neil Day, for reading sections of the manuscript and providing me with encouragement and constructive feedback. Margot Maurice for her guidance on publishing and belief in this project. Thanks to Jeny Ruelo and her team at The Fast Fingers Book Formatting Service.

Invaluable support and encouragement was also gratefully received from: Michelle and Lee Sommer, David Shneider, Andrew Rudzki, Dr Anthony Sommer and Maggie Kryk, Becky Sommer, Rosina and Mike Teichmann, Carol and Mike Hancock, Natalie and Paul Banks, Tania Haimon, Marcel Haimovici, Mitzi and Amos Lang and Catherine Chang, Mark Parker, Peter and Maria Saunders, Dr Daniel and Bev Lewis, Laurie Lacey, Dr Craig and Deirdre Hassed, Drs Ian and Ruth Gawler, Siegfried Gutbrod, Drs Andrew and Anita Davis, Dr Leon and Linda Chapman, Dr Katie Moss, Dr Marita Smith, Philip and Rae Rayner, Monica Winston, Robert and Ingrid Hindell, Fi Bisko, Anne Beischer, Kate Ellis and Peter Long, the Clark family, the Gador family, the Gray family, the Laird family, the Haimovici family, the Fisterman family, the Rosenstrauss family, Dr Sandra Palmer and Dr Nick Kafieris, Dr Dale and Jacqui Wilson, Dr Joe and Jean Di Stefano, Dr Ross Knight, Prof Neil Carson, Prof John Murtagh, Prof Marc Cohen, Prof Leon Piterman, Dr George Halasz, Dr Michael Axtens, John Coleman, Justine Day, Pam Garrity, Fran and Frank O'Reilly, Anne Thompson, Liz and Alan Flaherty, Max Polke, Michael Black, my other Bialik classmates, Rachel and Yohai Weiss, Drs Shirley and Doug Winter, the WHI core group, Sister Pat O'Brien, Liz and Scott Manning, Danita Harrison, Sue Streat, Nathan Dabkowski, Alan and Anne Randall, Janelle Humphries, Dinah Keary, Robyn Venables, Eva and Joe Shneider, Norelle Gross, Ingrid von Diebitsch and Steve Kontjonis, Alan and Arlette Eastgate, Dr Peter Hill, Joan McLagan, Jan Cahill, Dr Steve Mitchell, Ron and Di King, Dr James Bennett-Levy, David and Samantha McRae, John Gallagher, Lance Willis, Kirsten and Adrian Wojtowicz, Ron Phelan and John O'Connor.

For the most part, the names and identifying details of the patients and friends mentioned within the body of the text have been changed to preserve anonymity. The clinical stories are from public hospitals and general practice clinics I've worked in across the state of Victoria, Australia.

ABOUT THE AUTHOR

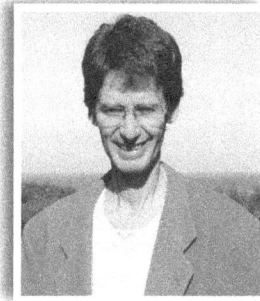

Steven Sommer M.B.,B.S FRACGP graduated from medical school in 1984, worked in hospital settings and successfully completed his general practice training to become a Fellow of the Royal Australian College of General Practitioners in 1991.

He began teaching stress management in the early 90's whilst working as a GP and senior lecturer at Monash University's Department of General Practice. Recognizing the need amongst his patients and medical students, he began by teaching them techniques to manage their stress. Soon he found himself presenting to groups of doctors, nurses, high school students and people from all walks of life. He has also been an invited Grand Round presenter on this topic at several major teaching hospitals.

In 1993 he took on the role of president of the Whole Health Institute of Australasia; a non-profit educational organization. A major health crisis in 1996 led to him relinquishing all of his roles. In 2007 he returned to general practice and teaching at Deakin University Medical School. Further health crises in 2011 left him unable to continue as a practitioner. This opened up the space for a lifetime ambition to share his ideas and insights through writing, he has found it to be a most rewarding activity.

He lives in Geelong, Australia, with his wife, Tori, and their two cats, Claude and Pip.

REFERENCES

INTRODUCTION

1. Pert C B. Molecules of Emotion. Simon & Schuster, New York 1999.
2. Coulehan J. Deep hope: A song without words. Theoretical Medicine and Bioethics, June 2011;32(3):143-60.

CHAPTER 1: CHANGING THE ODDS

1. Kiely BE, Tattersall MH, Stockler MR. Certain death in uncertain time: informing hope by quantifying a best case scenario. J Clin Oncol. 2010 Jun 1;28(16):2802-4.
2. Ibid
3. Pinquart M, Duberstein P R. Associations of Social Networks with Cancer Mortality: A Meta-Analysis. Critical Reviews in Oncology/Hematology August 2010;75(2):122-37.
4. Spiegel D, Bloom JR, Kraemer HC, et al. Effect of psychosocial treatment on survival of patients with metastatic breast cancer. Lancet. 1989 Oct 14;2(8668):888-91.
5. Fawzy FI, Fawzy NW, Hyun CS, et al. Malignant melanoma. Effects of an early structured psychiatric intervention, coping, and affective state on recurrence and survival 6 years later. Arch Gen Psychiatry. 1993 Sep;50(9):681-9.
6. Hirschberg C, Barasch M I. Remarkable Recovery – What Extraordinary Healings Tell Us About Getting Well and Staying Well. Riverhead Books, New York 1995:14.
7. Ibid. 6, pxiv.
8. Ibid. 6, pxiii.

9. Novack DH, Plumer R, Smith RL, et al. Changes in physicians' attitudes toward telling the cancer patient. JAMA. 1979 Mar 2;241(9):897-900.

10. Baade PD, Youlden DR, Chambers SK. When do I know I am cured? Using conditional estimates to provide better information about cancer survival prospects. Med J Aust. 2011 Jan 17;194(2):73-7.

11. Cousin-Frannel J, Cancer Immunotherapy. Science 2013 Dec 20;342(6165):1432-3.

12. Ibid. 6, p7-11.

13. Ibid. 6, p10-11.

14. Mayo C. Tumor Clinic Conference, Cancer Bulletin 1963;15:78-9.

15. Ibid. 6, p11.

16. Hagerty RG, Butow PN, Ellis PA, et al. Cancer patient preferences for communication of prognosis in the metastatic setting. J Clin Oncol 2004;22:1721–1730

17. Osborne RH, Sali A, Aaronson NK, et al. Immune function and adjustment style: do they predict survival in breast cancer? Psychooncology. 2004 Mar;13(3):199-210.

18. Turner KA. Radical Remission: Surviving Cancer Against All Odds. HarperOne, New York, 2014.

19. Ibid. 1, p2804.

20. Kaiser HE, Bodey B Jr, Siegel SE, et al. Spontaneous neoplastic regression: the significance of apoptosis. In Vivo 2000 Nov-Dec; 14(6): 773-788.

21. Thomas JA, Badini M. The role of innate immunity in spontaneous regression of cancer. Indian J Cancer 2011;48:246-51.

22. Ibid. 6, p17.

23. Gutbrod S, Rumbold G, Gruettke C. Remarkable recovery and exceptional disease course in cancer an overview. Healthy Living 2012;12:4-7.

24. Ibid. 18, p1.

25. Everson TC. Spontaneous regression of cancer. Prog Clin Cancer 1967;3:79-95. Http://www.noetic.org/research/project/spontaneous-remission/faqs/ (accessed February 2016)

26. Papac RJ. Spontaneous regression of cancer: possible mechanisms. In Vivo. 1998 Nov-Dec;12(6):571-8. Review.

27. Oquiñena S, Guillen-Grima F, Iñarrairaegui M, et al. Spontaneous regression of hepatocellular carcinoma: a systematic review. Eur J Gastroenterol Hepatol. 2009 Mar;21(3):254-7. Review.

28. Ghatalia P, Morgan CJ, Sonpavde G. Meta-analysis of regression of advanced solid tumors in patients receiving placebo or no anti-cancer therapy in prospective trials. Crit Rev Oncol Hematol 2016;98:122-36.

29. Ibid., p129.

30. Kraus P. Surviving Cancer – Inspiring stories of hope and healing. Michelle Anderson Publishing, Melbourne 2008. See also Gawler I, Inspiring People. The Gawler Foundation 1995.

31. Allenby G. Ian Gawler - The Dragons Blessing. Allen & Unwin 2008, p294.

32. Ibid. 6, pxiii-xiv.

33. Ibid. 6, p170.

34. Ibid. 18, p1-13.

35. Ibid. 18, p282.

36. Ibid. 18, p29.

37. http://theconversation.com/why-exercise-should-be-added-to-cancer-treatment-plans-12288 (accessed May 2016)

38. http://www.abc.net.au/catalyst/stories/4459555.htm (accessed May 2016)

39. Ornish D, Weidner G,Fair WR et al. Intensive lifestyle changes may affect progression of prostate cancer, the Journal of Urology September 2005; Vol. 174, 1065–1070.

40. Frattaroli J, Weidner G, Dnistrian AM, et al. Clinical events in prostate cancer lifestyle trial: results from two years of follow-up. Urology. 2008 Dec;72(6):1319-23.

41. Ornish D, Magbanua MJ, Weidner G et al. Changes in prostate gene expression in men undergoing an intensive nutrition and lifestyle intervention. Proc Natl Acad Sci U S A. 2008 Jun 17;105(24):8369-74.
42. Ornish D, Lin J, Chan JM et al. Effect of comprehensive lifestyle changes on telomerase activity and telomere length in men with biopsy-proven low-risk prostate cancer: 5-year follow-up of a descriptive pilot study, Lancet Oncol. 2013 Oct;14(11):1112-20.
43. Ibid. 4.
44. Ibid. 5.
45. Ibid. 18, p1-13.
46. Ibid. 6, p61-67.
47. http://cim.ucsd.edu/documents/IO2013Program_Final.pdf (see p29, accessed May 2016)
48. https://colascchamber.wordpress.com/tag/palmetto-health/ (accessed January 2016)

CHAPTER 3: MEDICINE AN INEXACT SCIENCE

1. Arbesman S. The Half-Life of Facts: Why Everything We Know Has an Expiration Date. Penguin Group USA 2012.
2. https://www.psychologytoday.com/blog/hide-and-seek/201209/brief-history-schizophrenia (accessed August 2016)
3. Wilson C. Out of the Shadows. New Scientist 8 February 2014:32-35.
4. Wunderink L, Nieboer RM, Wiersma D, et al. Recovery in remitted first-episode psychosis at 7 years of follow-up of an early dose reduction/discontinuation or maintenance treatment strategy: long-term follow-up of a 2-year randomized clinical trial. JAMA Psychiatry. 2013 Sep;70(9):913-20.
5. Leff J, Williams G, Huckvale MA, et al. Computer-assisted therapy for medication-resistant auditory hallucinations: proof-of-concept study. Br J Psychiatry. 2013 Jun;202:428-33.
6. Makary MA, Daniel M. Medical error -- the third leading cause of death

in the US. BMJ. 2016;353:i2139. http://www.bmj.com/content/353/bmj. i2139. (Accessed June 2016.)

7. Deutsch D. The Fabric of Reality. Penguin Great Britain 1997:30.

8. Méjean C, Droomers M, van der Schouw YT, et al. The contribution of diet and lifestyle to socioeconomic inequalities in cardiovascular morbidity and mortality. Int J Cardiol. 2013 Oct 15;168(6):5190-5.

9. Kotsirilos V, Vitetta L, Sali A. A guide to evidence-based integrative and complementary medicine. Elsevier Australia 2011:10.

10. Ulrich R S. View through a Window May Influence Recovery from Surgery. Science 1984;224 (4647): 420-1.

11. Headache Study Group, Predictors of outcome in headache patients presenting to family physicians--a one year prospective study. The Headache Study Group of The University of Western Ontario.(No authors listed) Headache. 1986 Jun;26(6):285-94.

12. Bösner S, Hartel S, Diederich J, et al. Diagnosing headache in primary care: a qualitative study of GPs' approaches. Br J Gen Pract. 2014 Sep;64(626):e532-7.

13. Jospe M. The Placebo Effect Healing. Lexington Books Toronto 1978.

14. Moerman D E. Meaning, Medicine and the Placebo Effect. Cambridge 2002:32-46.

CHAPTER 4: EPIGENETICS

1. Spector T. Identically different - Why you can change your genes. Weidenfeld & Nicholson 2012:9,10.

2. https://en.wikipedia.org/wiki/Genomics (accessed February 2016)

3. Ibid, 1, p11.

4. http://www.pbs.org/wgbh/nova/body/epigenetics.html (accessed February 2016)

5. http://learn.genetics.utah.edu/content/epigenetics/ (accessed February 2016)

6. Ibid, 1, p35.

7. Richardson K, The Making of intelligence. New York: Columbia University Press 2000. (Reference by Rossi EL, The Psychobiology of Gene Expression: Neuroscience and Neurogenesis in Hypnosis in the Healing Arts. New York: WW Norton and Co. 2002:50.)

8. Dispenza J. You Are the Placebo: Making Your Mind Matter. Hay House 2014:93.

9. http://www.epigenome.org (accessed February 2016)

10. http://nutrigenomics.ucdavis.edu (accessed February 2016)

11. DeBusk R, Joffe Y. It's Not Just Your Genes! Your diet, your lifestyle, your genes. BKDR Inc. USA 2006:21-2.

12. DeBusk R, Genetics: The Nutrition Connection. Chicago IL: The American Dietetic Association, 2003.

13. Menendez JA, Vellon L, Colomer R, et al. Effect of gamma-linolenic acid on the transcriptional activity of the Her-2/neu (erbB- 2) oncogene. J Natl Cancer Inst 2005;97(21):1611-1615.

14. Ibid 9,p.33,4.

15. National Health and Medical Research Council. Direct-to-consumer DNA genetic testing and information resource for consumers. Available at www.nhmrc.gov.au/_files_nhmrc/publications/attachments/ps0004_dna_direct_to_consumer pdf (accessed May 2014)

16. Ibid 10.

17. Lamarck JB. Philosophie Zoologique. Dentu Paris 1809.

18. Ibid. 1, p27-30.

19. Packard AS. Lamarck, The Founder of Evolution: His Life and Work, Longmans New York 1901.

20. Ibid. 1, p38,9.

21. Waterland RA, Jirtle RL. Transposable elements: targets for early nutritional effects on epigenetic gene regulation. Mol Cell Biol. 2003 Aug;23(15):5293-300.

22. Dolinoy DC, Weidman JR, Waterland RA, Jirtle RL. Maternal genistein alters coat color and protects Avy mouse offspring from obesity

by modifying the fetal epigenome. Environ Health Perspect. 2006 Apr;114(4):567-72.

23. Jirtle RL, Skinner MK, Environmental epigenomics and disease susceptibility.Nat Rev Genet. 2007 Apr;8(4):253-62. Review.

24. Whitelaw NC, Whitelaw E, Transgenerational epigenetic inheritance in health and disease. Curr Opin Genet Dev. 2008 Jun;18(3):273-9.

25. Jablonka E, Raz G. Transgenerational epigenetic inheritance: prevalence,mechanisms, and implications for the study of heredity and evolution. Q Rev Biol.2009 Jun;84(2):131-76. Review.

26. Qiu J. Epigenetics: unfinished symphony. Nature. 2006 May 11;441(7090):143-5.

27. Lumey LH, Stein AD, Kahn HS, et al. Cohort profile: the Dutch Hunger Winter families study. Int J Epidemiol. 2007 Dec;36(6):1196-204.

28. Roseboom TJ, van der Meulen JH, Osmond C, et al. Coronary heart disease after prenatal exposure to the Dutch famine, 1944-45. Heart. 2000 Dec;84(6):595-8.

29. Roseboom TJ, van der Meulen JH, Osmond C, et al. Plasma lipid profiles in adults after prenatal exposure to the Dutch famine. Am J Clin Nutr. 2000 Nov;72(5):1101-6.

30. Painter RC, Roseboom TJ, Bleker OP. Prenatal exposure to the Dutch famine and disease in later life: an overview. Reprod Toxicol. 2005 Sep-Oct;20(3):345-52. Review.

31. Kaati G, Bygren LO, Edvinsson S. Cardiovascular and diabetes mortality determined by nutrition during parents' and grandparents' slow growth period. Eur J Hum Genet Nov 2002 10 (11): 682–8.

32. Pembrey ME, Bygren LO, Kaati G et al. ALSPAC Study Team. Sex-specific, male-line transgenerational responses in humans. Eur J Hum Genet. 2006 Feb;14(2):159-66.

33. Bygren LO, Tinghög P, Carstensen J, et al. Change in paternal grandmothers' early food supply influenced cardiovascular mortality of the female grandchildren. BMC Genet. 2014 Feb 20;15:12.

34. Kral JG, Biron S, Simard S, et al. Large maternal weight loss from obesity surgery prevents transmission of obesity to children who were followed for 2 to 18 years. Pediatrics. 2006. Dec;118(6):e1644-9.

35. Benyshek DC. The "early life" origins of obesity-related health disorders: new discoveries regarding the intergenerational transmission of developmentally programmed traits in the global cardiometabolic health crisis. Am J Phys Anthropol. 2013 Dec;152 Suppl 57:79-93.

36. Spencer SJ. Perinatal nutrition programs neuroimmune function long-term: mechanisms and implications. Front Neurosci. 2013 Aug 12;7:144.

37. http://drchromo.wordpress.com/2014/03/11/epigenetics-from-greeks-to-geeks-and-leaks/ (accessed September 2014)

38. http://www.mrc-leu.soton.ac.uk/dohad/index.asp (accessed September 2014)

39. http://learn.genetics.utah.edu/content/epigenetics/rats/ (accessed September 2014)

40. Hellstrom IC, Dhir SK, Diorio JC, Meaney MJ. Maternal licking regulates hippocampal glucocorticoid receptor transcription through a thyroid hormone-serotonin-NGFI-A signalling cascade. Philos Trans R Soc Lond B Biol Sci. 2012 Sep 5;367(1601):2495-510.

41. Zhang TY, Labonté B, Wen XL, et al. Epigenetic mechanisms for the early environmental regulation of hippocampal glucocorticoid receptor gene expression in rodents and humans. Neuropsychopharmacology. 2013 Jan;38(1):111-123.

42. Ibid. 1, p278-80.

43. Ibid. 1, p280-1.

44. Ibid. 1, p1-5.

45. MacGregor AJ, Snieder H, Rigby AS, et al. Characterizing the quantitative genetic contribution to rheumatoid arthritis using data from twins. Arthritis Rheum 2000 Jan;43(1):30-7.

46. Roos L, van Dongen J, Bell CG, et al. Integrative DNA methylome analysis of pan-cancer biomarkers in cancer discordant monozygotic

twin-pairs. Clin Epigenetics. 2016 Jan 20;8:7. doi: 10.1186/s13148-016-0172-y. eCollection 2016.

47. Liu F, Wollstein A, Hysi PG, Ankra-Badu GA et al., Digital quantification of human eye color highlights genetic association of three new loci. PLoS Genet. 2010 May 6;6(5):e1000934.

48. http://www.theglobeandmail.com/life/parenting/why-identical-twins-can-look-different/article4186733/(accessed February 2016)

49. Ibid. 1, p20.

50. Ibid. 1, p293.

51. Benson H, The Relaxation Response: HarperCollins 1975.

52. Benson H, Proctor W. Relaxation Revolution: Simon & Schuster 2011.

53. Dusek JA, Otu HH, Wohlhueter AL, et al. Genomic counter-stress changes induced by the relaxation response. PLoS One. 2008 Jul 2;3(7):e2576.

54. Bhasin MK, Dusek JA, Chang BH et al. Relaxation response induces temporal transcriptome changes in energy metabolism, insulin secretion and inflammatory pathways. PLoS One. 2013 May 1;8(5):e62817.

55. Ornish D, Magbanua MJ, Weidner G, et al. Changes in prostate gene expression in men undergoing an intensive nutrition and lifestyle intervention. Proc Natl Acad Sci U S A. 2008 Jun 17;105(24):8369-74.

56. Ornish D, Lin J, Chan JM, et al. Effect of comprehensive lifestyle changes on telomerase activity and telomere length in men with biopsy-proven low-risk prostate cancer: 5-year follow-up of a descriptive pilot study, Lancet Oncol. 2013 Oct;14(11):1112-20.

57. Turner KA. Radical Remission: Surviving Cancer Against All Odds. HarperOne, New York, 2014.

CHAPTER 5: MEDITATION AS MEDICINE

1. Sommer SJ. Mind-body medicine and holistic approaches: the scientific evidence. Australian Family Physician 1996;25(8):1233–1244.

2. Hassed C, Mind-Body Medicine: Science, Practice and Philosophy.

At - http://www.lifestyleandculturelectures.org/lectures/mindfulness/ MindBodyMedicine/ (accessed March 2016)

3. Dunn AJ, Swiergiel AH, de Beaurepaire R. Cytokines as mediators of depression: what can we learn from animal studies? Neuroscience & Biobehavioral Reviews. 2005;29(4-5):891-909.

4. Benson H. The Relaxation Response. HarperCollins 1975.

5. Ibid. 2.

6. Kesterton J. Metabolic rate, respiratory exchange ratio and apneas during meditation. American J of Physiology 1989;256(3):632-8.

7. Benson H. The relaxation response and norepinephrine: a new study illuminates mechanisms. Australian J of Clinical Hypnotherapy and Hypnosis 1989;10(2):91-6.

8. Mills P, Schneider R, Hill D, et al. Beta-adrenergic receptor sensitivity in subjects practicing TM. J Psychosomatic Research 1990;34(1):29-33.

9. Delmonte M. Physiological responses during meditation and rest. Biofeedback and Self-regulation 1984;9(2):181-200.

10. Vyas R, Dikshit N. Effect of meditation on respiratory system, cardiovascular system and lipid profile. Indian Journal of Physiology & Pharmacology. 2002;46(4):487-91.

11. Bagga O, Gandhi A, Bagga S. A study of the effect of TM and yoga on blood glucose, lactic acid, cholesterol and total lipids. J of Clinical Chemistry and Clinical Biochemistry 1981;19(8):607-8.

12. Echenhofer F, Coombs M. A brief review of research and controversies in EEG biofeedback and meditation. The Journal of Transpersonal Psychology 1987;19(2):161-71.

13. Deepak K, Manchanda SK, Maheshwari MC. Meditation improves clinico-electroencephalographic measures in drug-resistant epileptics. Biofeedback and self-regulation 1994;19:(1)25-40.

14. Bujatti M, Riederer P. Serotonin, noradrenaline, dopamine metabolites in TM technique. Journal of Neural Transmission. 1976;39:257-67.

15. Jevning R, Anand R, Biedebach M, et al. Effects on regional cerebral blood flow of TM. Physiology and Behavior 1996;59(3):399-402.

16. Werner O, Wallace RK, Charles B, et al. Long-term endocrine changes in subjects practicing the TM and TM-siddhi program. Psychosomatic Medicine 1986;48(1-2):59-65.

17. Jedrczak A, Toomey M, Clements G. The TM-siddhi program, age, and brief tests of perceptual motor speed and non-verbal intelligence. Journal of Clinical Psychology 1986;42(1):161-4.

18. Brown D, Forte M, Dysart M. Visual sensitivity and mindfulness meditation. Perceptual and Motor Skills 1984;58:775-84.

19. Carlson LE, Speca M, Patel KD, et al. Mindfulness-based stress reduction in relation to quality of life, mood, symptoms of stress, and immune parameters in breast and prostate cancer outpatients. Psychosomatic Medicine. 2003;65(4):571-81.

20. Coehlo R, Silva C, Maia A, et al. Bone mineral density and depression: a community study in women. J of Psychosomatic Research 1999;46(1):29-35.

21. Kabat-Zinn J, Burney L, Sellers R, et al. Four year follow-up of a meditation based program for the self-regulation of chronic pain; treatment outcomes and compliance. Clinical Journal of Pain 1987;2:159-73.

22. Wilson A, Honsberger R, Chiu JT, et al. Transcendental meditation and asthma. Respiration 1975;32:74-80.

23. Cerpa H. The effects of clinically standardized meditation on type 2 diabetics. Dissertation Abstracts International 1989;499(8b):3432.

24. Kabat-Zinn J, Massion AO, Kristeller J, et al. Effectiveness of a meditation based stress reduction program in the treatment of anxiety disorders. Am J Psychiatry 1992;149:936-43.

25. Eppley K, Abrams AI, Shear J. Differential effects of relaxation techniques on trait anxiety: a meta-analysis. Journal of Clinical Psychology 1989;45(6):957-74.

26. Teasdale J, Segal Z, Williams J. How does cognitive therapy prevent depressive relapse and why should attention control (mindfulness) training help? Behavior Research and Therapy. 1995;33(1):25-39.

27. Bujatti M, Riederer P. Serotonin, noradrenaline, dopamine metabolites in TM technique. J of Neural Transmission. 1976;39(3):257-67.

28. Alexander CN, Rainforth M, Gelderloos P. TM, self-actualization, and psychological health: a conceptual overview and statistical meta-analysis. Journal of Social Behavior and Personality 1991;6(5):189-248.

29. Kornfield J. Intensive insight meditation: a phenomenonological study. Journal of Transpersonal Psychology 1979;11(1):48-51.

30. Kutz I, Lerserman J, Dorrington C, et al. Meditation as an adjunct to psychotherapy. An outcome study. Psychotherapy and Psychosomatics 1985;43(4):209-18.

31. Gelderloos P, Walton KG, Orme-Johnson DW, et al. Effectiveness of the TM program in preventing and treating substance misuse: a review. Int J Addict 1991;26:293-325.

32. Mason L, Alexander C, Travis F, et al. Electrophysiological correlates of higher states of consciousness during sleep in long-term practitioners of the TM program. Sleep 1997;20(2):102-10.

33. Abrams AI, Siegel LM. The TM program and rehabilitation at Folsom Prison: a cross-validation study. Criminal Justice and Behavior 1978;5(1):3-20.

34. Carrington P, Collings G, Benson H, et al. The use of meditation and relaxation techniques for the management of stress in a working population. J of Occupational Medicine 1980;22(4):221-31.

35. Fiebert MS, Mead TR. Meditation and academic performance. Perceptual and Motor Skills 1981;53(2):447-50.

36. Rani N, Rao PV. Effects of meditation on attention processes. Journal of Indian Psychology 2000;18:5260.

37. Delmonte M, Kenny V. Conceptual models and functions of meditation in psychotherapy. Journal of Contemporary Psychotherapy

1987;17(1):38-59.

38. Lucassen P, Assendelft W, Gubbels J, et al. Effectiveness of treatment for infantile colic: a systematic review. BMJ 1998;316(7144):1563-9.

39. www.drstevensommer.com

CHAPTER 6: LIFESTYLE AS THERAPY – HEART DISEASE AND BEYOND

1. lifestylemedicine.com.au (accessed February 2016)

2. lifestylemedicine.org (accessed February 2016)

3. http://www.calmlifestylemedicine.ca/ (accessed September 2016)

4. eu-lifestyle medicine.org (accessed February 2016)

5. Egger GJ, Binns AF, Rossner SR. The emergence of 'lifestyle medicine' as a structured approach for management of chronic disease. Medical Journal of Australia 2009;190(3):143-145.

6. http://www.medicalsciencenavigator.com/physiology-of-self-renewal (accessed February 2016)

7. Robbins J. Still Healthy at 100. Hodder & Stoughton 2006.

8. Ibid,p146.

9. Moritani T, Akamatsu Y. J Effect of Exericse and Nutrition upon Lifestyle-Related Disease and Cognitive Function. Nutr Sci Vitaminol (Tokyo). 2015;61 Suppl:S122-4.

10. Pedersen BK, Saltin B. Exercise as medicine - evidence for prescribing exercise as therapy in 26 different chronic diseases. Scand J Med Sci Sports. 2015 Dec;25 Suppl 3:1-72. doi: 10.1111/sms.12581. Review.

11. http://www.britannica.com/biography/Edward-Stanley-3rd-earl-of-Derby/article-supplemental-information (accessed February 2016)

12. Ibid.7,p72.

13. http://www.ctsu.ox.ac.uk/~china/monograph/ (accessed February 2016)

14. Campbell TC, Campbell TM. The China study: the most comprehensive study of nutrition ever conducted. Startling implications for diet, weight loss, and long-term health. BenBella Books 2004.

15. Madhavan TV, Gopalan C. The Effect of Dietary Protein on Carcinogenesis of Aflatoxin. Archives of Pathology 1968;85(2):133-7.

16. Schulsinger DA, Root MM, Campbell TC. Effect of Dietary Protein Quality on Development of Aflatoxin B1-induced Hepatic Pre-Neoplastic Lesions. Journal of the National Cancer Institute 1989;81:1241–1245.

17. Campbell TC. Dietary protein, growth factors, and cancer. Am J Clin Nutr. 2007 Jun;85(6):1667. Free article available at: http://ajcn.nutrition.org/content/85/6/1667.long ttps://wwwv=9atch?v=9RcQCQ0VS54

18. Le LT, Sabaté J. Beyond meatless, the health effects of vegan diets: findings from the Adventist cohorts. Nutrients. 2014 May 27;6(6):2131-47.

19. http://www.mayoclinic.org/healthy-lifestyle/nutrition-and-healthy-eating/in- depth/mediterranean-diet/art-20047801 (accessed April 2016)

20. Martinez-Gonzalez MA, Martin-Calvo N. Mediterranean diet and life expectancy; beyond olive oil, fruits, and vegetables. Curr Opin Clin Nutr Metab Care. 2016 Aug 23. (Epub ahead of print)

21. Bloomfield HE, Kane R, Koeller E, et al. Benefits and Harms of the Mediterranean Diet Compared to Other Diets (Internet).Washington (DC): Department of Veterans Affairs (US); 2015 Nov. free text at http://www.ncbi.nlm.nih.gov/pubmed/27559560 (accessed September 2016)

22. Oyebode O, Gordon-Dseagu V, Walker A, et al. Fruit and vegetable consumption and all-cause, cancer and CVD mortality: analysis of Health Survey for England data. J Epidemiol Community Health. 2014 Sep;68(9):856-62

23. Wang X, Ouyang Y, Liu J, et al. Fruit and vegetable consumption and mortality from all causes, cardiovascular disease, and cancer: systematic review and dose-response meta-analysis of prospective cohort studies. BMJ. 2014 Jul 29;349:4490.

24. Nguyen B, Bauman A, Gale J, et al. Fruit and vegetable consumption and all-cause mortality: evidence from a large Australian cohort study. Int J Behav Nutr Phys Act. 2016 Jan 25;13:9.

25. Wang X, Lin X, Ouyang Y, et al. Red and processed meat consumption and mortality: dose-response meta-analysis of prospective cohort studies. Public Health Nutr. 2016 Apr; 19(5):893-905.

26. Ornish D, Brown SE, Scherwitz L W et al. Can lifestyle changes reverse coronary heart disease? Lancet 1990:336: 129-133.

27. Moyers B. Healing and the Mind. Doubleday New York 1993:87-113.

28. News. US insurance company covers lifestyle therapy. Br Med J 1993;307:465.

29. Ornish D. Dr Dean Ornish 's program for reversing heart disease. New York: Random House, 1990; 119-121.

30. Zeng W, Stason WB, Fournier S et al. Benefits and costs of intensive lifestyle modification programs for symptomatic coronary disease in Medicare beneficiaries, Am Heart J. 2013 May;165(5):785-92.

31. Razavi M, Fournier S, Shepard DS, et al. Effects of Lifestyle Modification Programs on Cardiac Risk Factors PLoS One. 2014; 9(12): e114772.

32. http://www.dresselstyn.com/reversal01.htm (accessed February 2016)

33. Ibid.,14,p79.

34. DuBroff R, de Lorgeril M. Cholesterol confusion and statin controversy. World J Cardiol. 2015 Jul 26;7(7):404-9. (Free full text available at http://www.ncbi.nlm.nih.gov/pmc/articles/PMC4513492/) (accessed February 2016)

35. Esselstyn CB Jr, Gendy G, Doyle J et al. A way to reverse CAD? J Fam Pract. 2014 Jul;63(7):356-364b.

36. Myasaka Y, Barnes ME, Gerst BJ, et al. Secular trends in incidence of atrial fibrillation in Olmsted county, Minnesota 1980 to 2000 and implications on the projections for future prevalence. Circulation 2006;114(2):119-125.

37. Sritzke J, Markus MR, Duderstadt S, et al. MONICA/KORA Investigators. The ageing process of the heart: obesity is the main risk factor for left atrial enlargement during ageing the MONICA/KORA (monitoring of trends and determinations in cardiovascular disease/

cooperative research in the region of Augsburg) study. J Am Coll Cardiol 2009;54(21):1982-1989.

38. Abed HS,Wittert GA, Leong DP, et al. Effect of weight reduction and cardio metabolic risk factor management on symptom burden and severity in patients with atrial fibrillation - a randomised clinical trial. JAMA 2013:310(19);2050-2060.

CHAPTER 7: LIFESTYLE AS THERAPY – CANCER AND BEYOND

1. http://theconversation.com/why-exercise-should-be-added-to-cancer-treatment-plans-12288 (accessed May 2016)

2. http://www.abc.net.au/catalyst/stories/4459555.htm (accessed May 2016)

3. Ornish D, Weidner G,Fair WR et al. Intensive lifestyle changes may affect progression of prostate cancer, the Journal of Urology September 2005; Vol. 174, 1065–1070.

4. Frattaroli J, Weidner G, Dnistrian AM, et al. Clinical events in prostate cancer lifestyle trial: results from two years of follow-up. Urology. 2008 Dec;72(6):1319-23.

5. Ornish D, Magbanua MJ, Weidner G et al. Changes in prostate gene expression in men undergoing an intensive nutrition and lifestyle intervention. Proc Natl Acad Sci U S A. 2008 Jun 17;105(24):8369-74.

6. Ornish D, Lin J, Chan JM et al. Effect of comprehensive lifestyle changes on telomerase activity and telomere length in men with biopsy-proven low-risk prostate cancer: 5-year follow-up of a descriptive pilot study, Lancet Oncol. 2013 Oct;14(11):1112-20.

7. Jellinek G. Taking Control of Multiple Sclerosis -- Natural and Medical Therapies to Prevent its Progression. Melbourne: Hyland House Publishing 2005.

8. Esparza ML, Sasaki S, Kesteloot H. Nutrition, latitude and Multiple Sclerosis mortality: an ecologic study. Am J Epidemiol 1995;142:733-7.

9. Swank RL, Dugan BB. Effect of low saturated fat diet in early and late cases of Multiple Sclerosis. Lancet 1990;336:37-9.

10. Swank RL. Multiple Sclerosis: fat-oil relationship. Nutrition 1991;7:368-76.

11. Hadgkiss EJ, Jelinek GA, Weiland TJ et al. Health-related quality of life outcomes at 1 and 5 years after a residential retreat promoting lifestyle modification for people with multiple sclerosis, Neurol Sci. 2013 Feb;34(2):187-95.

12. lifestylemedicine.com.au (accessed February 2016)

13. lifestylemedicine.org (accessed February 2016)

14. http://www.calmlifestylemedicine.ca/ (accessed September 2016)

15. eu-lifestyle medicine.org (accessed February 2016)

CHAPTER 8: MIND-BODY WEAVING

1. Charlton M. Psychiatry and Ancient Medicine: in Galdston, Historic Derivations of Modern Psychiatry, McGraw-Hill 1967:12–16.

2. http://www.systemic-medicine.eu/subchap/2.3.a.Cartesian_split.html (accessed March 2016)

3. Gawler I, The Mind That Changes Everything. Brolga Publishing, Melbourne 2011:18,19.

4. Ibid.,p8.

5. Hackmann A, Bennett-Levy J, Holmes EA. Oxford Guide to Imagery in Cognitive Therapy. Oxford University press 2011:151-166.

6. Cumming J, Ramsey R. Sport imagery interventions. In Mellalieu S, Hanson S (eds.) Advances in applied sport psychology: a review. London Routledge 2008:5-36.

7. Nicklaus J, with Dowden K, Golf My Way. Simon & Schuster New York 2005:79.

8. Ehrsson HH, Geyer S, Naito E, Imagery of voluntary movement of fingers, toes, and tongue activates corresponding body-part-specific motor representation. Journal of Neurophysiology 2003;90(5):3304-3316.

9. Pasqual-Leone A, Nguyet D, Cohen L G, et al., Modulation of muscle responses evoked by transcranial magnetic stimulation during

the acquisition of new fine motor skills. Journal of Neurophysiology 1995;74(3):1037-1045.

10. Ranganathan V K, Siemionow V, Liu J Z, et al., From Mental Power to Muscle Power: gaining strength by using the mind. Neuropsychologia 2004;42(7):944-956.

11. Yue G, Cole K J, Strength Increases from the Motor Program: Comparison of training with maximal voluntary and imagined muscle contraction. Journal of Neurophysiology 1992; 67 (5):1114-1123.

12. Cohen P, Mental Gymnastics Increase Bicep Strength. New Scientist 2001;172(2318):17.

13. Guillot A, Lebon F, Rouiffer D, et al., Muscular responses during motor imagery as a function of muscle contraction types. International Journal of Psychophysiology 2007;66(1):18-27.

14. Preston C, Newport R, Analgesic Effects of Multisensory Illusions in Osteoarthritis. Rheumatology (Oxford) 2011;50(12):2314-15.

15. Greenleaf M, Mind Styles and The Hypnotic Induction Profile: Measure and Match to Enhance Medical Treatment. American Journal of Clinical Hypnosis. July 2006;49:1.

16. Spiegel H, Greenleaf M, Spiegel D. Hypnosis: An adjunct for psychotherapy.

17. Chapter in: Kaplan & Sadock Comprehensive textbook of psychiatry, 8th Ed., Virginia: Lippincott, Williams & Wilkins 2005:2548-2568.

18. Spiegel, H. The neural trance: A new look at hypnosis. Invited address: The Herbert Spiegel Lectureship, Department of Psychiatry, Columbia University, College of Physians & Surgeons 2006.

19. Spiegel, H. The grade 5 syndrome: The highly hypnotizable person. International Journal of Clinical and Experimental Hypnosis 1974;22:303-319.

20. Spiegel H, Greenleaf M, Spiegel D. Hypnosis: An adjunct for psychotherapy. Chapter in: Kaplan & Sadock Comprehensive textbook of psychiatry, 8th Ed. 2005:2548-2568. Virginia: Lippincott, Williams & Wilkins.

21. Greenleaf M, Fisher S, Miaskowski C, DuHamel, K. Hypnotizability and recovery from cardiac surgery. American Journal of Clinical Hypnosis 1992;35(2):119-128.

22. Spiegel, H. Nocebo: the power of suggestibility. Preventive Medicine 1997;26(5):616-621. American Society of Clinical Hypnosis. Annual Meeting, Scientific Session 1976; Panel on Medical Hypnosis, Dabney Ewin, Bertha Roger, Eric Wright, Chicago.

23. Greenleaf, M. (1994). Cancer and women: redefining the self. Gynecologic Oncology Nursing, 4(2),

24. Ewin D. Hypnosis in the emergency room. In Temes, R. (Ed.) Medical hypnosis: An introduction and clinical guide. Philadelphia: Churchill Livingston 1999:59–6.

25. Cannon, Walter B, The Wisdom of the Body. New York: Norton 1932.

26. Cannon WB, The mechanical factors of digestion, published in an international medical monograph series in London by Edward Arnold and in New York by Longmans, Green & Co., 1911.

27. Cannon WB, Bodily changes in pain, hunger, fear and rage. D Appleton and co-New York 1915.

28. Szabo S, Hans Selye and the development of the stress concept. Special reference to gastroduodenal ulcerogenesis. Ann N Y Acad Sci. 1998 Jun 30;851:19-27.

29. Benson H, The Relaxation Response: HarperCollins 1975.

30. Ader R, Cohen N. Behaviorally conditioned immunosuppression. Psychosom Med. 1975 Jul-Aug;37(4):333-40.

31. Felten DL, Overhage JM, Felten SY, Schmedtje JF. Noradrenergic sympathetic innervation of lymphoid tissue in the rabbit appendix: further evidence for a link between the nervous and immune systems. Brain Res Bull. 1981 Nov;7(5):595-612.

32. Ader R, Felten D, Cohen N, Psychoneuroimmunology. Academic press 1981.

33. Pert CB, Ruff MR, Weber RJ, Herkenham M. Neuropeptides and

their receptors: a psychosomatic network. J Immunol. 1985 Aug;135(2 Suppl):820s-826s.

34. Cohen S, Tyrell DAJ, Smith AP. Psychological stress and susceptibility to the common cold. N Engl J Med 1991;26:309–322.

35. Doidge N. The Brain That Changes Itself: Stories of Personal Triumph from the Frontiers of Brain Science. Viking Press 2007.

36. Mayo K R, Support from neurobiology for spiritual techniques for anxiety: a brief review. J Health Care Chaplain. 2009;16(1-2):53-7.

37. Rosas-Bailina M, Tracey KJ, The Neurology of the Immune System: Neural Reflexes Regulate Immunity. Neuron 2009; 64:28-32.

38. Routledge FS, Campbell TS, McFetridge-Durdle JA, Bacon SL. Improvements in heart rate variability with exercise therapy. Can J Cardiol. 2010 Jun-Jul;26(6):303-12. Review.

39. Kok BE, Coffey KA, Cohn MA, et al., How positive emotions build physical health: perceived positive social connections account for the upward spiral between positive emotions and vagal tone. Psychol Sci. 2013 Jul 1;24(7):1123-32.

40. Kok BE, Fredrickson BL. Upward spirals of the heart: autonomic flexibility, as indexed by vagal tone, reciprocally and prospectively predicts positive emotions and social connectedness. Biol Psychol. 2010 Dec;85(3):432-6.

41. Azam MA, Katz J, Fashler SR, et al., Heart rate variability is enhanced in controls but not maladaptive perfectionists during brief mindfulness meditation following stress-induction: A stratified-randomized trial. Int J Psychophysiol. 2015 Jun 25. pii: S0167-8760(15)00215-9.

42. Koopman FA, Schuurman PR, Vervoordeldonk MJ, et al., Vagus nerve stimulation: a new bioelectronics approach to treat rheumatoid arthritis? Best Pract Res Clin Rheumatol. 2014 Aug;28(4):625-35.

43. http://mosaicscience.com/story/hacking-nervous-system(accessed March 2016)

44. http://www.scientificamerican.com/article/electronic-medicine-fights-disease/ (accessed March 2016)

CHAPTER 9: MEANING

1. Brooks MV. Health-related hardiness and chronic illness: a synthesis of current research. Nurs Forum. 2003 Jul-Sep;38(3):11-20.
2. Gordon W Allport in Frankl V, Man's Search for Meaning. Pocketbooks 1984:11.
3. Pennebaker J W, Opening Up. The Healing Power of the Confiding in Others. First edition New York 1990: Wm. Morrow and Co.
4. Petrie K J, Booth R J, Pennebaker J W, et al., Disclosure of Trauma and Immune Response to . Hepatitis B Vaccination Program. Journal of Consulting and Clinical Psychology 1995; 63(5): 787-92.
5. Pennebaker J W, Barger S D, Tiebout J, Disclosure of Traumas and Health Among Holocaust Survivors. Psychosomatic Medicine 1989;51(5): 577-89.
6. Moerman D E, Meaning, Medicine and the Placebo Effect. Cambridge 2002.
7. Moerman D E, Cultural Variations in the Placebo Effect: Ulcers, Anxiety, and Blood Pressure. Medical Anthropology Quarterly 2000;14(1): 1-22.
8. de Craen A J, Moerman D E, Heisterkamp S H, et al., Placebo Effect in the Treatment of Duodenal Ulcer. British Journal of Clinical Pharmacology 1999;48(6):853-60.
9. Grenfell RF, Briggs AH, Holland WC, A Double-Blind Study of the Treatment of Hypertension. Journal of the American Medical Association 1961; 176:124-8.
10. de Craen A J, Tijssen J G, de Gans J, et al., Placebo Effect in the Acute Treatment of Migraine: Subcutaneous Placebos Are Better Than Oral Placebos. Journal of Neurology 2000; 247 (3): 183-8.
11. Braithwaite A, Cooper R, Analgesic Effects of Branding in Treatment of Headache. British Medical Journal (Clinical Research Ed.) 1981;282(6276):1576-8.

12. Blackwell B, Bloomfield S S, Buncher C B, Demonstration in Medical Students of Placebo Responses and Non-drug Factors. Lancet 1972;1(763):1279-82.

13. Cattaneo A D, Lucchelli P E, Filippucci G, Sedative Effects of Placebo Treatment. European Journal of Clinical Pharmacology 1970;43-45.

14. Lucchelli P E, Cattaneo A D, Zattoni J, Effect of Capsule Colour and Order of Administration of Hypnotic Treatments. European Journal of Clinical Pharmacology 1978;(2): 153-5.

15. Ibid.,6,p49.

16. Ibid.,6,p81,2.

17. Ibid.,7.

18. http://www.lrb.co.uk/v26/n01/carl-elliott/scriveners-palsy (accessed March 2016)

19. Dispenza J. You Are the Placebo: Making Your Mind Matter. Hay House 2014:23,4.

20. Beecher HK, The Powerful Placebo. Journal of the American Medical Association 1955;159 (17):1602-1606.

21. Mayberg HS, Arturo Silva J, Branna SK, et al. Functional neuroanatomy of the placebo effect. Am J Psychiatry 2002; 159 (3): 728-737.

22. Kirsch I, Moore TJ, Scoboria A et al. The emperor's new drugs: an analysis of antidepressant medication data submitted to the US Food and Drug Administration. Prev Treat 2002; 5(1):ArtID 23. Online: available: http://journals.apa.org/prevention/volume 5/Pre0050023 a.html (accessed March 2016)

23. Kirsch I, Deacon BJ, Huedo-Medina TB et al. Initial severity and antidepressant benefits: a meta-analysis of data submitted to the Food and Drug Administration PLoS medicine 2008; 5 (2): e45.doi: 10.1371/journal.pmed.0050045

24. Wager TD, Rilling J K, Smith EE et al. Placebo-induced changes in FMRI in the anticipation and experience of pain. Science 2004; 303 (5661): 1162-1167.

25. Ibid.,6,p105-6.

26. Benedetti F, The Opposite Effects of the Opiate Antagonist Naloxone and the Cholecystokinin Antagonist Proglumide on Placebo Analgesia. Pain 1996; 64(3): 535-43.

27. Mayberg HS. Modulating dysfunctional limbic-cortical circuits in depression: towards development of brain-based algorithms for diagnosis and optimised treatment. Br Med Bull 2003; 65:193-207.

28. Goldapple K, Segal Z, Garson C, et al. Modulation of cortical-limbic pathways in major depression: treatment specific effects of cognitive behaviour therapy. Arch Gen Psychiatry 2004; 61 (1): 34-41.

29. Phelps K and Hassed C, General Practice the Integrative Approach. Churchill Livingstone NSW 2011:56.

30. Shapiro A K, Shapiro E, The Powerful Placebo: From Ancient Priest to Modern Physician. Baltimore. Johns Hopkins University Press 1997:39.

31. Hall KT, Loscalzo J, Kaptchuk TJ. Genetics and the placebo effect: the placebome. Trends Mol Med 2015;21:285-294.

32. Ibid.6,p35-39.

33. Benson H, McCallie D P Jr, Angina Pectoris and the Placebo Effect. New England Journal of Medicine 1979; 300 (25):1424-9.

34. Ibid.,7.

35. Amanzio M, Pollo A, Maggi G, et al., Response Variability to Analgesics: A Role for Non-Specific Activation of Endogenous Opioids. Pain 2001; 90 (3):205-15.

36. Ibid.,6,p155.

37. Moseley J B Jr, Wray N P, Kaykendall D, et al., Arthroscopic Treatment of Osteoarthritis of the Knee: A Prospective Randomised Placebo-Controlled Trial. Results of a Pilot Study. American Journal of Sports Medicine 1996; 24(1):28-34.

38. Talbot M, The Placebo Prescription. New York Times Magazine January 9, 2000: 34-39.

39. Kaptchuk TJ, Friedlander E, Kelley JM, et al., Placebos without

Deception: A Randomized Controlled Trial in Irritable Bowel Syndrome. PLoS One 2010 Dec 22;5(12):e15591.

40. Kam-Hansen S, Jakubowski M, Kelley JM, et al. Altered placebo and drug labeling changes the outcome of episodic migraine attacks. Sci Transl Med 2014;6:218ra5-218ra5.

41. Kelley JM, Kaptchuk TJ, Cusin C, Lipkin S, Fava M. Open-label placebo for major depressive disorder: a pilot randomized controlled trial. Psychother Psychosom. 2012;81(5):312-4.

42. Ibid, 38.

43. Tilburt JC, Emanuel EJ, Kaptchuk TJ, et al., Prescribing "placebo treatments:" results of a national survey of US internists and rheumatologists. BMJ 2008; 337: a1938.

44. Fassler M, Meissner K, Schneider A, et al. Frequency and circumstances of placebo use in clinical practice – a systematic review of empirical studies. BMC Medicine 2010;8: 15.

45. http://www.ourcivilisation.com/medicine/usamed/deaths.htm (accessed March 2016)

46. Lazarou J, Pomeranz BH, Corey PN. Incidence of adverse drug reactions in hospitalized patients: a meta-analysis of prospective studies. JAMA. 1998 Apr 15;279(15):1200-5.

47. Ibid.,43.

48. http://blogs.trusttheevidence.net/category/blog-keywords/placebo (accessed March 2016)

49. http://blogs.webmd.com/all-ears/2012/07/placebos.html (accessed March 2016)

CHAPTER 10: HUMOR THAT HEALS

1. http://www.patchadams.org/gesundheit/ (accessed March 2016)

2. Cousins N, Anatomy of an illness as perceived by the patient. New England Journal of Medicine 1976; 295 (26): 1458 – 1463.

3. Cousins N. Anatomy of an illness as perceived by the patient: Reflections on Healing and Regeneration, WW Norton and co-New York 1979.

4. Ozonoff S, Miller J. An exploration of right-hemisphere contributions to the pragmatic impairments of autism. Brain and Language 1996;52(3):411-34.

5. Abel M. Interaction of humour and gender in moderating relationships between stress and outcomes. Journal of Psychology 1998;132(3):267-76.

6. Hayashi T, Tsujil S, Iburi T, et al., Laughter Up-regulates the genes related to NK cell activity in diabetes. Biomedical research 2007; 28 (6): 281–285.

7. Hassed C, Mind-Body Medicine: Science, Practice and Philosophy. At - www.lifestyleandculturelectures.org/.../MindBodyMedicine.pdf (accessed March 2016)

8. Abel M. Interaction of humour and gender in moderating relationships between stress and outcomes. Journal of Psychology 1998;132(3):267-76.

9. Moran C, Massam M. Differential influences of coping humour and humour bias on mood. Behavioural Medicine 1999;25(1):36-42.

10. Moran C. Short-term mood change, perceived funniness, and the effect of humour stimuli. Behavoural Medicine 1996;22(1):32-8.

11. Showalter S, Skobel S. American Journal of Hospice and Palliative Care 1996;13(4):8-9.

12. Saper B. The therapeutic use of humour for psychiatric disturbances of adolescents and adults. Psychiatric Quarterly 1990;61(4):261-72.

13. Perlini A, Nenonen R, Lind D. Effects of humour on test anxiety and performance. Psychological Reports 1999;84(3 part 2):1203-13.

14. Kurtz S. Humour as a perioperative nursing management tool. Seminars in perioperative Nursing 1999;8(2):80-4.

15. Beitz J. Keeping them in stitches: humour in perioperative education. Seminars in Perioperative Nursing 1999;8(2):71-9.

16. Vergeer G, MacRae A. Therapeutic use of humour in occupational therapy. Americal Journal of Occupational Therapy 1993;47(8):678-83.

17. Bain L. The place of humour in chronic or terminal illness. Professional Nurse 1997;12(10):713-5.

18. Savage L, Canody C. Life with a left ventricualr assist device: the patient's perspective. American Journal of Critical Care 1999;8(5):340-3.

19. Thorson J, Powell F. Sense of humour and dimensions of personality. Journal of Clinical Psychology 1993;49(6):799-809.

20. Hampes W. Relations between humour and generativity. Psychological Reports 1993;73(1):131-6.

21. Deaner S, McConatha J. The relation of humour to depression and personality. Psychological Reports 1993;72(3 Pt1):755-63.

22. Thorson J, Powell F, Sarmany-Schuller I et al. Psychological health and sense of humour. Journal of Clinical Psychology 1997;53(6):605-19.

23. Weisenberg M, Tepper I, Schwartzwald J. Humour as a cognitive technique for increasing pain tolerance. Pain 1995;63(2):207-12.

24. Weisenberg M, Raz T, Hener T. The influence of film-induced mood on pain perception. Pain 1998;76(3):365-75.

25. Matz A, Brown S. Humour and pain management. A review of current literature. Journal of Holistic Nursing 1998;16(1):68-75.

26. Prerost F. Presentation of humour and facilitation of a relaxatio response among internal and external scorers on Rotter's scale. Psychological Reports 1993;72(3 Pt2):1248-50.

27. Buchanan T, al'Absi M, Lovallo W. Cortisol fluctuates with increases and decreases in negative affect. Psychoneuroendocrinology 1999;24(2):227-41.

28. Lambert R, Lambert N. The effects of humour on secreatory immunoglobulin A levels in school-aged children. Pediatric Nursing 1995;21(1):16-9.

29. Berk L, Bittmen B, Covington T. et al. A video presentation of music, nature's imagery and positive affirmations as a combined eustress paradigm modulates neuroendocrine hormones. Annals of Behavioural Medicine 1997;19:201.

30. Berk L, Tan S, Fry W et al. Neuroendocrine and stress hormone changes during mirthful laughter. American Journal of Medical Science 1989;298:390-6.

31. Koh K. Emotion and immunity. Journal of Psychosomatic Research 1998;45(2):107-15.

32. Kamei T, Kumano H, Masumura S. Changes of immunoregulatory cells associated with psychological stress and humour. Perceptual and Motor Skills 1997;84(3 Pt2):1296-8.

33. Dillon K, Minchoff B, Baker K. Positive emotional states and enhancement of the immune system. International of Psychiatry in Medicine 1985;15:13-18.

34. Fry W. The physiological effects of humour, mirth and laughter. JAMA 1992;267(13):1857-8.

35. Peterson C, Seligman MEP. Character strengths and virtues: A handbook and classification. Oxford: Oxford University Press 2004. ISBN 0-19-516701-5

36. http://blogs.scientificamerican.com/beautiful-minds/which-character-strengths-are-most-predictive-of-well-being/ (accessed March 2016)

37. Seligman MEP. Flourish. New York: Free Press 2011. ISBN 9781439190760

38. Ibid 36.

39. Ibid 36.

40. Maurice M. Six Months to Live: An amazing true story of mind over medicine. Zeus Publications 2004.

41. Ibid

42. Ibid

CHAPTER 11: COMPLEMENTARY MEDICINE

1. World Health Organization media center fact sheets. Online. Available: http//www.who.int/media center/fact sheets/fs 134/EN/

2. Cassidy CM et al. Commentary on terminology and therapeutic

principles: challenges in classifying complementary and alternative medicine practices. J Altern Comp Med 2002; 8:893.

3. Douglas G, Altman J, Bland M. Absence of evidence is not evidence of absence. BMJ 1995; 311:19 August: 485.

4. Kotsirilos V, Vitetta L, Sali A. A guide to evidence-based integrative and complementary medicine. Elsevier Australia 2011: 3-13.

5. National Centre for Complementary and Alternative Medicine (NCCAM). What is Complementary and Alternative Medicine? May 2002, USA. http//nccam.nih.gov/health/whatiscam/

6. Easton K. Complementary medicine: attitudes and information needs of consumers and health care professionals. Prepared for the National Prescribing Services Limited (NPS). July 2007.

7. Patricia M, Barnes MA, Powell-Greiner E, et al. Complementary and alternative medicine use among adults: United States. Seminars in Integrative Medicine. July 2004; 2 (2): 54-71.

8. Germov J. Second Opinion: An introduction to health sociology. Oxford University press, Melbourne 1999:276.

9. Sali A, Vitetta L. Integrative medicine. In the mix. Australian doctor 2007, 20 April: 39-40.

10. Maclennan A, Wilson D, Taylor A. The escalating costs and prevalence of alternative medicine. Prev Med. 2002; 35:166-73.

11. Potiriadis M, Chondros P, Gilchrist G, et al. How do Australian patients rate their general practitioner? A descriptive study using the general practice assessment questionnaire. MJA 2008;189(4): 215 -19.

12. Spector T. Identically different - Why you can change your genes. Weidenfeld & Nicholson 2012:215.

13. http://www.grazetech.com.au/sites/default/files/BFJ%20Mayer_minerals_nutrients_0.pdf (accessed May 2014)

14. Campbell TC, Jacobson H. Whole - Rethinking the Science of Nutrition. BenBella Books, Inc. 2013:151-3.

15. Eberhardt MV, Lee CY, Liu RH. Antioxidant Activity of Fresh Apples. Nature June 22, 2000;405 (6789): 903-4.

16. Boyer J, Liu RH. Review: Apple Phytochemicals and Their Health Effects. Nutrition Journal 2004; (5). http://www.nutritionj.com/content/3/1/5.

17. Ibid 15.

18. http://summaries.cochrane.org/CD007176/antioxidant-supplements-for-prevention-of-mortality-in-healthy-participants-and-patients-with-various-diseases (accessed May 2014)

19. Omenn GS, Goodman GE, Thornquist MD, et al. Risk factors for lung cancer and for intervention effects in CARET, the Beta-Carotene and Retinol Efficacy Trial. J Natl Cancer Inst. 1996 Nov 6;88(21):1550-9.

20. Omenn G S. Chemoprevention of lung cancers: lessons from CARET, the beta-carotene and retinol efficacy trial, and prospects for the future. Eur J Cancer Prev. 2007 Jun;16(3):184-91.

21. http://www.ncbi.nlm.nih.govpubmed/?term=Vitamin+E%2C+cardiovascular+disease+Ann+Intern+Med+2014 (accessed June 2016)

22. Sobiecki JG, Appleby PN, Bradbury KE, Key TJ. High compliance with dietary recommendations in a cohort of meat eaters, fish eaters, vegetarians, and vegans: results from the European Prospective Investigation into Cancer and Nutrition-Oxford study. Nutr Res. 2016 May;36(5):464-77.

23. Bruinvels G, Burden R, Brown N, et al. The Prevalence and Impact of Heavy Menstrual Bleeding (Menorrhagia) in Elite and Non-Elite Athletes. PLoS One. 2016 Feb 22;11(2):e0149881.

24. https://ods.od.nih.gov/factsheets/VitaminD-HealthProfessional/#h6 (accessed October 2016)

25. Mridha MK, Matias SL, Chaparro CM, et al. Lipid-based nutrient supplements for pregnant women reduce newborn stunting in a cluster-randomized controlled effectiveness trial in Bangladesh. Am J Clin Nutr. 2016 Jan;103(1):236-49.

26. Moro K, Nagahashi M, Ramanathan R, et al. Resolvins and omega three polyunsaturated fatty acids: Clinical implications in inflammatory diseases and cancer.World J Clin Cases. 2016 Jul 16;4(7):155-64. doi: 10.12998/wjcc.v4.i7.155. Review.

27. Bagis S, Karabiber M, As I, et al. Is magnesium citrate treatment effective on pain, clinical parameters and functional status in patients with fibromyalgia? Rheumatol Int. 2013 Jan;33(1):167-72.

28. Hemilä H, Petrus EJ, Fitzgerald JT, Prasad A. Zinc acetate lozenges for treating the common cold: an individual patient data meta-analysis. Br J Clin Pharmacol. 2016 Jul 5.

29. summaries.cochrane.org/CD000980/ARI_vitamin-c-for-preventing-and-treating-the-common-cold (accessed January 2016)

30. http://www.ncbi.nlm.nih.gov/pubmed/?term=Am+J+Clin+Nutr.+2010+Aug%3B92(2)%3A330-5 (accessed June 2016)

31. Schmidt RJ, Hansen RL, Hartiala J, et al. Prenatal vitamins, one-carbon metabolism gene variants, and risk for autism. Epidemiology. 2011 Jul;22(4):476-85.

32. Smith-Spangler C, Brandea M, Hunter G, et al., Are organic foods safer or healthier than conventional alternatives? A systematic review. Annals of Internal Medicine 2012;157:348-66.

33. Brandt K, Leifert C, Sanderson R et al., Agroecosystem Management and Nutritional Quality of Plant Foods: The case of organic fruits and vegetables. Critical Reviews in Plant Sciences 2011; 30:1-2, 177-97.

34. Ibid. 27.

35. Lockie S, Lyons K, Lawrence G, et al., Choosing Organics: a path analysis of factors underlying the selection of organic food among Australian consumers. Appetite 2004; 43:135-46.

36. Lu C, Toepel K, Irish R, et al., Organic diets significantly lower children's dietary exposure to organophosphorus pesticides. Environmental Health Perspectives 2006; 114:260-63.

37. http://www.aap.org/en-us/about-the-aap/aap-press-room/Pages/American-

Academy-of-Pediatrics-Weighs-In-For-the-First-Time-on-Organic-Foods-for-Children.aspx (accessed February 2016)

38. Lourie B and Smith R, Toxin Toxout: Getting harmful chemicals out of our bodies and our world. University of Queensland press 2013:74.

39. Ibid., p76.

40. http://www.soilassociation.org/news/newsstory/articleid/6455/comment-organic-farming-the-scientifically-proven-way-of-saving-bees (accessed February 2016)

41. Seufert V, Ramankutty N, Foley J, Comparing the yields of organic and conventional agriculture. Nature 2012; 485: 229-32.

42. Ibid. 33, p77.

43. Mattson MP, What doesn't kill you... Chemicals that plants make to ward off pests stimulate nerve cells in ways that may protect the brain against diseases such as Alzheimer's and Parkinson's. Scientific American July 2015:29 – 33.

44. Merry TL, Ristow M. Mitohormesis in exercise training. Free Radic Biol Med. 2015 Nov 30. pii: S0891-5849(15)01141-7. doi: 10.1016/j.freeradbiomed.2015.11.032. (Epub ahead of print)

45. Valter D Longo; Luigi Fontana. Calorie restriction and cancer prevention: metabolic and molecular mechanisms. Trends in pharmacological sciences. 2010. 10.1016/j.tips.2009.11.004

46. Efeyan A, Comb WC, Sabatini DM. Nutrient-sensing mechanisms and pathways. Nature. 2015 Jan 15;517(7534):302-10.

47. Mattson MP, Allison DB, Fontana L et al. Meal frequency and timing in health and disease. Proc Natl Acad Sci U S A. 2014 Nov 25;111(47):16647-53.

48. Lee P, Brvchta RJ, Linderman J et al. Mild cold exposure modulates fibroblast growth factor 21 (FGF21) diurnal rhythm in humans: relationship between FGF21 levels, lipolysis, and cold-induced thermogenesis. J Clin Endocrinol Metab. 2013 Jan;98(1):E98-102.

49. Ibid. 38.

50. Brophy E. Informed consent and complementary medicine. J Comp Med 2003:223-8.

51. Reavley N, The New Encyclopaedia of Vitamins, Minerals, Supplements and Herbs. Bookman press Melbourne 1998:370.

52. http://www.fda.gov/ohrms/dockets/dailys/02/May02/052902/02p-0244-cp (accessed March 2016)

53. Cicero AF, Borghi C, Evidence of clinically relevant efficacy for dietary supplements and nutraceuticals. Curr Hypertens Rep. 2013 Jun;15(3):260-7.

54. Rosenfeldt F, Morasco S, Lyon W, et al., Coenzyme Q10 therapy before cardiac surgery improves mitochondrial function and in vitro contractility of myocardial tissue. The Journal of Thoracic and Cardiovascular Surgery 2005 Jan;129 (1):25-32.

55. Leong J, van der Merwe J,Pepe S, et al., Perioperative metabolic therapy improves redox status and outcomes in cardiac surgery patients: A randomized trial. Heart, Lung and Circulation 2010;19:584–591.

56. http://www.alfredhealth.org.au/icwg (accessed February 2016)

CHAPTER 12: THE COMPLEMENTARY CATCH

1. Germov J. Second Opinion: An Introduction to Health Sociology, Revised Ed., Oxford University Press Melbourne 1999:275.

2. Sackett D, Straus S, Richardson W et al. Evidence Based Medicine: how to practice and teach EBM. Second EBM Edinburg: Churchill Livingstone, 2000.

3. National Health and Medical Research Council (NHMRC). A guide to the development, implementation and evaluation of clinical practice guidelines. Commonwealth of Australia, Canberra, 1999. (Simplified model)

4. http://summaries.cochrane.org/CD004816/statins-for-the-primary-prevention-of-cardiovascular-disease (accessed March2015)

5. http://www.cochrane.org/CD000448/DEPRESSN_st.-johns-wort-for-treating-depression (accessed August 2016).

6. http://www.appliedclinicaltrialsonline.com/cost-develop-approved-new-drug-now-exceeds-25b (accessed September 2016)

7. Harper M. The truly staggering cost of inventing new drugs. 2012. http://www.forbes.com/sites/matthewherper/2012/02/10/the-truly-staggering-cost-of-inventing-newdrugs/#2ce906714477. (Accessed September 2016)

8. Light DW, Warburton R.N. Drug R&D Costs Question: widely quoted average costs to bring drugs to market doesn't appear to hold up to scrutiny. Genetic Engineering and Biotechnology News 2011;31(13). http://www.genengnews.com/gen-articles/drug-r-d-costs-questioned/3707/.

9. Capricorn JE, Blood E, Winer de SL. Association between pharmaceutical involvement and outcomes in breast cancer clinical trials. Cancer 2007;109(7):1239-1246.

10. Rising K, Bacchetti P, Bero L. Reporting bias in drug trials submitted to the Food and Drug Administration: review of publication and presentation. PLoS 2008; 5(11): e217.doc10.1371/journal.pmed.005 0217.

11. Ibid. 4.

12. http://www.abc.net.au/catalyst/heartofthematter/ (accessed March2016)

13. DuBroff R, de Lorgeril M. Cholesterol confusion and statin controversy. World J Cardiol. 2015 Jul 26;7(7):404-9. (Free full text available at http://www.ncbi.nlm.nih.gov/pmc/articles/PMC4513492/) (accessed March 2016)

14. http://www.fda.gov/Drugs/DrugSafety/ucm293101.htm (accessed March 2016)

15. http://www.theguardian.com/business/2014/apr/10/tamiflu-saga-drug-trials-big-pharma (accessed March 2016)

16. http://community.cochrane.org/features/tamiflu-and-relenza-getting-full-evidence-picture (accessed March2016)

17. www.alltrials.net (accessed March 2016)

18. Winstein K J, Top Pain Scientist Fabricated Data in Studies, Hospital Says. The Wall Street Journal. March 11, 2009.

19. Phelps K, Hassed C. General Practice the Integrative Approach. Churchill Livingstone NSW 2011:3-11.

20. Rutten L, Mathie RT, Fisher P, et al. Plausibility and evidence: the case of homeopathy. Med Health Care and Philos 2013; 16:525–532.

21. http://www.ncbi.nlm.nih.gov/pmc/articles/PMC2248601/ (accessed September 2014)

22. Ibid. 13.

23. Belon P, Cumps J, Ennis M, et al. Histamine dilutions modulate basophile activation. Inflammation Research 2004; 53: 181–188.

24. Endler PC, Thieves K, Reich C, et al. Repetitions of fundamental research models for homeopathically prepared dilutions beyond 10-23. Homeopathy 2010;99: 25–36.

25. Aguejouf O, Eizayaga FX, Desplat V, et al. Prothrombotic and hemorrhagic effects of aspirin. Clinical and Applied Thrombosis/ Hemostas 2008.

26. Gerber R. Vibrational Medicine 3rd Ed, Simon & Schuster NY 2001.

27. Kleijnen J, Knipschild P, ter Riet G. Clinical trials of homeopathy. British Medical Journal 1991;302: 316–323.

28. Linde K, Clausius N, Ramirez G, et al. Are the clinical effects of homeopathy placebo effects? A meta-analysis of placebo controlled trial. Lancet 1997;350: 834–843.

29. Cucherat M, Haugh MC, Gooch M, et al. Evidence of clinical efficacy of homeopathy—A meta-analysis of clinical trials. European Journal of Clinical Pharmacology 2000; 56: 27–33.

30. Shang A, Huwiler-Muntener D, Nartey L, et al. Are the clinical effects of homeopathy placebo effects? Comparative study of placebo controlled trials of homeopathy and allopathy. Lancet 2005;366:726–732.

31. http://www.publications.parliament.uk/pa/cm200910/cmselect/ cmsctech/45/4502.htm. (Accessed September 2014)

32. http://www.nhmrc.gov.au/_files_nhmrc/file/your_health/complementary_ medicines/nhmrc_homeopathy_overview_report_october_2013_140407. pdf (accessed September 2014)

33. Ibid. 13.

34. Ibid. 25.

35. Kaliora AC, Stathopoulou MG, Triantafillidis JK et al. Chios mastic treatment of patients with active Crohn's disease. World J Gastroenterol 2007 February 7; 13 (5): 748-753.

36. Al-Said MS, Ageel AM, Parmar NS et al. Evaluation of mastic, a crude drug obtained from Pistacia lentiscus for gastric and duodenal anti-ulcer activity. J Ethnopharmacol 1986; 15:271 – 287.

37. Ibid. 26, p753.

38. Papalois A, Gioxari A, Kaliora AC, et al. Chios mastic fractions in experimental colitis: implication of the nuclear factor ⬛B pathway in cultured HT29 cells. J Med Food. 2012 Nov;15(11):974-83.

39. Dimas KS, Pantazis P, Ramanujam R. Review: Chios mastic gum: a plant-produced resin exhibiting numerous diverse pharmaceutical and biomedical properties. In Vivo. 2012 Sep-Oct;26(5):777-85. Review.

CHAPTER 13: DESCENT

1. http://sacfs.asn.au/download/consensus_overview_me_cfs.pdf (accessed March 2016)

2. Hoffman E, After Such Knowledge - a Meditation on the Aftermath of the Holocaust. Vintage London 2004.

3. Grinblat K (ed), Children of the Shadows: Voices of the Second- Generation. University of Western Australia Press, Crawley WA, 2002:61-6.

CHAPTER 14: A CFS CLINIC

1.   Emerge Summer 2013, Vol 32 No (4):18.

2.   Bested AC, Marshall LM. Review of Myalgic Encephalomyelitis/ Chronic Fatigue Syndrome: an evidence-based approach to diagnosis and management by clinicians. Rev Environ Health. 2015;30(4):223-49. doi: 10.1515/reveh-2015-0026.

3.   Yancey JR, Thomas SM, Chronic fatigue syndrome: diagnosis and treatment. Am Fam Physician. 2012 Oct 15;86(8):741-6.

4.   McIntyre, A, M.E.- Chronic Fatigue Syndrome: a practical guide. Thorsons, London 1998:1-33.

5.   Darbishire L, Ridsdale L, Seed PT. Distinguishing patients with chronic fatigue from those with chronic fatigue syndrome: a diagnostic study in UK primary care. Br J Gen Pract. 2003;53(491):441-445.

6.   Ibid 2.

7.   Ibid 3.

8.   Clauw DJ. Perspectives on fatigue from the study of chronic fatigue syndrome and related conditions. PM&R 2010; 2 (5): 414-430.

9.   Walitt B, Ceko M, Gracely JL, Gracely RH. Neuroimaging of Central Sensitivity Syndromes: Key Insights from the Scientific Literature. Curr Rheumatol Rev. 2016;12(1):55-87.

10. Nisenbaum R, Jones A, Jones J, Reeves W. Longitudinal analysis of symptoms reported by patients with chronic fatigue syndrome. Ann Epi 2000;10(7):458.

11. Reynolds KJ, Vernon SD, Bouchery E, Reeves WC. The economic impact of chronic fatigue syndrome. Cost Effect Res Alloc 2004;2:4.

12. Cairns RH. Systematic review describing the prognosis of chronic fatigue syndrome. Occup Med (Oxford, England) 2005;55(1):20–31.

13. March D. The Natural Course of Chronic Fatigue Syndrome: Evidence from a Multi-Site Clinical Epidemiology Study. Presentation IACFS San Francisco Conference 2014.

14. https://www.betterhealth.vic.gov.au/health/conditionsandtreatments/ chronic-fatigue-syndrome-cfs (accessed March 2016)

15. Brown MM, Bell DS, Jason LA, Christos C, Bell DE. Understanding long-term outcomes of chronic fatigue syndrome. J Clin Psychol 2012;68(9):1028–35.

16. Joyce J, Hotopf M, Wessely S. The prognosis of chronic fatigue and chronic fatigue syndrome: a systematic review. Q J Med 1997;90(3):223–33.

17. Ciccone DS, Chandler HK, Natelson BH. Illness trajectories in the chronic fatigue syndrome: a longitudinal study of improvers versus non-improvers. J Nerv Ment Dis 2010;198(7):486–93.

18. Pheby D, Saffron L. Risk factors for severe ME/CFS. Biol Med 2009;1(4):50–74.

19. Bell DS. Twenty-five year follow-up in chronic fatigue syndrome: Rising Incapacity. Mass CFIDS Assoc. Continuing Education Lecture April 16, 2011.

20. Rusu C, Gee ME, Lagacé C, Parlor M. Chronic fatigue syndrome and fibromyalgia in Canada: prevalence and associations with six health status indicators. Health Prom Chron Dis Prev Can 2015;35(1):3–11.

21. Taylor RR, Kielhofner GW. Work-related impairment and employment-focused rehabilitation options for individuals with chronic fatigue syndrome: A review. J Mental Health 2005;14(3):253–267.

22. Crawley EM, Emond AM, Sterne JAC. Unidentified chronic fatigue syndrome/myalgic encephalomyelitis (CFS/ME) is a major cause of school absence: surveillance outcomes from school-based clinics. BMJ Open 2011;1(2):e000252.

23. Halapy E, Parlor, M. The Quantitative Data: Environmental Sensitivities/ Multiple Chemical Sensitivity (ES/MCS), Fibromyalgia (FM), Myalgic Encephalomyelitis/ Chronic Fatigue Syndrome (ME/CFS), October 2013. http://www.meao.ca/files/Quantitative_Data_Report.pdf.

24. Rusu C, Gee ME, Lagacé C, Parlor M. Chronic fatigue syndrome and

fibromyalgia in Canada: prevalence and associations with six health status indicators. Health Prom Chron Dis Prev Can 2015;35(1):3–11.

25. Jason LA, Benton MC, Valentine L, Johnson A, Torres-Harding S. The economic impact of ME/CFS: Individual and societal costs. Dynamic Med 2008;7:6.

26. Ibid

27. Ibid.,4.

28. Fremont, Coomans D, Massart S, et al. High-throughput 16S rRNA gene sequencing reveals alterations of intestinal microbiota in myalgic encephalomyelitis/chronic fatigue syndrome patients. 2013 Aug; 22:50-6.

29. Rao AV, Bested AC, Beaulne TM, et al. A randomized double-blind placebo-controlled pilot study of a probiotic and emotional symptoms of chronic fatigue syndrome. Gut Pathogens 2009;1(1):6.

30. Abokrysha NT. Vitamin D deficiency in women with fibromyalgia in Saudi Arabia. Pain Med 2012 Mar; 13 (3): 452-8.

31. Bierl C, Nisenbaum R, Hoaglin DC, et al. Regional distribution of fatiguing illnesses in the United States: a pilot study. Popul Health Metr. 2004;2(1):1.

32. Reeves WC, Jones JF, Maloney E, et al. Prevalence of chronic fatigue syndrome in metropolitan, urban, and rural Georgia. Popul Health Metr. 2007;5:5.

33. Nacul LC, Lacerda EM, Pheby D, et al. Prevalence of myalgic encephalomyelitis/chronic fatigue syndrome (CFS) in three regions of England: a repeated cross-sectional study in primary care. BMC Med. 2011 Jul 28;9:91.

34. Ramsay AM, Post Viral Fatigue Syndrome: The Saga of Royal Free Disease. Gower Medical Publishing 1988:12.

35. McEvedy CP, Beard AW, Concept of benign myalgic encephalömyelitis. Br Med J; 1 1967:11-15.

36. Morris G, Maes M. Mitochondrial dysfunctions in myalgic encephalomyelitis/chronic fatigue syndrome explained by activated

immuno-inflammatory, oxidative and nitrosative stress pathways. Metab Brain Dis. 2014 Mar;29(1):19-36.

37. Cevik R, Gur A, Acar S, et al., Hypothalamic-pituitary-gonadal axis hormones and cortisol in both menstrual phases of women with chronic fatigue syndrome and effect of depressive mood on these hormones. BMC Musculoskelet Disord. 2004;5:47.

38. Cleare AJ, Miell J, Heap E, et al. Hypothalamo-pituitary-adrenal axis dysfunction in chronic fatigue syndrome, and the effects of low-dose hydrocortisone therapy. J Clin Endocrinol Metab. 2001;86(8):3545-3554.

39. Nijs J, Nees A, Paul L, et al., Altered immune response to exercise in patients with chronic fatigue syndrome/myalgic encephalomyelitis: a systematic literature review. Exerc Immunol Rev. 2014;20:94-116.

40. White AT, Light AR, Hughen RW, Bateman L, Thomas B, et al. Severity of symptom flare after moderate exercise is linked to cytokine activity in chronic fatigue syndrome. Psychophysiology 2010;47(4):615–24.

41. Whistler T, Jones JF, Unger ER, Vernon SD. Exercise responsive genes measured in peripheral blood of women with chronic fatigue syndrome and matched control subjects. BMC Physiol. 2005;5(1):5.

42. Buchwald D, Buchwald D, Hererell R, Ashton BS, Belcourt M, et al. A twin study of chronic fatigue. Psychosomatic Med 2001;63:936–43.

43. Schur E, Afari N, Goldberg J, Dedra B, Sullivan PF. Twin analyses of fatigue. Twin Res Hum Genet 2007;10(5):729–33.

44. Hickie IB, Bansal AS, Kirk KM, Lloyd AR, Martin, NG. A twin study of the etiology of prolonged fatigue and immune activation. Twin Res 2001;4(2):94–102.

45. Kaiser J, Biomedicine. Genes and chronic fatigue: how strong is the evidence? Science 2006;312(5774):669–71.

46. Siegel SD, Antoni MH, Fletcher MA, Maher K, Segota MC, et al. Impaired natural immunity, cognitive dysfunction, and physical symptoms in patients with chronic fatigue syndrome: Preliminary evidence for a subgroup? J Psychosom Res 2006;60(6):559–66.

47. Hornig M, MOntoya JG, Klimas NG, Levine S, Felsenstein D, et al. Distinct plasma immune signatures in ME/CFS are present early in the course of illness. Sci Adv 2015;1:e1400121.

48. Broderick G, Fuite J, Kreitz A, Vernonb SD, Klimas N, et al. A formal analysis of cytokine networks in chronic fatigue syndrome. Brain Behav Immun 2010;24(7):1209–17.

49. Fletcher MA, Zeng XR, Barnes Z, Leivs S, Klimas NG. Plasma cytokines in women with chronic fatigue syndrome. J Transl Med 2009;7:96.

50. Fletcher MA, Zeng XR, Maher K, Levis S, Hurwitz B, et al. Biomarkers in chronic fatigue syndrome: Evaluation of natural killer cell function and dipeptidyl peptidase IV/CD26. PLoS ONE 2010;5(5):e10817.

51. Klimas NG, Salvato FR, Morgan R, Fletcher MA. Immunologic abnormalities in chronic fatigue syndrome. J Clin Microbiol 1990;28(6):1403–10.

52. Brenu EW, Huth TK, Hardcastle SL, Fuller K, Kaur M, et al. Role of adaptive and innate immune cells in chronic fatigue syndrome/ myalgic encephalomyelitis. Int Immun 2014;26(4):233–42.

53. Hardcastle SL, Brenu EW, Johnston S, Nguyen T, Huth T, et al. Characterisation of cell functions and receptors in Chronic Fatigue Syndrome/Myalgic Encephalomyelitis (CFS/ME). BMC Immunology 2015;16:35.

54. Stringer EA, Baker KS, Carroll IR, Montoya JG, Chu L, et al. Daily cytokine fluctuations, driven by leptin, are associated with fatigue severity in chronic fatigue syndrome: evidence of inflammatory pathology. J Translat Med 2013;11:93.

55. Morris G, Maes M, Myalgic encephalomyelitis/chronic fatigue syndrome and encephalomyelitis disseminata/multiple sclerosis show remarkable levels of similarity in phenomenology and neuroimmune characteristics. BMC Med. 2013 Sep 17;11:205.

56. Ibid 9.

57. Nakatomi Y, Mizuno K, Ishii A, Wada Y, Tanaka M, et al.

Neuroinflammation in patients with chronic fatigue syndrome/myalgic encephalomyelitis: an 11C-(R)-PK11195 PET study. J Nucl Med 2014;55:945–50.

58. Ibid.,4,p30.

59. Jason LA, Benton M. The impact of energy modulation on physical functioning and fatigue and severity among patients with ME/CFS. Patient Educ Couns 2009;77(2):237–41.

60. Larun L, Brurberg KG, Odgaard-Jensen J, Price JR. Exercise therapy for chronic fatigue syndrome. Cochrane Database Syst Rev. 2016 Feb 7;2:CD003200. doi: 10.1002/14651858.CD003200.pub4. Review.

61. Price JR, Mitchell E, Tidy E, Hunot V. Cognitive behavior therapy for chronic fatigue syndrome in adults. Cochrane Database Syst Rev. 2008;(3):CD001027.

62. Action for M.E. Severely neglected: M.E. in the U.K.—membership survey. London Action for M.E. Mar.2001 2:1–8. Available from: http://www.actionforme.org.uk/Resources/Action%20for %20ME/Documents/get-informed/Severely%20Neglected%202001. (Accessed July 2016)

63. Kindlon T. Reporting of harms associated with graded exercise therapy and cognitive behavioral therapy in myalgic encephalomyelitis/chronic fatigue syndrome. Bulletin of IACFS/ ME. 2011; 9(2):59–111.

64. Action for ME and Association of Young People with ME. ME 2008: What progress?. May. 2008 Available at: http://www.actionforme.org.uk/Resources/Action%20for %20ME/Documents/get-informed/ME%20 2008%20%20What%20progress.pdf (accessed July 2016)

CHAPTER 15: VALIDITY AND SOCIAL SUPPORT

1. House JS, Landis KR, Umberson D. Social relationships and health. Science 1988;241(4865):540–5.

2. Orth-Gomer K, Johnson J V, Social network interaction and mortality. A six year follow-up study of a random sample of the Swedish population. Journal of Chronic Diseases 1987;40(10):949–57.

3. Berkman LA, Syme SL. Social networks, host resistance, and mortality: a nine year follow-up study of Alameda County residents. American Journal of Epidemiology 1979;109:186–204.

4. Ibid

5. Prins JB, Bos E, Huibers MJ, et al. Social support and the persistence of complaints in chronic fatigue syndrome. Psychother Psychosom. 2004;73(3):174-182.

6. Chalder T, Godfrey E, Ridsdale L, King M, Wessely S. Predictors of outcome in a fatigued population in primary care following a randomized controlled trial. Psychol Med. 2003;33(2):283-287.

7. Band R, Wearden A, Barrowclough C. Patient Outcomes in Association With Significant Other Responses to Chronic Fatigue Syndrome: A Systematic Review of the Literature. Clin Psychol (New York). 2015 Mar;22(1):29-46. Epub 2015 Mar 14.

8. http://www.cdc.gov/media/transcripts/t061103.htm (accessed March 2016)

9. Hoffman E, After Such Knowledge - a Meditation on the Aftermath of the Holocaust. Vintage London 2004.

10. Bentall RP, Powell P, Nye FJ, Edwards RH. Predictors of response to treatment for chronic fatigue syndrome. Br J Psychiatry 2002;181:248-252.

11. Friedberg F, Leung DW, Quick J. Do support groups help people with chronic fatigue syndrome and fibromyalgia? A comparison of active and inactive members. J Rheumatol. 2005 Dec;32(12):2416-20.

12. Savica R, Rocca WA, Ahlskog JE. When does Parkinson disease start? Arch Neurol. 2010 Jul;67(7):798-801. doi: 10.1001/archneurol.2010.135.

13. Green J, Romei J, Natelson BJ. Stigma and chronic fatigue syndrome. Journal of Chronic Fatigue Syndrome. 1999; 5:63–75.

14. Twemlow SW, Bradshaw SL Jr, Coyne L, Lerma BH. Patterns of utilization of medical care and perceptions of the relationship between

doctor and patient with chronic illness including chronic fatigue syndrome. Psychological Reports. 1997; 80:643–659.

CHAPTER 16: A NEARLY DEAD EXPERIENCE

1. Geiger J, The Third Man Factor. Toronto: Viking Canada 2009.
2. Gonzalez-Huix, F., de Leon, R., Fernandez-Banares, F. et al. Polymeric enteral diets as primary treatment of active Crohn's disease: A prospective steroid controlled trial. Gut. 1993; 34: 778–782.
3. Jones, V.A. Comparison of total parenteral nutrition and elemental diet in induction of remission of Crohn's disease. Dig Dis Sci. 1987; 32: S100–S107.
4. Dalessandro T, What to Eat with IBD: A Comprehensive Nutrition and Recipe Guide for Crohn's Disease and Ulcerative Colitis. CMG publishing 2006.
5. Harper V, Controlling Crohn's Disease: The Natural Way. Kensington Publishing Corporation 2002.
6. Dietary and other risk factors of ulcerative colitis. A case control study in Japan. Epidemiology Group of the Research Committee of Inflammatory Bowel Disease in Japan. J Clin Gastroenterol 1994; 19: 166-171.
7. Morita N, Minoda T, Munekiyo M, et al., Case-control study of ulcerative colitis in Japan. In: Ohno Y, editor. Annual report of Research Committee on Epidemiology of Intractable Diseases, the Ministry of Health and Welfare of Japan. Nagoya: The Department of Preventive Medicine, School of Medicine, Nagoya University, 1996:153-158. (Abstract in English)
8. Morita N, Ohnaka O, Ando S, et al., Case-control study of Crohn's disease in Japan. In: Ohno Y, editor. Annual report of Research Committee on Epidemiology of Intractable Diseases, the Ministry of Health and Welfare of Japan. Nagoya: The Department of Preventive Medicine, School of Medicine, Nagoya University, 1997: 58-64. (Abstract in English)

9. Thornton JR, Emmett PM, Heaton KW. Diet and Crohn's disease: characteristics of the pre-illness diet. Br Med J 1979;2: 762-764.

10. Tragnone A, Valpiani D, Miglio F, et al., Dietary habits as risk factors for inflammatory bowel disease. Eur J Gastroenterol Hepatol 1995; 7: 47-51.

11. Riordan AM, Ruxton CH, Hunter JO. A review of associations between Crohn's disease and consumption of sugars. Eur J Clin Nutr 1998; 52: 229-238.

12. Sakamoto N, Kono S, Wakai K, et al., Dietary risk factors for inflammatory bowel disease: a multicenter case control study in Japan. Inflamm Bowel Dis 2005; 11: 154-163.

13. Sartor RB. Key questions to guide a better understanding of host-commensal microbiota interactions in intestinal inflammation. Mucosal immunology 2011;4(2): 127–32.

14. Dylag K, Hubalewska-Mazgaj M, Surmiak M,et al. Probiotics in the mechanism of protection against gut inflammation and therapy of gastrointestinal disorders. Curr Pharm Des. 2014;20(7):1149-55.

15. Shen J, Zuo ZX, Mao AP. Effects of probiotics on inducing remission and maintaining therapy in ulcerative colitis, Crohn's disease and pouchitis: a meta-analysis of randomized controlled trials. Inflamm Bowel Dis 2014; 20 (1): 21-35.

16. Hou JK, Lee D, Lewis J. Diet and inflammatory bowel disease: review of patient-targeted recommendations. Clin Gastroenterol Hepatol. 2014 Oct;12(10):1592-600.

17. Spooren CE, Pierik MJ, Zeegers MP, et al., Review article: the association of diet with onset and relapse in patients with inflammatory bowel disease. Aliment Pharmacol Ther. 2013 Nov;38(10):1172-87.

18. Chiba, M., Abe, T., Tsuda, H. et al. Lifestyle-related disease in Crohn's disease: Relapse prevention by a semi-vegetarian diet. World J Gastroenterol. 2010; 16: 2484–2495.

19. Kakodkar S, Farooqui AJ, Mikolaitis SL, et al.,The Specific Carbohydrate Diet for Inflammatory Bowel Disease: A Case Series. J Acad Nutr Diet.

2015 Aug;115(8):1226-32.

20. Haas, S.V. and Haas, M.P. Management of Celiac Disease. Lippincott, Philadelphia, PA 1951.

21. Golden Jubilee world tribute to Dr Sidney V Haas 1949. Story of Dr Sidney V Haas New York Academy of Medicine, New York.

22. Gottschall, E. Breaking the Vicious Cycle. 2012 ed. The Kirkton Press, Baltimore, Ontario, Canada; 2012.

23. Ibid., 17.

24. Ibid., 17.

25. Kakodkar, S., Mikolaitis, S.L., Engen, P. et al. The effect of the Specific Carbohydrate Diet (SCD) on gut bacterial fingerprints in inflammatory bowel disease. Gastroenterology. 2012; 142: S395

26. Kakodkar, S., Mikolaitis, S., Engen, P. et al. The bacterial microbiome of inflammatory bowel disease patients on the Specific Carbohydrate Diet (SCD). Gastroenterology. 2013; 144: S552

27. Ibid., 20.

28. Ibid., 20, p1.

29. Martinez-Gonzalez MA, Martin-Calvo N. Mediterranean diet and life expectancy; beyond olive oil, fruits, and vegetables. Curr Opin Clin Nutr Metab Care. 2016 Aug 23. (Epub ahead of print)

30. Bloomfield HE, Kane R, Koeller E, et al. Benefits and Harms of the Mediterranean Diet Compared to Other Diets (Internet).Washington (DC): Department of Veterans Affairs (US); 2015 Nov. free text at http://www.ncbi.nlm.nih.gov/pubmed/27559560 (accessed September 2016)

31. http://www.mayoclinic.org/healthy-lifestyle/nutrition-and-healthy-eating/in-depth/mediterranean-diet/art-20047801 (accessed April 2016)

CHAPTER 17: SEARCHING FOR THE BOTTOM LINE

1. Neff K, Self Compassion. Hodder and Stoughton 2011.
2. Peterson CT, Sharma V, Elmén L et al., Immune homeostasis, dysbiosis and therapeutic modulation of the gut microbiota. Clin Exp Immunol. 2015 Mar;179(3):363-77.
3. Bakhed F, Ley RE, Sonnenburg JL, et al., Host–bacterial mutualism in the human intestine. Science 2005;307:1915–20.
4. Strachan DP. Hay fever, hygiene, and household size. BMJ 1989;299:1259-60.
5. Rook GA. Regulation of the immune system by biodiversity from the natural environment: an ecosystem service essential to health. Proc Natl Acad Sci U S A 2013;110:18360-7.
6. Wold AE. The hygiene hypothesis revised: is the rising frequency of allergy due to changes in the intestinal flora? Allergy 1998;53:20-5.
7. Fraher MH, O'Toole PW, Quigley EM. Techniques used to characterize the gut microbiota: a guide for the clinician. Nat Rev Gastroenterol Hepatol 2012;9:312-22.
8. Ibid 2.
9. Biedermann L, Rogler G. The intestinal microbiota: its role in health and disease. Eur J Pediatr. 2015 Feb;174(2):151-67.
10. Qin J, Li R, Raes J et al. A human gut microbial gene catalogue established by metagenomic sequencing. Nature 2010; 464:59–65.
11. Gosalbes MJ, Llop S, Valles Y, Moya A, Ballester F, Francino MP. Meconium microbiota types dominated by lactic acid or enteric bacteria are differentially associated with maternal eczema and respiratory problems in infants. Clin Exp Allergy 2013;43:198-211.
12. Rautava S, Luoto R, Salminen S, Isolauri E. Microbial contact during pregnancy, intestinal colonization and human disease. Nat Rev Gastroenterol Hepatol 2012;9:565-76.
13. Dominguez-Bello MG, Costello EK, Contreras M, et al. Delivery mode shapes the acquisition and structure of the initial microbiota

across multiple body habitats in newborns. Proc Natl Acad Sci U S A 2010;107:11971-5.

14. Karlstr€om A, Lindgren H, Hildingsson I. Maternal and infant outcome after caesarean section without recorded medical indication: findings from a Swedish case-control study. BJOG 013;120:479-86.

15. Kolokotroni O, Middleton N, Gavatha M, et al. Asthma and atopy in children born by caesarean section: effect modification by family history of allergies—a population based cross-sectional study. BMC Pediatr 2012;12:179.

16. Li H, Ye R, Pei L, Ren A, Zheng X, Liu J. Caesarean delivery, on maternal request and childhood overweight: a Chinese birth cohort study of 181,380 children. Pediatr Obes 2014;9:10-6.

17. Stene LC, Gale EA. The prenatal environment and type 1 diabetes. Diabetologia 2013;56:1888-97.

18. Roberts CL, Nippita TA. International caesarean section rates: the rising tide. Lancet Glob Health. 2015 May;3(5):e241-2.

19. Vogel JP, Betrán AP, Vindevoghel N, et al. WHO Multi-Country Survey on Maternal and Newborn Health Research Network. Use of the Robson classification to assess caesarean section trends in 21 countries: a secondary analysis of two WHO multicountry surveys. Lancet Glob Health. 2015 May;3(5):e260-70.

20. Claesson MJ, Cusack S, O'Sullivan O et al. Composition, variability,and temporal stability of the intestinal microbiota of the elderly. Proc Natl Acad Sci USA 2011; 108 (Suppl. 1):4586–91.

21. http://www.abc.net.au/catalyst/stories/4070977.htm (accessed April 2016)

22. David LA, Maurice CF, Carmody RN, et al., Diet rapidly and reproducibly alters the human gut microbiome. Nature 2014;505(74847484):559–563.

23. Alcock J, Maley CC, Aktipis CA. Is eating behavior manipulated by the gastrointestinal microbiota? Evolutionary pressures and potential mechanisms. Bioessays. 2014 Oct;36(10):940-9.

24. Duca FA, Sakar Y, Lepage P, et al., Replication of obesity and associated signaling pathways through transfer of microbiota from obese-prone rats. Diabetes. 2014 May;63(5):1624-36.

25. Lin A, Bik EM, Costello EK, et al., Distinct Distal Gut Microbiome and Diversity and Composition in Healthy Children from Bangladesh and the United States. PLoS ONE 2013;8(1):e53838.

26. De Filippo C, Cavalieri D, Di Paola M, et al.,Impact of diet in shaping gut microbiota revealed by a comparative study in children from Europe and rural Africa. Proceedings of the National Academy of Sciences 2010;107(33):14691-14696.

27. Leach JD. Rewild -a collection of essays from the human food project.2015:102–104.

28. Ley RE, Turnbaugh PJ, Klein S, Gordon JI. Microbial ecology: human gut microbes associated with obesity. Nature 2006;444:1022–3.

29. Keeney KM, Yurist-Doutsch S, Arrieta MC, Finlay BB. Effects of antibiotics on human microbiota and subsequent disease. Annu Rev Microbiol 2014; 68:217–35.

30. Bailey LC, Forrest CB, Zhang P, et al. Association of antibiotics in infancy with early childhood obesity. JAMA Pediatr. 2014 Nov;168(11):1063-9.

31. Turnbaugh PJ, Backhed F, Fulton L, Gordon JI. Diet-induced obesity is linked to marked but reversible alterations in the mouse distal gut microbiome. Cell Host Microbe 2008; 3:213–23.

32. http://www.bbc.com/news/health-29572670 (accessed April 2016)

33. Giongo A, Gano KA, Crabb DB et al. Toward defining the autoimmune microbiome for type 1 diabetes. ISME J 2011; 5:82–91.

34. Brugman S, Klatter FA, Visser JT et al. Antibiotic treatment partially protects against type 1 diabetes in the Bio-Breeding diabetes prone rat. Is the gut flora involved in the development of type 1 diabetes? Diabetologia 2006; 49:2105–8.

35. Scher JU, Sczesnak A, Longman RS, et al., Expansion of intestinal

Prevotella copri correlates with enhance susceptibility to arthritis. Elife2013;2:e01202.

36. Kang DW, Park JG, Ilhan ZE, et al., Reduced incidence of Prevotella and other fermenters in intestinal microflora of autistic children. Curtis PLoS ONE 2013;8(7):e68322.

37. Krajmalnik-Brown R, Lozupone C, Kang DW, et al., Gut bacteria in children with autism spectrum disorders: challenges and promise of studying how a complex community influences a complex disease. Microb Ecol Health Dis. 2015 Mar 12;26:26914.

38. Siener R, Bangen U, Sidhu H, et al., The role of Oxalobacter formigenes colonization in calcium oxalate stone disease. Kidney Int. 2013 Jun;83(6):1144-9.

39. Qin J, Li R, Raes J, et al. A human gut microbial gene catalogue established by metagenomic sequencing. Nature 2010;464:59–65.

40. Frank DN, Robertson CE, Hamm CM, et al. Disease phenotype and genotype are associated with shifts in intestinal-associated microbiota in inflammatory bowel diseases. Inflamm Bowel Dis 2011;17:179–184.

41. Ott SJ, Musfeldt M, Wenderoth DF, et al. Reduction in diversity of the colonic mucosa associated bacterial microflora in patients with active inflammatory bowel disease. Gut 2004;53:685–693.

42. Boleij A, Tjalsma H. Gut bacteria in health and disease: a survey on the interface between intestinal microbiology and colorectal cancer. Biol Rev Camb Phil Soc 2012;87:701–30.

43. Rutter M, Saunders B,Wilkinson K et al. Severity of inflammation is a risk factor for colorectal neoplasia in ulcerative colitis. Gastroenterology 2004;126:451–9.

44. Sokol H, Pigneur B, Watterlot L, et al. Faecalibacterium prausnitzii is an anti-inflammatory commensal bacterium identified by gut microbiota analysis of Crohn disease patients. Proc Natl Acad Sci USA 2008;105:16731–6.

45. Schwabe RF, Wang TC. Cancer. Bacteria deliver a genotoxic hit. Science 2012;338:52–3.

46. Boleij A, Muytjens CM, Bukhari SI, et al., Novel clues on the specific association of Streptococcus gallolyticus subsp. gallolyticus with colorectal cancer. J Infect Dis 2011; 203:10(3):235-43.

47. Scheperjans F, Aho V, Pereira PA, et al. Gut microbiota are related to Parkinson's disease and clinical phenotype. Mov Disord. 2015 Mar;30(3):350-8. doi: 10.1002/mds.26069. Epub 2014 Dec 5.

CHAPTER 18: FECAL MICROBIAL TRANSPLANT (FMT)

1. Zhang F, Luo W, Shi Y, et al. Should we standardize the 1,700-year old fecal microbiota transplantation? Am J Gastroenterol 2012;107:1755.

2. Sbahi H, Di Palma JA. Fecal Microbiota Transplantation: Applications and Limitations in Treating Gastrointestinal Disorders. BMJ Open Gastro. 2016;3(e000087)

3. Sekirov I, Russell SL, Antunes LC, et al. Gut microbiota in health and disease. *Physiol Rev* 2010;90:859–904.

4. Lewis A. Merde: excursions in scientific, cultural, and socio-historical coprology. New York, NY: Random House, 1999.

5. Vindigni SM, Surawicz CM. C. difficile Infection: Changing Epidemiology and Management Paradigms. Clin Transl Gastroenterol. 2015 Jul 9;6:e99. doi: 10.1038/ctg.2015.24.

6. http://www.cdc.gov/HAI/organisms/CDifff/CDifff_infect.html (accessed December 2015)

7. Eiseman B, Silen W, Bascom GS, et al. Fecal enema as an adjunct in the treatment of pseudomembranous enterocolitis. Surgery 1958;44:854–859.

8. Schenck LP, Beck PL, MacDonald JA. Gastrointestinal dysbiosis and the use of fecal microbial transplantation in Clostridium difficile infection. World J Gastrointest Pathophysiol. 2015 Nov 15;6(4):169-180. Review.

9. http://www.ddw.org/news/articles/2016/05/23/transplanting-healthy-stool-might-be-an-answer-to-ulcerative-colitis (accessed May 2016)

10. Ananthaswamy A, Bugs from Your Gut to Mine. New scientist January 22, 2011:8,9.

11. Borody TJ, Leis S, Campbell J, et al. Fecal microbiota transplantation (FMT) in multiple sclerosis (MS). Am J Gastroenterol 2011;106:S352.

12. Andrews P, Borody TJ, Shortis NP, et al. Bacteriotherapy for chronic constipation—long term follow-up. Gastroenterology 1995;108:A563.

13. Le Roy T, Llopis M, Lepage P, et al. Intestinal microbiota determines development of non-alcoholic live disease in mice. Gut 2013;62:1787–1794.

14. Borody T, Brandt LJ, Paramsothy S. Therapeutic fecal microbiota transplantation: current status and future developments. Curr Opin Gastroenterol. 2014;30:97–105.

15. Borody TJ, Campbell J, Torres M, et al. Reversal of idiopathic thrombocytopenic purpura (ITP) with fecal microbiota transplantation (FMT). Am J Gastroenterol. 2011;106:S352.

16. Borody TJ, Rosen DM, Torres M, et al. Myoclonus-dystonia (M-D) mediated by GI microbiota diarrhea treatment improves M-D symptoms. Am J Gastroenterol. 2011;106:S352.

17. Vrieze A, van Nood E, Holleman F, et al. Transfer of intestinal microbiota from lean donors increases insulin sensitivity in individuals with metabolic syndrome. Gastroenterology 2012;143:913–916.

18. Borody TJ, Nowak A, Torres M, et al. Bacteriotherapy in chronic fatigue syndrome: a retrospective review. Am J Gastroenterol. 2012;107(suppl 1):S591–S592.

19. Adams JB, Johansen LJ, Powell LD, et al. Gastrointestinal flora and gastrointestinal status in children with autism—comparisons to typical children and correlation with autism severity. BMC Gastroenterol. 2011;11:22–35.

20. Foster JA, McVey Neufeld K-A. Gut–brain axis: how the microbiome influences anxiety and depression. Trends Neurosci 2013;36:305–312.

21. Huang E, Wells CA. The ground state of innate immune responsiveness

is determined at the interface of genetic, epigenetic, and environmental influences. J Immunol. 2014 Jul 1;193(1):13-9. doi: 10.4049/jimmunol.1303410. Review.

22. Holmqvist S, Chutna O, Bousset L, et al. Direct evidence of Parkinson pathology spread from the gastrointestinal tract to the brain in rats. Acta Neuropathol. 2014 Dec;128(6):805-20.

23. Ibid 7.

24. Ibid 2.

25. Scheperjans F, Aho V, Pereira PA, et al. Gut microbiota are related to Parkinson's disease and clinical phenotype. Mov Disord. 2015 Mar;30(3):350-8. doi: 10.1002/mds.26069. Epub 2014 Dec 5.

26. Brandt LJ. Fecal Microbiota Transplant: Respice, Adspice, Prospice. J Clin Gastroenterol. 2015 Nov-Dec;49 Suppl 1:S65-8.

27. Pandey KR, Naik SR, Vakil BV. Probiotics, prebiotics and synbiotics- a review. J Food Sci Technol. 2015 Dec;52(12):7577-7587. Epub 2015 Jul 22.

28. Tannock GW, Munro K, Harmsen HJ, et al. Analysis of the fecal microflora of human subjects consuming a probiotic product containing Lactobacillus rhamnosus DR20. Appl Environ Microbiol. 2000 Jun;66(6):2578-88.

29. Szajewska H, Kołodziej M. Systematic review with meta-analysis: Lactobacillus rhamnosus GG in the prevention of antibiotic-associated diarrhea in children and adults.Aliment Pharmacol Ther. 2015 Nov;42(10):1149-57. doi: 10.1111/apt.13404. Epub 2015 Sep 13. Review.

30. Szajewska H, Kołodziej M. Systematic review with meta-analysis: Saccharomyces boulardii in the prevention of antibiotic-associated diarrhea. Aliment Pharmacol Ther. 2015 Oct;42(7):793-801. doi: 10.1111/apt.13344. Epub 2015 Jul 27.

31. Barnes D, Yeh AM. Bugs and Guts: Practical Applications of Probiotics for Gastrointestinal Disorders in Children. Nutr Clin Pract. 2015 Dec;30(6):747-59. doi: 10.1177/0884533615610081.

CHAPTER 19: PARKINSON'S DISEASE – MY EXPERIENCE

1. Maidan I, Rosenberg-Katz K, Jacob Y, et al. Altered brain activation in complex walking conditions in patients with Parkinson's disease. Parkinsonism Relat Disord. 2016 Apr;25:91-6. doi: 10.1016/j.parkreldis.2016.01.025. Epub 2016 Feb 2.

2. Weiner WJ, Shulman LM, Lang AE. Parkinson's disease: A Complete Guide for Patients and Families 3rd Ed. The John Hopkins University Press, Baltimore 2013:288.

3. http://www.pdf.org/environment_parkinsons_tanner (accessed May 2016)

4. Martino R, Candundo H, Lieshout PV, et al. Onset and progression factors in Parkinson's disease: A systematic review. Neurotoxicology. 2016 Apr 5. pii: S0161-813X(16)30049-3. doi: 10.1016/j.neuro.2016.04.003. (Epub ahead of print)

5. http://www.greenpeace.to/publications/carpet.pdf (accessed May 2016)

6. Lock EA, Zhang J, Checkoway H. Solvents and Parkinson disease: a systematic review of toxicological and epidemiological evidence. Toxicol Appl Pharmacol. 2013 Feb 1;266(3):345-55. doi: 10.1016/j.taap.2012.11.016. Epub 2012 Dec 7. Review.

7. Goldman SM, Quinlan PJ, Ross GW et al. Solvent exposures and Parkinson's disease risk in twins. Annals of Neurology June 2012;71(6):776–784.

8. http://medicalxpress.com/news/2016-12-protein-secret-parkinson-disease.html (accessed January 2017)

9. http://www.bbc.com/news/health-15639440 (accessed May 2016)

10. Haoyang Lu, Xinzhou Liu, Yulin Deng et al. DNA methylation, a hand behind neurodegenerative diseases. Front Aging Neurosci. 2013; 5: 85.

11. https://www.youtube.com/watch?v=_akIWiUIjoU (accessed May 2016)

12. Cortese C, Motti C. MTHFR gene polymorphism, homocysteine and cardiovascular disease. Public Health Nutr. 2001 Apr;4(2B):493-7.

13. Vallelunga A, Pegoraro V, Pilleri M, et al. The MTHFR C677T polymorphism modifies age at onset in Parkinson's disease. Neurol Sci.

2014 Jan;35(1):73-7. doi: 10.1007/s10072-013-1545-z. Epub 2013 Sep 20.

14. Tan YY, Wu L, Zhao ZB, et al. Methylation of α-synuclein and leucine-rich repeat kinase 2 in leukocyte DNA of Parkinson's disease patients. Parkinsonism Relat Disord. 2014 Mar;20(3):308-13.

15. Katzenschlager R, Evans A, Manson A, et al. Mucuna pruriens in Parkinson's disease: a double blind clinical and pharmacological study. J Neurol Neurosurg Psychiatry. 2004 Dec;75(12):1672-7.

16. Cassani E, Cilia R, Laguna J, et al. Mucuna pruriens for Parkinson's disease: Low-cost preparation method, laboratory measures and pharmacokinetics profile. J Neurol Sci. 2016 Jun 15;365:175-80. doi: 10.1016/j.jns.2016.04.001. Epub 2016 Apr 16.

17. Crosby NJ, Deane K, Clarke CE, et al. Amantadine in Parkinson's disease. Cochrane Database of Systematic Reviews, 2003. doi:10.1002/14651858. CD003468

18. http://list.wada-ama.org/by-substance/ (accessed July 2016)

CHAPTER 20: PARKINSON'S – LOOKING BEYOND MEDICATION

1. http://www.ninds.nih.gov/disorders/deep_brain_stimulation/detail_deep_brain_stimulation.htm (accessed October 2016)

2. Dams J, Balzer-Geldsetzer M, Siebert U et al; EARLYSTIM-investigators. Cost-effectiveness of neurostimulation in Parkinson's disease with early motor complications. Mov Disord. 2016 Aug;31(8):1183-91. doi: 10.1002/mds.26740.

3. http://www.mayoclinic.org/tests-procedures/deep-brain-stimulation/details/risks/cmc-20156104 (accessed October 2016)

4. Ibid 1.

5. Nassery A, Palmese CA, Sarva H, et al. Psychiatric and Cognitive Effects of Deep Brain Stimulation for Parkinson's Disease. Curr Neurol Neurosci Rep. 2016 Oct;16(10):87. doi: 10.1007/s11910-016-0690-1.

6. Ibid 3.

7. Papageorgiou PN, Deschner J, Papageorgiou SN. Effectiveness and Adverse Effects of Deep Brain Stimulation: Umbrella Review of Meta-Analyses. J Neurol Surg A Cent Eur Neurosurg. 2016 Sep 19. (Epub ahead of print)

8. Doidge N. The Brain's Way of Healing. Scribe Publications Melbourne 2015.

9. Ibid,p226-279.

10. Danilov Y, Kaczmarek K, Skinner K, Tyler M. Cranial Nerve Noninvasive Neuromodulation: New Approach to Neurorehabilitation. In: Kobeissy FH, editor. Brain Neurotrauma: Molecular, Neuropsychological, and Rehabilitation Aspects. Boca Raton (FL): CRC Press/Taylor & Francis; 2015. Chapter 44. Free text available at: http://www.ncbi.nlm.nih.gov/pubmed/26269928 (accessed January 2016)

11. Ibid

12. http://www.jci.org/articles/view/80822 (accessed January 2016)

13. Marxreiter F, Regensburger M, Winkler J. Adult neurogenesis in Parkinson's disease. Cell Mol Life Sci. 2013 Feb;70(3):459-73.

14. http://stemcells.nih.gov/info/basics/pages/basics1.aspx (accessed January 2016)

15. https://www.ted.com/talks/sandrine_thuret_you_can_grow_new_brain_cells_here_s_how?language=en (accessed January 2016)

16. http://www.hindawi.com/journals/np/2014/454696/ (accessed January 2016)

17. Ibid.,12.

18. Smith AD, Zigmond MJ, Can the brain be protected through exercise? Lessons from an animal model of Parkinsonism. Experimental Neurology 2003;184(1):31–39.

19. Faherty CJ, Raviie Shepherd K, Herasimtschuk A, Smeyne RJ. Environmental enrichment in adulthood eliminates neuronal death

in experimental Parkinsonism. Brain Res Mol Brain Res. 2005 Mar 24;134(1):170-9.

20. Sathiya S, Ranju V, Kalaivani P, et al. Telmisartan attenuates MPTP induced dopaminergic degeneration and motor dysfunction through regulation of -synuclein and neurotrophic factors (BDNF and GDNF) expression in C57BL/6J mice. Neuropharmacology. 2013 Oct;73:98-110.

21. Lau YS, Patki G, Das-Panja K, et al. Neuroprotective effects and mechanisms of exercise in a chronic mouse model of Parkinson's disease with moderate neurodegeneration. Eur J Neurosci. 2011 Apr;33(7):1264-74.

22. Shulman LM, Katzel LI, Ivey FM, et al. Randomized clinical trial of 3 types of physical exercise for patients with Parkinson disease. JAMA Neurol. 2013 Feb;70(2):183-90.

23. Reynolds GO, Otto MW, Ellis TD, Cronin-Golomb A. The Therapeutic Potential of Exercise to Improve Mood, Cognition, and Sleep in Parkinson's Disease. Mov Disord. 2015 Dec 30. doi: 10.1002/mds.26484. (Epub ahead of print) Review.

24. Shen X, Wong-Yu IS, Mak MK. Effects of Exercise on Falls, Balance, and Gait Ability in Parkinson's Disease: A Meta-analysis. Neurorehabil Neural Repair. 2015 Oct 21. pii: 1545968315613447. (Epub ahead of print) Review.

25. Morberg BM, Jensen J, Bode M, et al. The impact of high intensity physical training on motor and non-motor symptoms in patients with Parkinson's disease (PIP): a preliminary study. NeuroRehabilitation. 2014 Jan 1;35(2):291-8. doi: 10.3233/NRE-141119.

26. Herman T, Giladi N, Gruendlinger L, et al. Six weeks of intensive treadmill training improves gait and quality of life in patients with Parkinson's disease: a pilot study. Arch Phys Med Rehabil. 2007 Sep;88(9):1154-8.

27. Lötzke D, Ostermann T, Büssing A. Argentine tango in Parkinson disease--a systematic review and meta-analysis. BMC Neurol. 2015 Nov 5;15:226.

28. Hashimoto H, Takabatake S, Miyaguchi H, et al. Effects of dance on motor functions, cognitive functions, and mental symptoms of Parkinson's disease: a quasi-randomized pilot trial. Complement Ther Med. 2015 Apr;23(2):210-9.

29. Boulgarides LK, Barakatt E, Coleman-Salgado B. Measuring the effect of an eight-week adaptive yoga program on the physical and psychological status of individuals with Parkinson's disease. A pilot study. Int J Yoga Therap. 2014;24:31-41.

30. Sharma NK, Robbins K, Wagner K, Colgrove YM. A randomized controlled pilot study of the therapeutic effects of yoga in people with Parkinson's disease. Int J Yoga. 2015 Jan;8(1):74-9.

31. Zhou J, Yin T, Gao Q, Yang XC. A Meta-Analysis on the Efficacy of Tai Chi in Patients with Parkinson's Disease between 2008 and 2014. Evid Based Complement Alternat Med. 2015;2015:593263.

32. Johnson JA, Pring TR. Speech therapy and Parkinson's disease: a review and further data. Br J Disord Commun. 1990 Aug;25(2):183-94.

33. Martens H, Van Nuffelen G, Dekens T, et al. The effect of intensive speech rate and intonation therapy on intelligibility in Parkinson's disease. J Commun Disord. 2015 Nov-Dec;58:91-105.

34. Leung IH, Walton CC, Hallock H, et al. Cognitive training in Parkinson disease: A systematic review and meta-analysis. Neurology. 2015 Nov 24;85(21):1843-51.

35. Ibid 1.,p221-32.

36. Hirsch MA, Iyer SS, Sanjak M. Exercise-induced neuroplasticity in human Parkinson's disease: What is the evidence telling us? Parkinsonism Relat Disord. 2016 Jan;22 Suppl 1:S78-81. doi: 10.1016/j.

37. Ibid 5.,p33-100.

38. Ibid 5.,p55-7.

39. Ibid 5.,p77.

40. Pepper J. Reverse Parkinson's Disease. Pittsburg: Rose Dog Books, 2011.

41. Ibid 18.

42. Ibid 19.

43. Ibid 20.

44. Ibid 21.

CHAPTER 21: JUDGEMENT AND ENLIGHTENMENT

1. http://www.oprah.com/spirit/The-Law-of-Attraction-Real-Life-Stories_1/ (accessed September 2015)

2. Byrne R. The Secret the Power. Simon & Schuster Sydney 2010.

3. Antonovsky, A. Unraveling The Mystery of Health - How People Manage Stress and Stay Well, San Francisco: Jossey-Bass Publishers, 1987.

4. https://fwb.rickhanson.net/ (accessed September 2015)

5. http://www.jci.org/articles/view/80822 (accessed January 2016)

CHAPTER 22: DYING WELL

1. https://www.mja.com.au/journal/2015/202/1/ what-can-we-do-help-australians-die-way-they-want

2. Foreman LM, Hunt RW, Luke CG, Roder DM. Factors predictive of preferred place of death in the general population of South Australia. Palliat Med 2006; 20: 447-453.

3. Broad JB, Gott M, Kim H, et al. Where do people die? An international comparison of the percentage of deaths occurring in hospital and residential care settings in 45 populations, using published and available statistics. Int J Public Health 2013; 58: 257-267.

4. Parsons W B. The Enigma of the Oceanic Feeling. Revisioning the Psychoanalytic Theory of Mysticism. Oxford University Press, New York 1999.

5. Jennifer S. Temel, M.D., Joseph A. Greer, Ph.D., et al. Early Palliative Care for Patients with Metastatic Non–Small-Cell Lung Cancer. N Engl J Med 2010; 363:733-742.

6. Smith R. A good death. An important aim for health services and for us all. BMJ 2000; 320: 129-130.

7. Bernhard J. Final Chapters – How Famous Authors Died, Sky Horse Publishing, Delaware 2015:xi.

8. http://www.thegroundswellproject.com/ (accessed October 2016)

9. http://www.deathtalker.com/ (accessed October 2016)

FINDING HOPE – SUMMING UP

1. Bedson P. Hope empowers patients towards recovery. Living Well Spring 2015;25:4,5.

INDEX

W

Y

www.ingramcontent.com/pod-product-compliance
Lightning Source LLC
Chambersburg PA
CBHW022050210326
41519CB00054B/290